To Ma... ...y

The world's _GREATEST_ smile !)

Thanks for your wonderful
Friendship over the years since

LIFE ROW

We first met on the track
at WSHS. Good luck as

you proceed toward even greater

challenges ahead .

God Bless !,

Red Li...

LIFE ROW

A Case Study of How a Family
Can Survive a Medical Crisis

ED LINZ

Exchange Publishing
Spokane

LIFE ROW
A Case Study of How A Family
Can Survive a Medical Crisis

by Ed Linz

Published by:

Exchange Publishing
P.O. Box 14347
Spokane, WA 99214 U.S.A.
(800) 326-2223

All rights reserved. No part of this book may be reproduced or transmitted in any form or by any means, electronic or mechanical, including photocopying, recording, or by any information storage and retrieval system without written permission from the author or the Publisher, except for the inclusion of brief quotations in a review.

Copyright © 1997 by Ed Linz
First Printing 1997

Publisher's Cataloging in Publication
(Prepared by Quality Books Inc)

Linz, Ed
    Life Row : a case study of how a family can survive a medical crisis / Ed Linz.
    p. cm.
    Includes index.
    Preassigned LCCN: 97-60095.
    ISBN 0-9656895-0-6

    1. Linz, Ed--Health. 2. Heart--Transplantation--Patients--United States--Biography. 3. Sarcoidosis--Patients--United States--Biography. 4. Terminally ill--United States--Biography. I. Title.

RD598.35.T7L56 1997   362.1'97412'0592'092
                              QBI97-40299

NOTE

The information and suggestions presented in this book are not intended to substitute medical, legal, or other professional services. If expert medical, financial, or legal assistance is required, the services of a competent professional should be sought. The purpose of this book is to educate and entertain. The author and Exchange Publishing shall have neither liability nor responsibility to any person or entity with respect to any loss or damage caused, or alleged to be caused, directly or indirectly, by the information in this book.

Printed in the United States of America

For

Sharry, Aaron, Nelle, and Emily

and in memory of

Monica

CONTENTS

INTRODUCTION

I started to write this book while I lie dying in the hospital. I had requested that a laptop computer be brought to my room in the hope that typing my thoughts each day might somehow slew my mind away from the constant realization that I had been given a death sentence by the medical professionals. Writing became part of my survival therapy.

Several months later, after I had been given the gift of life, I realized that others faced with their own medical crisis might benefit from hearing the experiences of our family. As I worked to complete the story, I did not want to be so presumptive as to suggest that I could suddenly proclaim some simple formula to guarantee survival for anyone suffering from a terminal disease or life-threatening medical condition. What did become possible, however, was to relate our true story in a manner which would highlight those techniques which we felt were important in increasing our odds, not only for my own physical survival, but also for the psychological well-being of our family throughout this ordeal.

Although every disease cannot have a happy ending such as ours, what we have learned, both through our own situation and from discussions with other families, is that there are definite actions which can be taken to improve many situations, and possibly to shape a more favorable outcome. The final chapter, **10 Steps to Survive an Extended Medical Crisis,** beginning on page 301, lists specific suggestions for use by the patient, family members, and friends. This chapter can be read as a "stand-alone" segment, but I recommend that the reader save it to be used as a summary and review after the case study has been read. Each of the **10 Steps** contains several references to specific situations in various chapters of **Life Row** which illustrate the concept which we found to be useful.

Life Row

We would like to encourage feedback from readers concerning their experiences. Please photocopy the form on page 334 (at the end of the 10 steps chapter), or simply drop a note to me at the publisher's address listed on the form. It is our prayer that your results will be as encouraging as ours.

I have used the real names of most of the health care professionals, family members, and friends who have been so instrumental in guiding us through this entire process. For those few individuals whose identity may be embarrassing, I have used fictitious names. All locations, dates, and facilities are as accurate as I remember them. While I have attempted to use technically correct terms for the many medical devices and procedures involved, my goal has been to present medicine from a layman's perspective. If there are errors and omissions, I accept full responsibility.

I am very grateful to have had the assistance and wisdom of many professionals who have provided input and corrections throughout development of the manuscript. Mark Davis, M.D., and Kathleen Kimberlin, R.N., were particularly helpful in pointing out many technical errors. Many other readers offered thoughtful suggestions throughout several drafts. A fellow teacher, Helen Vance, and a meticulous former student of mine, Jessica Cunningham, were very generous with their time and expertise in this regard. Marcella Drula, of Spectrum Publishing, was incredibly patient and creative in her design of the cover. The ultimate assistance came from my editor, Aaron Spurway, of Exchange Publishing. Without his continuous encouragement and good judgment, this project would not have been possible.

Successfully confronting adversity alone would have been extremely difficult, but I was blessed with a loving family whose support never wavered and friends who remained steadfast throughout our ordeal. I will be forever grateful for their generosity, assistance and prayers.

The true heroes of our story are the medical professionals whose dedication, skill, and love gave **Life Row** a happy ending. Without their unending efforts to save my life and to provide constant encouragement, we would not be able to share our story with you.

Chapter 1

THE DIAGNOSIS

" *This is a difficult diagnosis. You have cardiac sarcoidosis. We do not know what causes it, there is no known cure, and it is usually fatal.* "

My wife, Sharry, and I were sitting in the office of Dr. Robert Matthews in Annandale, Virginia. We were stunned. We had been prepared for bad news, but neither of us had any indication that a potentially deadly situation would be confronting us.

I was the first to break the heavy silence. "How long does someone with this disease have to live?"

Dr. Matthews folded his hands and spoke softly, "Typically two, maybe three, years." Neither his face nor his somber demeanor changed. "There have been instances of over ten years. On the other hand, you could experience sudden death in the very near term. It is impossible to predict, Ed."

I suddenly realized that I had been given the medical equivalent of the death penalty.

Sharry, who is a registered nurse, asked Matthews how he could be so sure. Her voice was remarkably steady, but I could tell from her eyes that she was obviously shocked. It was as if she had been punched in the stomach.

Dr. Matthews, still in the same calm voice, replied, "During the heart catheterization, we took five biopsies from your heart tissue. All of your pressures and flow rates were essentially normal, and the tissue samples were almost an afterthought while we were in there. One of the biopsies showed an abnormal cell structure, commonly caused by a disease called sarcoidosis. The hospital lab spent considerable time analyzing the sample. I have looked at the sample myself. It appears that the cell structure is consistent with a formation unique to cardiac sarcoidosis."

By now Sharry and I were totally stunned. We both now knew what Matthews had meant when he used the term "a difficult diagnosis." The difficult part had not been the biopsy analysis, but determining how to tell a family that one member has a fatal disease.

The date was May 8, 1991.

As Sharry and I instinctively reached for the other's hand, our eyes met in mutual disbelief. It was obvious that both of our minds were racing to find further questions to ask Matthews. Sharry was the first to speak: "Tell us more about this disease. How does it affect the heart? Why is it dangerous?"

Dr. Matthews was sitting in his office in an expensive-looking chair with a very large desk separating us from him. Although we were at least eight feet from the doctor, his eyes seemed much closer and penetrating. He paused before giving us a rather detailed description of the mechanism of the disease and how it harmfully affects heart tissue.

Most of his words were rather meaningless to me, but Sharry, of course, understood much of what he was saying. Her face became ashen. She understood the gravity of our situation. Due to my engineering background I was able to form a layman's view of the effects of the disease on the heart, but it was only a general understanding of my condition. In the months ahead I was to become very knowledgeable about sarcoidosis (the term "sarcoid" has been used interchangeably by my doctors).

"Your situation, Ed, is extremely rare. I haven't been able to find any other case like it," Matthews explained. He was speaking slowly while rubbing his hands together slowly. He was definitely having difficulty with this conversation.

"Having sarcoid only in the heart and no where else....we just haven't seen this very often. Usually it affects several areas within the body - the kidneys, lungs, eyes, even your skin. Most of the time, the lungs are involved. That's a long term thing, and it generally doesn't kill you by itself. If the sarcoid is in the eyes, a person can lose sight. In general, the disease is not a killer. But when it gets in the heart....that's a problem."

I found my interest decreasing as he spoke of the typical effects on other body organs. At that moment I did not care what might be happening to people with sarcoid elsewhere in their body. I was still trying to handle the implications of my own situation. "How can this be happening to me?" I wondered. "I have been in perfect health, I have no noticeable symptoms, and I have never had any indication of a problem with any part of my body - especially my heart." Basically I felt cheated.

Sharry now asked what I also was thinking. "Dr. Matthews, is there anything that can be done?"

Her voice already had a touch of desperation to it. I was glad that she had asked, because I did not have the courage to ask a question for which the answer may be "No."

Matthews paused a moment, but it was obvious what his answer would be. He was simply searching for an appropriate way to tell us more bad news. Eventually he responded that there are no known treatments which would guarantee recovery, that sarcoidosis has been known to the medical community for nearly a century, and that the best method to show any significant effect was steroid treatment. He cautioned, however, that sarcoid remained a mysterious disease and that, even if it were to go dormant, damage to the heart would undoubtedly be significant due to scarring of the affected tissue.

Was there any good, or even semi-good, news available? I know that this was the thought in my own mind, and I suspected the same reaction was hitting Sharry. The look on her face and the increased pressure with which we were squeezing each other's hand told me that she was desperately searching for a silver lining.

Dr. Matthews broke the silence by turning around in his chair and picking up a stack of papers. "Both of you are intelligent. I think that it would be best for you to know as much as possible about this disease. I have made copies of several journal articles which have been written about sarcoidosis. I would like you to read them at your convenience. I also encourage you to feel free to use the library facilities at Fairfax Hospital to gather as much information as possible about your disease."

For some reason I became further upset by his use of the words "your disease." This nightmare at four in the afternoon seemed to be going from bad to worse. I chose not to press him on the life expectancy issue which he had stated earlier. At the moment I did not want to hear about probabilities or receive false hope.

After another long period of silence, Dr. Matthews told us that it would be very helpful to obtain a second, or even third, opinion concerning the diagnosis. Although we had known Matthews for only a month, he was obviously very concerned about our emotional state.

Sharry responded, "Whom do you recommend? Is there someone around this area? How soon should we do this?"

Dr. Matthews was well prepared for Sharry's questions. He told us of two cardiologists in particular whom he recommended. Both had considerable experience in sarcoid diagnosis and treatment. "I have known both of them for years. Although we do not get many opportunities to see each other, I talk to them fairly often. In terms of cardiac sarcoid, they are tops in the field."

Somehow this discussion of specialists was reassuring to both Sharry and me. Perhaps there was an escape route away from the terribly bad news which we had been receiving from Matthews.

As I silently stared at the doctor, my mind was searching desperately for any avenue of hope, "Maybe his diagnosis is incorrect. Both of the specialists, one at Johns Hopkins University Hospital in Baltimore and the other at Duke University Medical Center in North Carolina, are sufficiently close for us to reach in a day. We'll go there. Maybe someone having greater familiarity with sarcoidosis can give us a different diagnosis, perhaps something which is treatable. Or maybe they will know of some recently developed cure for sarcoidosis. Or maybe..." I was definitely grasping.

Dr. Matthews continued this somewhat optimistic hope for us by stating that he would telephone each of his two friends to brief them on my case and, more importantly, to ensure that I could receive an appointment in the near term.

Matthews then rose and requested that I accompany him to an examining room. Sharry remained in his office. She looked exhausted, but managed a smile as I left the room.

The examination was thorough, but unremarkable, in that nothing seemed to be different from previous ones by Matthews. In less than ten minutes we returned to Sharry. She again smiled at me as if to say, "Don't worry, we are in this together." I was too shocked to return her smile.

Following a brief period of rather uncomfortable small talk, we shook hands with the doctor, and left the building. Sharry and I had come to the doctor's office from our workplaces in separate cars, but we both walked directly to my pickup truck. Although we had not spoken, we were obviously very much in communication. Twenty years of marriage together will do that. As we sat silently on the bench seat in the front of the pickup, we stared intensely into each other's eyes. Both of us were obviously struggling to digest what we had just heard from Dr. Matthews. No words came out as we fought to hold back tears. Suddenly we lunged to hug one another.

My eyes were squeezing together intensely, as I felt both of us trembling. Sharry was the first to break the silence. "Don't worry, sweetheart. Somehow or other we will make it through this."

I was not as optimistic, but I did not voice my fear. I was 47 years old, in what I had thought was perfect health. I had recently run a marathon, and I was working daily as a high school teacher and coach. No serious problems had surfaced during physical exams during my 20 years in submarines in Navy nor in the six years since my retirement from the service. What could be happening? It all seemed so impossible.

We held each other for about 30 seconds, and then Sharry kissed me as she left to return to her car. She said that she would follow me home. I did not make an immediate move to place the key into the ignition. I just sat there stunned.

I did not realize at the time that I had just been placed on "Life Row." Instead of lawyers and judges maneuvering the legal system around a prisoner sentenced to death row, my family, friends, work colleagues, doctors, nurses and hundreds of others in the medical community worked with me in a process to save my life. This is the story, this is "Life Row."

Chapter 2

MERLINO

I first met Robin Merlino in the spring of 1988. It was a situation that some would call fate, others divine intervention, others luck. All I know is that I am alive today because of this person.

Actually, up to my sentence to Life Row, I had been blessed with good fortune throughout my life. My parents, Edwin David and Clarice Nello Linz, were wonderful, hard-working people. I was born in Dayton, Kentucky in 1943 in the same hospital in which my mother, a Registered Nurse, was working. My father, whom I called "Pop," was a third grade dropout, whose main goal in life was to ensure that I, his only child, received a good education. He worked as a molder in a foundry across the river in Cincinnati, Ohio. At the time of my birth, we were living in a second story flat of just three rooms, only one of which was heated. Both of my parents were from large Kentucky families and were survivors of the Great Depression. They saved every cent they earned. One of Mom's favorite expressions was, "We're poor, but we're clean."

My childhood was medically unremarkable. Like most of the other children my age in the late 1940's and early 50's, I had all the usual childhood diseases. I was fortunate to avoid polio, the terrible crippler of so many of my contemporaries of the time. Following the lead of many other mothers, Mom forbade me to go swimming in any public pool during the summer to avoid "the germs in the pool." Instead I sneaked down to the Ohio River and swam in the dangerous currents which probably killed more youngsters than the dreaded polio. In fact, swimming in the river was only one of the dangerous activities which my crowd of buddies did. We had little parental involvement or supervision in our play, whether it be jumping from tree to tree in a game of airborne chicken called "catcher-in-the-trees" or waging imaginary war by hurling rocks at each other from encampments on opposite sides of the railroad tracks which ran through town.

In retrospect, my greatest health hazard was probably in my own home. Pop was a heavy smoker - three packs of Lucky Strikes cigarettes a day - right up to the end when his lungs finally gave up in 1969 after a long battle with emphysema. As a result, my mother and I both inhaled large quantities of secondary smoke. Remarkably, neither of us had any apparent lung problems in spite of our daily submersion in Pop's nicotine cloud.

I attended local Catholic schools throughout grade school and high school. Although neither of my parents were Catholic, they chose this path because they had no confidence in the Kentucky public school system. I spent two years studying physics on scholarship at a local Catholic college before receiving an appointment to the Naval Academy at Annapolis.

I had never seen a ship, had rarely been outside Kentucky, and had no idea what I was getting into. As with my childhood, things worked out very well.

I loved the Academy. Although in 1961 it was still a male bastion of learning to survive, the Naval Academy did introduce me to an entirely different world. I felt as if I had simultaneously escaped the hills of Kentucky and a life of farming. The incredibly cruel acts of hazing meted out daily by the upperclassmen on us as plebes (first year midshipmen) seemed to me to be a very acceptable trade-off for my new-found thrills of adventure and independence. Aided by my two prior years of college, I did well academically and went into a career in nuclear submarines following graduation in 1965.

I had no significant medical problems while in the Navy, although I nearly killed myself several times due to crazy acts of poor judgment following frequent excessive drinking splurges as a young officer. It was fashionable for sailors to drink to excess at the time, and I was always **very** fashionable - and stupid. After Sharry and I were married in 1970, my social act improved slowly, but not without several periods of total indiscretion.

When I retired from 20 years of active duty in the Navy in 1985, I decided that I would receive a physical at least every three years. I considered using my retirement status to obtain a free physical at a military base or at the Veterans Administration (VA) hospital in nearby Washington, D.C. My immediate post-retirement experience with some dental work at this hospital convinced me that the VA was not for me, if I wanted a thorough physical examination conducted by the same doctor three years later. There was also the question of location. It took me over an hour drive to the VA hospital through some of the meaner streets of D.C.

My experience with the dental clinic there had not been favorable. Although the dentists had been pleasant and competent, some of the other support personnel were questionable at best. For example, during a work-up to receive crowns on several of my teeth, it was necessary to receive a panorex x-ray. The VA dental technician, a lady in her mid-40's, directed me to sit as a machine rotated about my head at mouth level exposing my teeth, head, and finally the film to the ionizing radiation of the x-rays.

During my twenty years in the Navy I had developed an appreciation of both the benefits and the hazards of radiation. The electromagnetic spectrum is a term which describes all types of energy waves ranging from harmless, low energy telephone waves, to radio waves, to microwaves, to infrared, to visible light, to ultraviolet, to x-rays, and finally to the very high energy gamma rays, which penetrate almost everything. X-rays are also strong penetrators of the human body. They are of a slightly lower frequency than the harmful gamma radiation typically emitted by an unshielded nuclear reactor or an atomic bomb. Because they do penetrate the body, x-rays can produce the same type of damage as gamma rays, although in lesser amounts. This potential damage is the reason why x-ray technicians wear dense lead aprons to shield themselves and stand behind a lead barrier when the x-ray machine is placed in the radiating mode.

Most doctors and dentists do not discuss this aspect of an x-ray with their patients. A fact which few wish to explain is that *no* x-ray is "good" for a human as it travels through the body. The high energy waves pass through everything in their path causing some cells to die or to mutate. If the person is unlucky, a cancer develops. I say "unlucky" because the damage which causes a cancer is a statistical phenomenon. Although cells in the x-ray path are always struck, the degree of harm is dependent on the specific component which was altered. If the person is lucky (as is usually the case), little or no permanent damage is done. Sometimes, however, a vital DNA link is altered or destroyed. The more radiation which a person receives, the higher the probability that damage will occur. This is the reason why radiation treatment can be used successfully to treat certain types of cancer. An intense beam of x-ray radiation is directed at a tumor causing a high percentage of the malignant cells to be destroyed. Of course, even in this "beneficial" use of an x-ray, other "good" cells are unavoidably damaged or destroyed, leading to possible negative side effects.

I have found that most doctors and dentists (particularly the latter) are reluctant to discuss the pro's and con's of receiving x-rays. They understandably do not wish to alarm patients unnecessarily, because for many people, the knowledge that **no** x-ray is physically "good for you" may generate reluctance to receive appropriate treatment. And then there have been some physicians and dentists who, because they have purchased expensive x-ray equipment for their office, push x-rays in order to pay for the equipment.

On many occasions I have asked technicians, nurses and doctors (even radiologists) how much radiation I would be receiving from a given x-ray, for example, a typical chest x-ray. Some stated quickly that they did not know, but that it was a negligible amount, and I should not be concerned. Others, particularly the technicians, had a standard analogy ready, "About the same amount you would receive during an airplane flight from New York to the West Coast." [The actual amount of radiation received in a chest or a dental x-ray varies, depending upon the power level setting of the machine, but is generally 10 times that absorbed by a passenger in a five hour transcontinental flight]. Another frequently heard response is, "About the same amount you would get by smoking one cigarette." To this one, I would generally respond, "I see...and just how much would that be in terms of some standard unit of radiation measurement, such as millirems?"

Of course, such a question was never answered satisfactorily, even by most radiologists. Typically I would receive the "OK, wise guy, do you want this x-ray or not?" expression on their face. Because the answer to this question was generally "Yes," I usually dropped the issue and allowed the x-ray to proceed.

There is an appropriate explanation to help patients make an informed decision on receiving an x-ray. It is simply a matter of costs and benefits. The cost is the potential damage to your body. Statistically a person who receives more ionizing radiation than another has an increased chance of dying earlier, all other factors being equal. The benefit is the increased information which the physician can receive from the x-ray to understand the illness and to develop a plan of treatment. Fractured bones are a good example of a situation when one should surely opt to receive an x-ray. Dental x-rays are also useful in detecting cavities; the question is how often the dentist requires this information to treat you effectively.

So I am relatively hyper about receiving unnecessary x-rays. Imagine my surprise when the VA dental technician told me that we would have to do the panorex over again. When I asked why, she replied, "The last one didn't come out." I then asked what was wrong with it. Rather sheepishly she responded, "Well, to tell you the truth, I forgot to put the film in." That, plus several other bad experiences at the VA hospital, convinced me that I would be wasting my time to try to obtain a meaningful physical examination there.

My experience with military medicine had been mixed. During my years in the Navy I had received many physicals, some better than others. I came to regard Navy medical care as very good in terms of its overall mission: to keep sailors healthy enough to go to sea, and to provide adequate medical services for their families. Our first child, Aaron, had been born in the naval hospital in Groton, Connecticut, and that had gone moderately well. The deliveries of our second and third children were in civilian hospitals, Nelle in England under the British national health care plan, and Emily in Pascagoula, Mississippi in a local hospital. We regarded these two experiences to have been considerably more pleasant, if only because I was not at sea and was able to assist Sharry using LaMaze childbirth techniques. Our only other occasion to use military facilities for other than "ear infection, etc." clinic visits was a surgery performed to remove a non-malignant tumor from Sharry's left leg.

Our main complaint with military medicine is the inherent lack of continuity in care. Military doctors are like every other serviceman, they are frequently transferred to a new assignment in a different part of the country or the world. This rotation of physicians is not terribly bothersome to a soldier or sailor who is himself likely to receive orders to a new assignment at two year intervals. A retired serviceman intending to remain in a given location for the foreseeable future has a different viewpoint. The doctor who is treating you and your family this year will probably be elsewhere shortly in the future. There is no continuity of care.

It was this reasoning which led Sharry and me to choose to seek a civilian doctor for my physicals, which I had decided to receive every three years. I was 41 years old at the time of my retirement in 1985 and my intentions were to obtain a thorough physical exam in 1988, 1991...

Not knowing any local doctors in the Washington, D.C. area, other than an orthopedic surgeon who had repaired my son's fractured right leg in 1984, we decided to ask others for their opinion. Since most of my friends and co-workers were just as unknowledgeable in medicine as I, it fell on Sharry to use her network of nurse and doctor friends to receive recommendations and opinions for an internal medicine doctor to conduct a physical. Several of her colleagues suggested Robin Merlino as a very competent doctor, who was young, with whom we could obtain an appointment, whose office was nearby, and who was known for thoroughness.

Sharry had always chosen to pay the additional premiums through her work for medical insurance which covered all of our family, in addition to the government coverage which we already had due to my status as retired military. "I'm not worried about the little stuff," she always explained. "What I want is to have plenty of options if something big ever happens."

When we learned that the cost of a typical physical exam would be at least $300 to $400, we were not concerned. Even if the entire bill was not covered by the two insurance plans, we saw periodic physicals as a prudent investment. With little further discussion, we decided on Dr. Merlino. Sharry made an appointment for me to receive a complete physical in late spring of 1988, about two months away.

It was not until the week before the exam that I asked Sharry just where Merlino's office was located. After giving me directions, she added, "You know that Dr. Merlino is a woman, don't you?"

Of course, I did not. I had never been examined by any female physician, and I was sufficiently stupid and chauvinistic to assume that any doctor giving me a physical was naturally a man.

Sharry asked, "Is that a problem for you?"

Having been married for over 20 years, I could tell from her tone that the only acceptable answer was, "No, of course not!" I chose this exact reply.

My mind, however, was not thinking the same thought. I immediately wondered just how some of the more "intimate" or "delicate" parts of the examination would be handled. (Of course, it never occurred to me at the time that women had been going through this process for centuries with male doctors.) I already had enough experience with doctors of my own gender trying to stick their fingers in various embarrassing places inside my body. The order "turn your head and cough" sends chills up most men's spines in anticipation of the forthcoming procedure in which the doctor uses his fingers to attempt to poke your testicles into your stomach while allegedly searching for a hernia. Then when the doctor puts on those flimsy plastic gloves for the rectal exam, many of us macho men really cringe in fear.

So how in the world would I react when this female doctor started these embarrassing parts of the exam? Would I be sexually aroused? Would I suffer incredible humiliation? Would I freeze up? Would I find it kinky? And worse, what if I liked it?!!

All of these fears turned out to be silly. Dr. Merlino gave me the best physical examination I had ever received. She began by asking me about myself and my family. She then elicited from me a very detailed medical history. This part of the examination took longer than any complete physical that I had ever received in the military. Of equal surprise to me was her professionalism and demeanor. Although she was an attractive woman, apparently in her early 30's, I quickly found myself totally oblivious to the fact that she was a female - she was simply a very good doctor. The parts of the examination which I had been fearing were total non-events. She put her fingers everywhere male doctors do, and I felt no different either physically or psychologically. She directed her nurse to give me an electrocardiogram (EKG) and obtain blood and urine samples. The nurse also handed me a kit to take home to use to sample my stool over a several day period (it was then mailed in for analysis).

After looking carefully at the results immediately available, Dr. Merlino called me into her own office and said that I appeared to be in fine health. The EKG indicated normal heart function. My blood pressure was somewhat elevated, but not sufficiently high to require corrective action. She concluded the exam by recommending that I remain active with respect to running and sports activities.

I went home feeling great. I could not remember when I had spent $350 more intelligently. I shared the good news with Sharry when she arrived home from work. A few days later Merlino telephoned me at home during the evening to inform me that all of my blood, urine, and stool samples indicated no problems. Life proceeded much as before the examination.

Immediately following my Navy retirement in August 1985, I had become a high school physics and mathematics teacher at a large suburban high school, Woodbridge Senior High School, about 11 miles south of our home in northern Virginia. I loved teaching and was happy that I had made the choice to do so. Although the pay was considerably less than I could have been making as a government consultant, I was also receiving a military retirement check monthly. With the addition of Sharry's salary as a nurse, we had no financial problems. More importantly, I could now be home with my children and wife each evening, as opposed to going to sea for extended periods of time or traveling frequently to other cities on business.

In the late fall of the year of my physical (1988), I had also become involved in coaching track as an assistant at West Springfield High School, near our home. Our oldest child, Aaron, was a sophomore there and was a runner. The head coach, an outgoing Italian named Fred Benevento, asked me to help with the female distance runners. Although Fred had been a sprinter and jumper, he had little personal experience with runners in events over 800 meters. When Aaron mentioned to Benevento that I regularly ran 10K

(10,000 meter) races and had run a marathon, Fred contacted me and asked if I would like to help out. Reluctantly I said yes.

It was a reluctant decision for several reasons. The first was that I had never run track in school and knew virtually nothing about the sport, other than what I had observed while watching Aaron run some races the previous year. And then there was the issue of surrendering the free time in the afternoons after I had finished teaching at Woodbridge. Was I about to replace the rat race of the Navy with an equally demanding life style?

However, coaching turned out to be very enjoyable. I learned from Fred and other coaches the essential elements of teaching track skills, and I was still able to be home before Sharry arrived each evening from her job at the Fairfax County Health Department. I felt as if I had a great life.

The year 1991 arrived quickly and, in keeping with our plan for me to receive a physical every three years, I scheduled one with Dr. Merlino.

This examination proceeded exactly like the one three years earlier. Robin Merlino remembered me and had all the results of my previous examination and tests available for comparison. I had just run several races, including another marathon, and felt great. I was certain that she would confirm my good health.

I was wrong.

After conducting a lengthy discussion of my activities during the preceding three years, Dr. Merlino gave me the other routine portions of the physical, including an EKG. As before, she told me to wait for about 10 minutes while she examined the results.

The mood during the discussion and examination parts of the physical had been very light and relaxing; for me it had been truly a "routine" physical. When Dr. Merlino asked me to come into her office, I could tell immediately that her demeanor had changed. She was very serious as she said, "Ed, there may be a problem indicated by your EKG. Also your blood pressure is slightly elevated. I'm going to start you on some Calan. It will help reduce your blood pressure."

I was dumbfounded. I was not bothered by the high blood pressure news; my mother had lived with this all her adult life and was still going strong at 77. But the EKG news really alarmed me. I had received numerous EKG's in my life, and all had been fine, including the earlier one in 1988 with Merlino. I replied, "Doctor, what's wrong?"

In a calm, deliberate voice she explained, "One of the waves on your EKG is inverted. It's the T wave. I have checked the previous one which we did three years ago. There has been a definite change."

Not grasping the medical significance of this silly little blip on a strip of chart paper, I asked in a rather exasperated voice, "So what? This is nothing important, is it?"

Continuing her quiet and patient manner, Merlino answered, "Well, it could be. What it tells us is that something has changed. Without further tests we cannot determine the seriousness of your condition. You should see a cardiologist."

"Condition, what condition?" I thought to myself. I tried to collect myself, but fear was beginning to scramble my thoughts.

Aloud I argued, "Why should I go see some other doctor? I feel fine. I run every day. I have no symptoms of a problem. I really don't have time for this unless it is really important."

Dr. Merlino remained calm. She responded, "Ed, I think that this is important. I cannot tell you specifically what may be wrong, but something has changed. It could be serious, but it may also not be serious. We need to find out. I know a very good cardiologist to recommend. The choice, of course, is yours. I recommend very strongly that you take the time to have someone else look at this."

"Who's the cardiologist?" I asked, still not certain exactly what a cardiologist does. There was no way that I was going to indicate my ignorance by asking, "Just what is a cardiologist?"

This was an incredibly stupid reaction, of course, but Merlino, not being a novice in dealing with patients with egos, politely finessed my dilemma, "I like Bob Matthews. He is very well respected and has extensive experience in dealing with heart problems. His office is located in one of the adjacent buildings to this. I can talk to him about your situation and arrange for you to obtain an appointment."

I tried to end our discussion on an upbeat note, "Thank you very much, Doctor. I am going to have to think about this and discuss the situation with my wife."

As I left the examining area, Dr. Merlino walked slightly behind me and said, "Ed, if it would be helpful, I would be glad to discuss this with Sharry." [Sharry had also been to her for a physical, and they liked each other.]

Without turning around I replied, "Thanks." I went directly to the receptionist's area to obtain a copy of the bill and the prescription for the Calan. I hurried to leave, fearing that if I lingered, I might receive more bad news.

For the first time in my life, I now had some serious medical problems on my mind. It was Wednesday, March 6, 1991, and I was worried.

As soon as Sharry arrived home, I told her about the physical and my discussion with Dr. Merlino. Her reaction was calm alarm tempered with professional concern. She asked me medical questions for which I had no answer. Having both a mother and a wife who were nurses, I was not exactly uninformed to many aspects of medicine, but I knew little about the heart, other than that it is basically a pump for the blood. Sharry said that she wanted to talk to Merlino. I said, "Fine, she also wants to talk to you." Knowing my wife, I understood that no matter what my response was, she would be talking to the doctor.

Later that evening I telephoned Mom in Kentucky to tell her the news. I could not, of course, see her facial expression as she said, "Don't worry, Edwin. It is probably something insignificant." The crack in her voice told me that she was very worried.

In retrospect, what was very unusual was that I made no immediate effort to learn more about EKGs or the heart itself. As a physics teacher I am typically interested in learning about anything remotely technical which might affect me, but I had no desire to learn more about this situation. Maybe I did not want to know.

By Monday I called Dr. Merlino's office and asked to speak to her. She called me back in the late afternoon. I said, "I've decided to take your advice. Can you please help me get an appointment with Dr. Matthews?"

I was not totally surprised by her response, "I've already talked to Bob Matthews about your situation. I think that he will probably be able to fit you in sometime later this week."

I saw Dr. Matthews at 2:45 PM on the following Friday. He was older looking than I expected, but was roughly my age, I estimated. After several minutes of small talk about our families and my medical history, he took me to an examining room. I was asked to remove my shirt and trousers so that he could listen with a stethoscope on several locations on my back and chest. He thoroughly checked my ankles and legs for signs of swelling and also poked several areas on my abdomen. He then measured my blood pressure and said that he would like to do his own EKG, even though he knew that I had received one just last week from "Robin." My only reaction was, "A lot of these doctors refer to others by their first names. I wonder if patients are supposed to do this also?"

The 10 leads of the equipment were attached to various places on my body, and the EKG was conducted without incident. Unfortunately when we returned to his office down the hall, he had the same news as Merlino, "Ed, your EKG indicates a potential problem. I would like you to obtain an echocardiogram."

"What's that?"

Matthews explained, "It's similar to a sonogram. It uses acoustical waves to map your heart shape and function. I would like you to schedule one with Dr. Bob O'Connell in the near future. The echo can be conducted in this same medical complex."

I had several reactions, all flippant: (1) Are all of these guys named Bob? , (2) How did we get to the medical slang so quickly, echocardiogram first, then 15 seconds later we are calling it an echo?, and (3) Hey, I know a lot about sonar from my days in the Navy when I had once been a Sonar Officer on a submarine. Maybe I will have a better shot at understanding this.

My verbal response was unrelated, "Do you have this Dr. O'Connell's phone number?"

Matthews concluded the visit by saying, "I will give you his number. And I'll call over there to ask them to get you on his schedule as soon as possible."

The echocardiogram was given the following Monday, March 28, by a technician in a darkened, cold room in a building immediately adjacent to Matthews' office. The procedure was not painful, but it was somewhat annoying. A young, gum-chewing technician directed me to remove my shirt and lie down on a flat, narrow table. After placing a white sheet over the upper portion of my body, she requested that I lie on my left side facing away from her and the equipment. I had a very good view of the blank wall directly in front of me.

After some small talk regarding Easter, the technician turned to business, "Stay on your side, please" and "please hold still." I felt some incredibly cold, gooey cream being applied to my chest. Before I could think up some appropriately clever comment, she had a metal probe about the size and shape of a small microphone, which she was attempting to push through my chest, - or at least that was the sensation from my perspective. This slow form of torture lasted approximately 30 minutes while the technician moved the probe to all points on my chest. From the corner of my eyes, I could tell that she was watching the resultant images on a television monitor. There was the occasional pushing of various buttons on the monitor, but in my position I could not participate, or even see, all the fun. I felt no sensation from the actual high frequency sound waves which were mapping my heart. Fortunately, I knew enough about physics to understand that I was not being microwaved.

Shortly after the technician finished, she left me alone in the still dark, still cold, room for about 15 minutes. At that time, Dr. O'Connell appeared. He exchanged a few "I see," "Uh Huh," and "Interesting" comments with the technician as he watched what appeared to be a video replay of her work on the monitor. He then proceeded to conduct Phase II of the echo, which was exactly like Phase I, except that he pressed harder. Occasionally he would say to the technician, "See that?"

When O'Connell finished his part, the technician handed me a paper towel to wipe off the now very cold cream as the doctor gave me a brief synopsis of his findings. He stated that the right ventricle of my heart was not working well and that both my right atrium and right ventricle were enlarged. He delivered this assessment in a congenial tone and said that he would forward a written report to Dr. Matthews, Dr. Merlino and me by the end of the week.

Although the words sounded serious and I had no idea what he was talking about, my only question was, "Is this really a problem?"

Dr. O'Connell patiently explained that my heart was not functioning normally, but that there may still be no serious problem. I chose to hear only the last part of his answer.

Upon Sharry's arrival home from work, I told her of my echo experience and the preliminary results. As a medical professional, she was worried and it showed.

I then said, "You know, I am not really worried about this. I feel fine, I am still running every day, there is nothing wrong with my heart. I think that these doctors are just trying to milk me for more tests and more money."

I actually believed this.

The written report from Dr. O'Connell arrived in Friday's mail. It was a more detailed explanation of his findings and included actual measurements and dimensions. To me, the results seemed the same as those which had been verbally presented to me on Monday. Sharry was more worried than ever, but I was sending strong signals that I did not want to discuss it further.

On Wednesday of the following week, Matthews called me at home late in the afternoon. He said that he had received the echo results and had talked to "Bob." He said that he recommended that I receive a heart catheterization procedure as an out-patient at Fairfax Hospital in order to clarify my situation. He could schedule this for me at my convenience.

I asked Matthews what would be involved. He explained that a small catheter would be inserted into the femoral artery in my groin area. It would then be directed up through the artery into the heart to take measurements of pressures and flow rates. I winced. He then told me that I would be sedated and would feel only "a little pressure" at the insertion site. Naturally I suspected that he was lying, or at least sugar-coating, the true sensation. I had been hit in the groin as a catcher in fast pitch softball, so I was very familiar with "a little pressure." I thanked Matthews and told him that I would talk this over with Sharry and get back to him.

Now I really dreaded talking to Sharry. I knew that she was going to want me to undergo the procedure. I could already feel the pressure building.

I was correct. Sharry said that we had no choice other than to learn what was happening to my heart. I became angry and said, "Thanks for your opinion, but there is nothing wrong with me."

Sharry does have a temper, and she did lose it. The kids went scurrying to other parts of the house as we had it out over the catheterization. Neither of us changed our minds. We continued being angry with each other for several days.

During the following week, the first in April, Dr. Merlino called me in the early evening. She said that she had talked to Bob. (I wondered which one.) It soon became apparent that she was referring to Matthews. She came quickly to the point, "Ed, you need to have this catheterization. I don't know what is wrong, but something is there. You need to find out."

I explained to Merlino that I really was not terribly interested in such a major step, at least until I had some symptoms. I appreciated her obvious concern, but it was my body. I wanted to remain in control. No number of "Bobs" was going to force this down my throat (or up my groin).

I did tell Sharry the content of Merlino's call, if only because we were having dinner at the time and she had overheard my side of the conversation. Predictably she was in total agreement with Merlino. A silence fell over the table. Our children finished their meal very quickly, and excused themselves to seek shelter. We did not, however, fight. Our battle positions had become hardened, and we both knew it.

During the next three weeks I sunk deeper into a state of denial, similar to that described by Elisabeth Kübler-Ross in her classic book, *On Death and Dying*. In fact, I now realize that her explanation of the first stage of the process, denial and isolation, was a perfect descriptor of my state of mind. I really had no interest in discussing the subject with anyone, including some of my long-time friends.

Dr. Merlino telephoned me again at the end of April to make another pitch. She was straightforward and to the point, "Ed, I have talked to Sharry. She tells me that you are still refusing the catheterization. I think that you are making a big mistake."

I again repeated my now familiar refrain that I had no symptoms of a heart problem. She was brutally blunt in her response, "The reason that I am so persistent is that I recently lost a patient who dropped dead in a similar circumstance. I do not know what is wrong with your heart, but it could be serious. I don't want to see you in the same situation as him. I recommend that you call Bob Matthews as soon as possible and allow him to schedule the catheterization."

I paused briefly and then said, "OK." I had been outgunned.

Sharry's astuteness in selecting, and then supporting, an exceptionally talented and conscientious doctor, such as Robin Merlino, was the first positive step in my medical salvation. I did not fully appreciate their combined contribution until several years later. Their roles, however, were real and significant. Essentially, I owe my continued life to these two women.

The heart catheterization was performed by Dr. Matthews the following week, on Thursday, May 2nd in the "cath lab" at Fairfax Hospital in Falls Church, Virginia. I entered the hospital at 7 AM. Prior to the "cath" (as all the nurses referred to it), I changed my clothes to a hospital gown, put everything in a plastic bag provided by the hospital, and sat in a large Lazy-Boy type chair in a small area facing an aquarium. Soft "elevator-type" music was playing in the background. There was a TV in the room, but I was not interested. One of the nurses took my blood pressure, asked me for a detailed medical history, and then started an intravenous (IV) in my arm. I could not recall ever having an IV, but it was not an unpleasant process. The nurse tied a short length of rubber tubing around the biceps area of my arm, asked me to make a fist, tapped my arm a few times to induce my veins to appear, and then successfully inserted a needle on the first try. It was only at this time that I felt as if I had entered the point of no return. I had.

After the IV had been started, one of the cath lab nurses located Sharry in the waiting area and invited her to join me. Sharry held my hand as we talked. At 8:30 AM other nurses came to take me to the cath lab in a wheel chair. Sharry kissed me, and we exchanged a long hug. She was then directed to another waiting room where Dr. Matthews would talk to her after the procedure.

From this point on I have only a vague recollection of what happened. I had apparently been heavily sedated with Valium. I do recall Matthews saying, "You may feel a little pressure," but everything else was a blur.

At 10 AM the procedure was finished and I was delivered to a recovery room, although it may have had a different name. Dr. Matthews had already talked to Sharry, but he also came to see me when I was more coherent. He explained that the initial results looked good, there was no blockage, and the heart valves were functioning properly. He added that five biopsies of heart tissue had been taken for laboratory analysis. He asked that we make an appointment to see him in his office the following Wednesday.

The immediate recovery phase for a heart catheterization is far more painful than the procedure itself. The patient must lie flat on his back for six hours with a tightly bandaged dressing covering the entrance area of the catheter in the groin artery. A nurse actually applied hand pressure for the first 15 minutes to the top of the dressing. Then a small sandbag of several pounds was positioned onto the entrance site to ensure that blood clotting occurs. If the wound were left untended, it could easily give way with the patient rapidly bleeding to death. Because the catheter entry is made through an artery, which contains "refreshed" blood being pumped directly from the heart, instead of a vein, which is returning "used" blood to the heart for recycling, the danger of bleeding is greater. At any rate, the patient must lie flat for at least six hours.

This position would not be very painful to maintain, except for the fact that the patient is also required to force fluids to flush out the dye which had been inserted into the blood stream during the catheterization (for enhanced viewing purposes). I soon learned that what goes in, also must come out. This basic law of nature became rapidly apparent as my bladder filled. The urge to urinate was incredible. Unfortunately my body was not designed to accomplish this act while lying in a perfectly flat position. I tried to use a urinal, but all the laws of nature seemed to be working against me, like gravity, for example. The pain was becoming serious.

By now, Sharry was at my side, and together we developed a plan of action. We asked the nurse to leave, and Sharry obtained a small pan of warm water. I inserted my right hand into the water and swished it around. Although the effect was not instantaneous, the flow did eventually begin. I was now relieved, in more ways than one!

This period of "water torture" ended in late afternoon. I was allowed to sit up, and by 7 PM we were home. Both of us were in reasonably good spirits. The news was not necessarily good, but it certainly had not been bad. We had a good weekend and looked forward to receiving favorable news from Dr. Matthews on the following Wednesday when we were to visit his office.

Once again our optimism was unfounded. The "following Wednesday" was May 8th - the day we learned from Matthews that I had cardiac sarcoidosis and might soon die. Just how long I might last on Life Row was not a topic anyone wanted to confront. We decided to approach it day-to-day and to pray for the best. We had no idea what lay ahead.

Chapter 3

SARCOID

In the weeks immediately following Dr. Matthews' diagnosis of sarcoidosis, my mood changed considerably. I found myself wanting to learn as much as possible about the disease. Perhaps my long years of Navy experience during the Cold War had conditioned me to try to know my adversary as well as possible. If I was going to have to fight this killer, I wanted to know what options were available.

First I needed to learn more about the heart itself. One evening at home I sat down with the Human Anatomy and Physiology textbook which we had used during one of my teacher certification courses at George Mason University. Chapter 18 had some graphic photographs and detailed explanations of the entire cardiovascular system. With Sharry helping me to translate from medical to layman lingo, I considerably increased my understanding of the heart.

Although the dimensions vary with body size, the human heart is generally about 5 to 6 inches long and 3 to 4 inches wide in an average adult. "Think of it as about the size of your fist," explained Sharry. "It's surrounded by your lungs on the sides with the backbone behind it and the sternum - that's the breast bone - in front. Its pointed end, the apex, is on the bottom and goes off toward the left somewhere near your fifth intercostal space."

"My what?"

In response, Sharry pointed to her left rib area as she continued the tutorial, "There is a sac, a membrane actually, which encloses the heart. It is called the pericardium. The heart sort of floats in a fluid which is inside this sac. The pericardium is what is attached to the diaphragm, the sternum and the veins and arteries going to and coming from the heart. Do you remember me talking about some patients who have had pericarditis?"

"Not really."

"Well, that's what it's called when the pericardium gets an infection. It can be fairly serious."

I was more interested in the plumbing aspects. "What is the difference between veins and arteries?"

"Veins carry blood back to your heart to be pumped to the lungs to receive a fresh supply of oxygen. They are the ones which look purple from the outside. Arteries carry freshly oxygenated blood out to various parts of your body. There is higher pressure in the arteries than in the veins."

I stopped asking questions and read some more. The textbook indicated that the heart is divided into four separate hollow chambers, two on the left and two on the right, separated by a thick tissue called the septum. The upper chambers are the atria and are referred to as the right and left atrium. I smiled as I noticed the singular and plural spellings of these Latin words, because my four years of high school Latin finally started to pay a few dividends.

The right atrium receives blood low in oxygen and high in carbon dioxide through large veins called the vena cavae. As the wall of the atrium contracts, the blood is pumped through a valve in the atrioventricular orifice into the chamber of the right ventricle. The ventricle is a strong pump which contracts to send the blood into the capillaries associated with the alveoli of the lungs where it receives a new supply of oxygen and nutrients. The blood then exits the lungs into the left atrium, which pushes it into the final pumping chamber, the left ventricle. When the left ventricular wall contracts, the blood now rich in oxygen passes out of the heart into the body's blood distribution system. Several internal valves open and shut in the proper sequence to make all of this pumping and flow possible. Basically, as with the rest of the body, it is a continuous miracle.

The highest pressure occurs in the left ventricle, because it must generate sufficient force to push the oxygenated blood throughout the body. This pressure is called the systolic and is the top number of a typical blood pressure reading. The lower number refers to the diastolic pressure, which is the force per unit area in the body's blood vessels between heart beats. I always got these two readings mixed up until, as a high school teacher, it suddenly dawned on me to associate them alphabetically with two of my favorite words: Snow Days.

The heart itself requires blood to perform all of this work. (In an average human, it "beats" over 35 million times a year!) If a branch of one of the arteries supplying blood to the heart itself becomes clogged or obstructed, the muscle cells become starved for oxygen and a severe chest pain, angina pectoris, results. If cells die in the process, the person is said to be having a heart attack, which may result in death.

I did not have this type of heart disease. The catheterization had shown that flow through my heart was fine. My problem was in the conduction system, that is, the intricate network of nerve paths which send signals telling each of these muscles when to squeeze and when to relax. In a healthy heart, there are clumps and strands of specialized tissue which send impulses throughout the heart. A key part of the conduction system is the sinoatrial (S-A) node, a small mass of muscle in the wall of the right atrium. The cells of the S-A node have the ability to excite themselves, initiating impulses that travel to the muscles which do the pumping. As if this were not sufficiently magical, the S-A node activity is rhythmic, about 70 to 80 times each minute. This is why it is sometimes called the heart's natural pacemaker.

The S-A signals eventually reach another mass of specialized muscle tissue called the atrioventricular (A-V) node, located near the bottom of the right atrium. After a short delay, the signal reaches the other side of the A-V node where it passes into some "human wiring" called the A-V bundle (also known as the "bundle of His"). This path stimulates larger pathways (Purkinje fibers) which transmit signals to the other muscle fibers in the walls of the ventricles. These fibers are arranged in irregular swirls causing the ventricular walls to contract with a twisting motion when stimulated, as if it were a mop being wrung out. The blood is thus squeezed out of the chambers of the ventricles into the arteries for its trip throughout the body. It is a **major** miracle.

Dr. Merlino and then Dr. Matthews had initially learned that something was not working properly in my heart by means of an EKG. Actually, in English, it should be called an ECG because the process is an electrocardiogram. All of my doctors and nurses used the term "EKG." Apparently the procedure, which is nothing more than a recording of the electrical changes in the heart during one complete pumping cycle, originated in Europe where the original Greek word for heart, καρδια, influenced the spelling of cardiac. Hence the k for kappa (κ) instead of c. Because I had always heard both Mom and Sharry use "EKG," I had never given the distinction much thought. Most current textbooks use ECG, but the authors are swimming against the tide of popular usage, - at least in this neck of the woods.

To conduct an EKG, the doctor, nurse, or technician places metal electrodes on certain designated locations on the skin. Most are on the chest area, but some are placed on the legs. The electrodes are connected by wires to a sensitive measuring device which can detect the very small electrical changes occurring within the body as a result of the rhythmic heart activity. These changes are recorded by a pen moving up and down on a strip of paper moving at a known speed. The distance between the pen deflections can be measured, providing a means to determine and analyze the time which elapses between various phases of the cardiac cycle.

Although a typical EKG trace is unintelligible to me, there are distinct waves which can be rather easily interpreted by a trained observer. For example, the time period between the beginning of the "P wave" and the beginning of the "QRS complex" tells how long it takes for the electrical impulse to travel from the S-A node through the A-V node into the walls of the ventricles. An abnormally high value for this time may indicate a specific type of heart problem. In my case, the "T wave" was inverted, i.e., upside down, suggesting that there was an abnormality in the repolarization of the fibers in my ventricles. The problem was that this information did not lead automatically to a diagnosis of what was causing the inversion.

Still, the EKG had served as an early warning "smoke detector" for my cardiac problem. It led to the echocardiogram, which led to the catheterization, which led to the biopsy, which led to the diagnosis of sarcoidosis. Dr. Merlino had been able to use her expertise to interpret the EKG to tell us that I had a problem before I suddenly dropped dead. Although the EKG had enabled me to be placed on Life Row rather than in a morgue, I was not particularly grateful at the time.

I still had no outward symptoms, but I did not want to wait until the sarcoid was in control before educating myself about this killer. Dr. Matthews had given me several articles to read, and I searched libraries, medical encyclopedias, and even old dictionaries to try to understand my problem.

Sarcoidosis, I learned, is basically a mystery disease. In many reference books it is characterized as "a multi-system granulomatous disorder of unknown etiology." Multi-system simply means that the disease can, and usually does, affect many different organs. Granulomatous, I learned, is an adjective describing the microscopic physical appearance of the sarcoid lesion. A granuloma is a defined area of tissue growth with the characteristics of small particles or pellets joined together. An open wound heals in this manner as the body repairs itself with rapidly growing cells. Disorder is just that - a growth pattern (such as a tumor) which is not part of a healthy body. Etiology is the medical term for cause.

Although sarcoidosis typically affects different parts of the body, it has a common cellular signature which can be readily identified by pathologists using microscopes and other common laboratory equipment. Identifying sarcoid is not the problem. Determining the cause and finding a cure have been the mystery.

Most of the cases of sarcoid involve more than one part of the body. I learned from the literature that Dr. Matthews was correct in his discussion with Sharry and me in his office. The lungs are the most frequent target; a standard chest x-ray will show an abnormality shortly after onset of the disease over 90 percent of the time. Other areas attacked are the skin (lesions), eyes (can ultimately lead to blindness), lymph nodes, liver, spleen, and the heart. In reality, almost any organ can be involved. Because symptoms are often not observable or are masked by other diseases, statistics on sarcoidosis are somewhat misleading. For example, while involvement of the heart has been observed clinically (by biopsies) in only about 5 % of sarcoid patients, over 5 times that number have the telltale granulomas in their heart tissue when an autopsy is performed following death.

Sarcoidosis is not, however, normally a killer. Less than 4 % of those afflicted with sarcoid die from the disease, but death rates vary dramatically depending on the specific organs affected. Whereas very few die from sarcoid skin lesions, most heart cases are fatal. Matthews' estimate that I might have two years to live seemed to be supported by the literature. There were instances of patients living over 10 years after being diagnosed with cardiac sarcoidosis, but the majority died quickly - often with no warning. In fact, as one doctor wrote, "sudden death is frequently the first manifestation of cardiac sarcoidosis." As I read this information, I took some consolation from the fact I had not fallen into that category. Maybe I could set a new record for longevity. That became my immediate goal. Perhaps a cure would be discovered in the interim.

The more I read about sarcoid, the unluckier I felt. Most studies have found that the disease affects approximately 2 per 10,000 in the overall world population, or 2/100 of one percent, roughly the percentage equivalent of having one bad day every 14 years!

Although sarcoidosis occurs everywhere, there is considerable variation among locales, and even within each region, there are unusual patterns of infection. The disease, for example, is much more prevalent in Scandinavia, Great Britain and North America than in Central and South American countries, Africa and China. In Sweden, based upon autopsy studies, the incidence has been reported as high as 64 in 10,000, whereas in Canada it is only 1 in 10,000. Cases involving Eskimos and Native American Indians have been extremely rare. In many areas of the world, such as most countries in South America and Africa, there simply is little reliable data for valid comparisons. What is clear is that there are wide variations in incidence of the disease and no one, yet, understands why.

There is also an apparent race factor, - at least in the U.S. and South Africa, where reliable data is available. Blacks, in both locations, are over 10 times more likely to contract sarcoidosis than whites in the same area. There is also a higher fatality rate for black patients. Black women are particularly at risk. Over twice as many black females have the disease compared to black men. This gender bias does not extend to the white population, where studies throughout the world have shown approximately a 50/50 split among the sexes. Sarcoidosis most frequently strikes people in the 30 to 50 year age bracket, but there are instances of children and the elderly being infected. Some studies have shown multiple cases of sarcoid within the same family, but a proven hereditary trait has not been established.

Within the United States, the disease occurs most often in the southeast, particularly the Carolinas. There has been some speculation that sarcoid was somehow caused by prolonged exposure to the pollen of southern pine trees, but this theory has been generally discredited. Correlation to other environmental factors, as widely different as beryllium and hair spray, have been suggested in studies involving subjects in various locations around the world, but, as with the pine tree theory, none that I am aware of have withstood detailed analysis. As of the mid 1990's, we do not understand the cause of this mysterious disease.

Originally sarcoidosis was thought to be a special type of tuberculosis. This premise was certainly plausible due to the similarity in lung symptoms between the two. As increasingly sophisticated methods of studying tuberculosis became available, it became apparent that sarcoid was a separate entity. The actual designation of the disease came not from a lung condition, but from skin lesions. In 1877 a British physician, Jonathan Hutchinson, wrote a paper detailing what is now considered the first description of sarcoidosis. Two of his patients had large, purple patches on their face, hands and feet. The disfiguration was not tender to the touch and did not exhibit the characteristics of a known skin disorder, lupus. He called the condition, "Mortimer's Malady," because one of the patients was named Mrs. Mortimer. As I read about Dr. Hutchinson's alliterative nomenclature, I wondered if Dr. Matthews was describing my sarcoid to his friends as "Linz's Lesions."

So I had a mysterious, deadly disease which had been around for at least a century. The lack of a cure is what bothered me. Some forms of sarcoidosis, according to the literature, seem to heal themselves, or at least go into remission. This is often the case when the skin is involved. The standard treatment for sarcoid is corticosteroids, such as Prednisone. Why these drugs sometimes help, but in other cases provide little relief, is as mysterious as the disease itself. Unfortunately, there is no consensus regarding the maximum effective dose, how long the drug should be given, or even how Prednisone alters the growth process of the granulomas. Controlled clinical studies have been very difficult to achieve because of the nature of the disease and unreliable methods of following its course, with and without treatment. Chest x-rays, for example, are a crude device to attempt to track cellular details. What is generally agreed is that steroids have been shown to be useful in some situations, with varying results, depending on the organs involved. In other cases, the steroid treatment has not been helpful.

There was one avenue of potential healing: pregnancy! Studies indicated that becoming pregnant has a beneficial effect on a patient with sarcoid. Presumably, this improvement is due to the body's natural increase in steroids during pregnancy. Before I could develop a detailed fantasy in which I made medical history by becoming pregnant, I read that the same studies showed, unfortunately, that the effect is only temporary and is lost following childbirth.

Another interesting finding from the reading which Dr. Matthews had provided us was that, believe it or not, smoking reduces the risk factor for contracting sarcoidosis. One study showed that non-smokers were four times more likely to develop the disease than smokers! I would not be surprised to see the results of this study appearing in the next series of "Joe Camel" ads. Since the end results of smoking (e.g., lung cancer, heart disease, etc.) are generally fatal, while sarcoid typically is not, I will let you decide. In my own situation, I had long ago made my decision as I watched Pop suffer an agonizing death due to his Lucky Strikes-induced emphysema.

My problem was that the sarcoid was in my heart. The granulomas are dangerous there, because they adversely affect the heart's natural electrical conduction system. As the body attempts to send the rhythmic signal from the S-A node to various sections of the heart causing it to pump, the granulomas disrupt the normal signal paths. The heart becomes confused, and the normally smooth pumping rhythm is erratic. The condition can last for a few seconds and then correct itself spontaneously, or the heart can proceed into a prolonged and dangerous arrhythmia, possibly leading to death. Although steroid treatment may halt or slow the formation of granulomas, scar tissue is often formed in the process, creating equally dangerous blockages for the electrical signals. Because the internal timing system in the heart is so critical to effective pumping action by the muscles involved, an electrical problem is a **major** problem.

Although I now knew much more about my condition, I also understood that my days on Life Row might be very few. I was in big trouble, and the clock was running.

Chapter 4

FIRST SYMPTOMS

After hearing Dr. Matthews' diagnosis in early May of 1991, Sharry and I were in a heightened level of awareness concerning my health. Although no definite symptoms were yet apparent, we were living a very concerned and nervous existence. Every time I thought that my heart had fluttered or acted in a strange manner, I became worried that this might be the beginning of the end, or that I might even keel over dead on the spot. Plenty of well known people, such as the runner and author, Jim Fixx, had suddenly died from a heart condition with little or no warning. Would the same happen to me?

There were several new issues to consider. What, if anything, should we tell our relatives and friends? We had kept my mother well informed, but others presented a different situation. We were absolutely straightforward with our three children. Aaron was now a senior in high school, Nelle was a sophomore, and Emily was in 7th grade. All, we felt, should know exactly what their father's medical condition was. From Day 1 of my time on Life Row, they were integral players in our lengthy ordeal. The decision to involve them was one which Sharry and I never regretted.

Although we had no conscious plan, we told a few close friends our disturbing news. To others, we said nothing. Sharry did write to her four sisters, but not on a priority basis. In general, we did not want to broadcast our predicament, - particularly since we did not yet understand the implications or timelines ourselves. I chose not to say anything to my colleagues or my classes at Woodbridge High, except that I did have a confidential discussion with our principal, Pam White. She was exceptionally cooperative and supportive. Sharry told a few of her close friends at her office at the Health Department, but it was a small number and those told proved to be very discrete.

On Thursday, May 9, I took off work and went to Dr. Merlino's office in the morning for a follow-up visit. She told me that she had spoken with Dr. Matthews at length the previous evening. I was to learn that Robin always went out of her way to discuss her patient's condition with colleagues who were specialists in applicable areas. Her mood was extremely somber. In addition to a normal office exam, she ordered blood work and scheduled a Pulmonary Function Test (PFT) at Fairfax Hospital for the following afternoon. Based on her conversation with Matthews, she started me on 50 mg of Dyazide to reduce my blood pressure and 60 mg of Prednisone for the sarcoidosis.

The benefit of taking Prednisone to combat sarcoid is dubious, at best. It seems to be a drug which is prescribed for a wide variety of situations in which little else will work. A friend of mine told me that her father, her son, and her dog were **all** on Prednisone at the same time a few years ago. Presumably they did not have the same ailment. The drug is a corticosteroid which has certain anti-inflammatory and immunosuppressant properties. It is often pre-scribed for bad cases of poison ivy. In my case, the desired result was a lessening of the inflammation of the tissue affected by the sarcoid. Prednisone treatment has been shown, in some instances, to stop the spread of sarcoid within a body organ. Unfortunately, when the heart is involved, scar tissue tends to form during the healing process, causing the same arrhythmias (rhythm distur-bances) as the sarcoid itself. All of my doctors were very straight-forward about Prednisone: it probably would not help, but maybe...

I certainly was willing to try.

Taking Prednisone for an extended period is no free lunch, be-cause the side effects are considerable. Dr. Merlino went over each with me so that I could recognize them as they appeared. As she discussed the side effects, I found myself only marginally interested, until she mentioned "moon face."

When I looked puzzled by this term, she explained, "Ed, many people on steroids such as Prednisone develop a condition called cushingoid. It's called that because the symptoms are very similar to a disease first described by a neurosurgeon in Boston named Cushing - Harvey Cushing, if I am remembering my med school stuff correctly. It is also sometimes referred to as Cushing's Syndrome and is caused by excess secretions of the pituitary gland. It's relatively rare and affects women far more than men. You don't have that problem, but continued doses of Prednisone create the same set of symptoms. The most noticeable change in men is a swelling of the body in certain areas, usually the abdomen. However, for most patients, it also causes a rounded, or "moon" face to develop after a period of time."

Dr. Merlino then showed me some photographs in one of her medical books. My only verbal reponse was a mumbled "I see," but I was simultaneously thinking, "That guy really does have a moon face!" He looked as if his face had been inflated and was about to explode. Surely this was an extreme case?

Ignoring my fascination with the rather graphic photographs in her medical book, Merlino went on to expain that the other side effects of Prednisone were not as visual. There is typically a weight gain, which may, or may not, be obvious to others. Some patients may also have difficulty sleeping, and experience mood changes, nervousness, or even rather serious emotional upheaval. I was to later learn that several of my friends had developed intense emotional swings when they were on high doses of Prednisone. After Dr. Merlino discussed each of these possibilities with me, she added that the drug also lessens the effectiveness of the body's natural immune system. If I were to develop an infection or show symptoms of a virus, I should contact her. I would probably have given this conversation more attention if I had been able to foresee the future.

Dr. Merlino had one more treat for me before I left her office. She wanted me to wear a Holter Monitor for the next 24 hours. This is a portable device to record heart function, developed, I presume, by a physician named Holter. Sometimes it is referred to as a dynamic electrocardiogram, a long term ECG, or an ambulatory ECG. All of my doctors used the Holter term. Regardless of the name, all perform the same function, that is, providing a continuous electrocardiogram which can be played back for later analysis. Because the Holter records every heart beat, it can detect various types of arrhythmias, such as bradycardia (abnormally slow heart rhythm), tachycardia (fast heart rhythm), pauses in heart action or extra heart beats.

The Holter Monitor looked like a small portable tape recorder, such as a Walkman. Instead of headphones, it had five color-coded wires (white, red, green, brown and black). Snaps on the ends of each of the wires were attached to patches which Dr. Merlino's office nurse stuck to various locations on my upper body. The "Walkman portion" was indeed simply a cassette tape recorder powered by a standard 9 volt battery. There was a carrying case with a belt and a shoulder harness so that I could wear it continuously, day and night. I was told to follow my normal daily routine, but to record my activities in a "patient diary."

The nurse told me that the success of the Holter depended on my cooperation in recording all activities and any possible symptoms, such as dizziness or shortness of breath. Her monologue began to get interesting as she gave examples of what type of activities I should record: eating, sleeping, exercising, drinking alcoholic or caffeine beverages, taking medications, bowel movements, and sexual activity. This last item intrigued me. I formed a mental picture of my explaining to Sharry, "This is all for science, Honey."

The Holter had an "event button" which is to be pressed by the patient whenever he thinks that "something big" is happening. In view of my lingering thoughts on the sexual stuff, I chose not to pursue a clarification of this last item.

I wore the Holter for the next 24 hours and was a very dutiful recorder. I noticed no unusual events and experienced no strange feelings from my body. What I did notice as I climbed into bed was a steady "whirl" sound coming from the recorder as it did its thing. I encouraged Sharry to ignore the impression that she was in bed with a bionic man. It certainly was **not** mood music for any intimate relationship. The diary of this night certainly made fairly boring reading. Thanks a lot, Dr. Holter!

I returned the entire unit to Merlino's office the next day. The tape and diary were sent to a local office of the manufacturer, where each of my approximately 110,000 heart beats from the 24 hour period was analyzed using specialized equipment. A report was then forwarded to Dr. Merlino. Her nurse called me near the end of following week to report that "everything looked good on the Holter." Over the next year I had occasion to wear the Holter several times. In each case the result was the same: nothing. It turns out that an "in joke" among doctors is that the best way to prevent arrhythmias in patients is to have them wear a Holter Monitor. This may be a medical equivalent of "a watched pot never boils."

The Pulmonary Function Test took place at nearby Fairfax Hospital on May 10. It lasted about an hour and was conducted by a technician. There are various types of PFTs, but mine required that I blow air from my lungs into a machine. This device is connected to, and controlled by, a computer system to analyze the results. The goal is to exhale all of the air possible to determine lung capacity and function. The technician acted as a coach/cheerleader encouraging me to keep blowing - even after there was obviously nothing left to exhale. I found myself wanting to please the guy. I also wanted desperately to prove that there was nothing wrong with me.

After a few runs, the patient receives an aerosol medication to inhale. A waiting period follows, and the entire test procedure is repeated. There is also a phase in which the patient is placed inside a plexiglass booth and told over a speaker system to "blow in" or "breathe normally." There is one part of this procedure in which I was told to breathe, but a valve had been shut and there is nothing to breathe. Hello, Claustrophobia City! In spite of all my submarine experience, I came very close to losing it on this one. I wanted to bang on the walls and yell, "Get me out of here!!!" with some choice profanity added for emphasis.

I hung around the PFT lab until the data was reviewed by the technician for preliminary analysis. He told me that my lungs lacked the capacity which the computer had calculated a male of my height, weight, and age should have, but that they were in reasonably good shape and did not indicate a problem. About one week later, I received a copy of the written report sent to Merlino and Matthews. It contained various graphs and data, but the text indicated the same thing which I had been told by the technician.

Over the following weekend I was very active. My track team had a meet on Saturday and, as usual, I ran just as much as the athletes. On Sunday, after church in the morning, Aaron and I mowed the grounds of one of the local swimming pools for which he had the contract. He had started a mowing business, Aaron's Lawn Service, four years earlier, when he was in junior high school. It had grown each year, and he now had several commercial mowing contracts with automobile dealerships and swim clubs. During the busy part of the mowing season, I would often help him. My son, the entrepreneur, normally hired friends to work, but I was his dream employee: I worked free. Driving a ride-on lawn tractor is one of the ultimate "guy things." I probably would have paid him to sit on that mower and cut grass.

That evening was a turning point. Although I went to bed around 10:30 PM, I could not get to sleep until after midnight. I awoke at 2:45 AM experiencing a shortness of breath and a noticeably strange heartbeat. I was frightened, but decided not to awaken Sharry. After a relatively short period, I went back to sleep, but was awake again at 4:30 AM with the same heart disturbance, plus a bad sweat in place of the shortness of breath.

In the morning I told Sharry what had happened. She was upset that I had not awoken her during the night. After thoroughly scolding me for being so macho (I think that her exact words were, "That was really stupid, Ed!"), she insisted that I promise to call Dr. Merlino as soon as her office opened. Since I now felt fine, I decided to go to work. I telephoned Merlino at 9AM to relay the events of the night. Her response was, "I think that we may have a problem. I will talk to Bob Matthews and get back to you."

Within an hour she called and left a message for me to talk to her as soon as possible. I waited until the end of my fifth period class to do so. I was dreading the conversation.

Robin told me that she had discussed my situation with Dr. Matthews and that they both felt that I should be admitted to Fairfax Hospital for additional tests and monitoring of my heart. I asked how long I might be in the hospital. She replied the obvious, "We don't know for sure. Probably several days."

I asked some of my colleagues to cover my 6th and 7th period classes, then left the school shortly. Feeling no sense of urgency, I stopped at the bank to take care of some financial matters. At home I picked up pajamas and some toiletry items to take with me. I was not certain about what else to pack, because I had not stayed overnight in a hospital in over 30 years. The main thing which I remembered about that experience, which was minor surgery to remove an undescended testicle prior to my admission to the Naval Academy, was how the doctor had laughed at me when I confided to him my fear of not being able to have children following the surgery. "Do you have any idea how many sperm you still have left in the other testicle?" he roared far too loudly for my young sensibilities. I think that I carried the resulting pyschic scar longer than the actual physical one from the surgery. I also remembered that hospital gowns were annoying, ill-fitted sacks which always left my rear end cold: hence my priority to take pj's with me.

I had telephoned Sharry before leaving the high school. She did not seem to be surprised that Robin wanted to admit me. In fact, her voice had a tone of relief. We decided to meet at the hospital at 3 PM.

As I backed out of our driveway to go to the hospital, I found myself taking a prolonged look at our yard and home. It was a sobering moment. I was now, for the first time, becoming very worried. "Would I ever return?" I wondered. I was definitely entering uncharted water.

Fairfax Hospital is a 656 bed regional medical center located in Falls Church, Virginia, approximately 20 minutes from our home. It is part of Inova Health System, a local network of several hospitals and medical facilities. Its medical reputation is superb, particularly in the field of oncology and cardiac treatment.

Dr. Merlino had called ahead authorizing my admission. The process went smoothly, primarily because we have two insurance plans. Admission has much to do with insurance, and little with illness. Actually, it is **all** insurance, as in, "What do you have?" rather than "What is ailing you?"

Our primary coverage was with Blue Cross/Blue Shield of Virginia through Sharry's employment with the Health Department. Our "backup," or secondary, insurance was CHAMPUS, a program for military personnel, both active duty and retired. As we sat in the admissions office that afternoon, we had no idea that we would become such experts in insurance matters over the next several years. If degrees were granted, both Sharry and I would have earned Ph.D.'s in health insurance long ago. We also did not realize that we were about to embark on a prolonged medical adventure costing well over one million dollars.

I was taken to a room on the second floor of the hospital. This floor was equipped with telemetry units to provide continuous monitoring of each patient's heart. I was wired with electrodes similar to the Holter, except that the wires were connected to a small transmitter (also the approximate size of a Walkman) which fit nicely into the front pocket of my pajamas. The signals from my heart were received as a trace on a TV monitor at the nursing station. A technician, backed up by an audible and visual alarm system, continuously observed the traces of all the patients.

I remained in the hospital for the next three days. On Tuesday, I was taken to a different part of the hospital for a "CAT scan" of my chest. I had taught my students the physics of this combined x-ray/computer process, but I had never experienced, or seen, the equipment or the procedure. CAT, computerized axial tomography, is conducted by a large machine in which a narrow beam of x-rays is scanned across a small slice of the designated area of the body. The amount of the beam received is measured by a row of detectors and the results are computer recorded. As the x-ray tube rotates in an arc of a circle around the patient, the radiation passing through the body is absorbed in differing amounts depending on the type of biological matter through which it passes. The computer is programmed to calculate the density of those portions of the body observed so that a three-dimensional image can be formed. Tumors are frequently detected more readily on a CAT scan than with a conventional x-ray. I was not told whether the intent was to use the CAT scan to detect evidence of sarcoid or to determine if there was another problem with my heart. At any rate, the results were negative. Nothing unusual was noted.

I also did not have rhythm disturbances during the 72 hours that I was on the hospital monitoring system. If I was having arrhythmia episodes, they were so infrequent and minor that they were undetected.

On Thursday morning I was discharged. We had learned essentially nothing from this four thousand dollar investment, except that hospital food was not as bad as I expected and that hospital gowns had not changed much in the past thirty years. I still did not have any documented instances of heart disturbances. Maybe this was all in my head. At least that was the line I was trying to sell to myself.

The next morning Sharry and I drove the 60 miles from our home in Virginia to Johns Hopkins University Hospital in Baltimore, Maryland to be seen by Bob Matthew's friend, Dr. Kenneth Baughman. The medical center is located in a "neighborhood in transition" in East Baltimore. We passed by the harbor area downtown, then took Pratt Street before turning left onto Broadway. It was not a pretty sight. My first impression was that the entire area surrounding the hospital had been bombed. The streets in the vicinity were torn up, apparently for construction of a subway, and the hospital itself was in a state of large-scale renovation. This sighting continued my unbroken streak of nearly 50 years, stretching back to my birth at Speers Hospital in Kentucky, of **never** being in a hospital or an airport which was not under construction.

Johns Hopkins actually consists of a large complex of buildings, some very old, and others quite modern in appearance, located on a 44-acre campus on a sloping hillside. The hospital opened in 1889 as the result of the will of the founder of the B&O Railroad, Mr. Johns Hopkins. Not being an expert on 19th century male first names, I always wondered if Hopkins' parents had made a typo on his birth certificate or if they had really been hoping for twins. At any rate, "Johns," having made a fortune, wanted to establish a university in Baltimore which would include a school of medicine and an associated hospital. I think that he would be pleased with the result of his donation.

Hopkins currently includes a 1036-bed hospital, a world-renowned school of medicine, a school of nursing and the oldest and largest school of public health in the U.S. There is also a large outpatient center and a huge medical library. More than 8000 physicians are alumni of the School of Medicine. Some of the highlights of Hopkins' contributions to the advancement of medical science include the first use of surgical rubber gloves, the discovery of vitamin D, development of gene mapping, the first use of drugs to prevent rheumatic fever, and the development of an implantable, rechargeable cardiac pacemaker. I felt that I was in good hands.

As Sharry and I walked toward the main entrance to the hospital, I noticed that the exteriors were brick. The mathematician in me suddenly wanted to try to calculate the total number of all the bricks at Johns Hopkins. Apparently my mind was trying to focus on anything other than our medical predicament. As we entered the building, we were confronted with a rather elaborate security checkpoint manned by two guards and a metal detector. Crowds of people were coming and going. From this perspective, Hopkins looked more like a busy airport terminal than a hospital.

After obtaining security badges to display on our clothing, Sharry and I found our way to the Clayton Heart Center on the 5th floor of the Blalock Building, an older part of the complex. We checked in with a rather disinterested clerk, who, after considerable shuffling of papers, found our appointment which had been made by Dr. Matthews when I was in Fairfax Hospital earlier in the week. While waiting for the next hour, we both read a special edition of *U.S. News and World Report* which rated Hopkins as "Best of the Best" in its annual rankings. I was not yet ready to join in the chorus of hosannas, but I was impressed.

The patients at Hopkins appeared to be from a distinctly different socio-economic group than those at I had seen at Fairfax. I doubt that many people in the waiting area that day had medical insurance. I wondered how many of these patients understood that they were being cared for by a staff which had a world-wide reputation for excellence. My own feeling was that we had journeyed to Mecca and were about to have an audience with the Supreme Cardiac.

Rather than resembling anything remotely divine, Dr. Baughman was a totally ordinary looking physician in a white lab coat. The examining room was equally plebeian. Upon meeting us, Baughman made several jokes and seemed to be going out of his way to be Mr. Casual Guy. He did give me a thorough examination and spent considerable time discussing my medical history. Suddenly a young resident entered the room and breathlessly proclaimed, "I would have been here sooner, but Mr. _____ just arrested and died in the E.R." Baughman took the news with little apparent emotion and then chastised the young doctor for being late. As the resident absorbed this rebuke, I was reminded of my own experiences as a junior officer aboard ship when confronted by a testy Commanding Officer. Life is not always fair when you are the new kid on the block.

Sharry had brought several items from Fairfax Hospital for Dr. Baughman to review. He gave the videotapes of my echocardiogram to the resident and asked him to prepare them for later viewing. He then looked closely at several of my recent EKGs. His demeanor had changed into total professionalism. I handed over the slides which contained the heart tissue samples which had been obtained by Dr. Mattthews during the cardiac catheterization two weeks earlier. Baughman's plan, he told us, was to look at the videotape and the slides later in the evening with several of his colleagues. He would call me on Monday to tell us his findings.

Before we left, Sharry asked Dr. Baughman what he thought based on the examination and the information which he had seen. Without hesitation he replied, "I think that it is highly unlikely that your husband has cardiac sarcoidosis. There simply is nothing in the literature to suggest a case like yours where there is no sarcoid except in the right side of the heart. It could be, but I really doubt it. This doesn't mean that there is not a problem. It's just that I don't think that we are talking sarcoid here. I won't know for sure until I see the slides. What I would really prefer is for us to do our own biopsy of your heart tissue here. That way we could be sure."

Dr. Baughman then walked us to the elevator. He seemed to have reverted to his joking mode. "You know," he said, " If you do die, and it's sarcoid, you could be great material for someone's journal article." Neither Sharry nor I laughed.

During the 75 minute drive back to our home in Springfield, Sharry and I went through several rationalizations about the usefulness of our visit with Baughman. We both thought that he was very knowledgeable and competent. His opinion that I probably did not have sarcoid was encouraging. Matthews had told us that I would die soon from the sarcoid - maybe if the condition was something else, as Baughman had suggested, there would be a cure for it. We remained generally optimistic throughout the weekend.

On Monday our world again collapsed.

Dr. Baughman telephoned and confirmed Matthews' original diagnosis of cardiac sarcoidosis. His voice was very sober as he said, "There is a remarkable amount of granulomas in one of the tissue samples. It is very intense. From the echo, it appears to be unique to the right ventricle. I have never seen anything like it."

Dr. Baughman went on for several minutes discussing his findings. I did not hear most of his words because I was in a daze. Once again, I was receiving a death sentence. I did hear him explain how he had spoken with a Dr. Margaret Billingham of Stanford University to confirm his diagnosis. Apparently she was another expert in cardiac sarcoidosis. He then told me that he wanted me to receive a gallium scan and a slit lamp eye exam, both at Hopkins, if possible. Weakly I said, "Sure."

In my shock upon hearing Baughman's confirmation of sarcoid, I failed to ask him exactly what a gallium scan was. It was not until I relayed the phone conversation to Sharry that I realized how little I understood what was about to happen. As a nurse, she knew that the procedure involved nuclear medicine, but that was it. The specifics were unclear. We decided to save our questions until my next scheduled appointment with Dr. Matthews.

All was normal throughout the week. Teaching and coaching posed no problems. Sometimes I would feel a pressure in my upper left chest area, but there was no sharp pain. I did not know whether this was real or imaginary.I decided to tell no one, including Sharry, until I saw Matthews.

My appointment with Dr. Matthews was after school on Friday, May 24, 1991. He gave me another EKG and a thorough examination. The EKG was unchanged; the T-wave was still inverted. The exam revealed nothing new. He had no explanation for the chest pain and did not seem terribly concerned about it.

Sharry and I had prepared a list of questions concerning the visit with Baughman. I was not surprised when Matthews told me in response that he had spoken with "Ken." By now, I was beginning to understand that word spreads quickly in the medical community when an unusual case like mine is encountered. A healthy exchange of professional opinions takes place. It did not make me feel better that I was becoming a celebrity, of sorts.

Dr. Matthews explained the purpose of the gallium scan and exactly how it would be done. I had already been scheduled by Baughman's secretary to go to Hopkins on the following Tuesday to be injected with a radioactive isotope of gallium. Forty-eight hours later I would return to Baltimore to have the actual scan performed using specialized equipment within their nuclear medicine facility. I would also receive the slit lamp eye exam on that same date to determine if the sarcoid had spread to my eyes. I asked whether the gallium might relieve or exacerbate the sarcoidosis. Matthews replied that the scan was meant to be diagnostic, not therapeutic. How it affected the sarcoid granulomas was "not in the literature." In closing the discussion, he added that he wanted Dr. O'Connell to do another echocardiogram on me during the first week of June to see if there had been any degradation in the condition of my heart. I said to myself, "Any other cheerful thoughts for the weekend, Bob?"

The following Tuesday I took a day of sick leave and drove by myself to Baltimore for the first phase of the gallium scan at Johns Hopkins. A British doctor, Petra Jeffrey, injected 10 microcuries of a radioactive isotope of gallium directly into a vein in my arm. When I asked Dr. Jeffrey which isotope of gallium she was using, she was startled. Apparently most patients do not ask such questions. She replied, "Gallium 67. Why do you want to know?"

I laughed and said, "I teach physics at a high school in Virginia. My students will be interested. What is the half life of this gallium-67 anyway? I assume that it is a gamma emitter, isn't it?"

To my surprise, she did not know for certain the half life (how long it takes for one half of the radioactivity of a substance to decay while emitting radiation). She did, however, immediately obtain the information for me from the literature enclosed with the gallium. The half life was 48 hours and it was a gamma emitter. She went on to explain that gallium has a tendency to "go to the sarcoid." Those areas with heavy concentrations of sarcoidosis absorb higher levels of the radioactive gallium, resulting in increased radiation coming from those areas. When I returned in two days, I would lie motionless on a table while specialized radiation detection equipment would slowly scan my chest region. Those regions with sarcoid should appear to be darker than unaffected areas.

I thanked Dr. Jeffrey for her patience and left the hospital. The next day I checked myself with a Geiger Counter (a radiation measurement device) in my classroom and found that I was incredibly hot, radiologically speaking. In fact, I could set off the automatic alarm on the equipment by simply walking into the classroom! For many of my students, this new development with Mr. Linz con-

firmed their belief that I was exceptionally weird. I took this opportunity to tell my classes that I had recently learned that I had a potentially serious heart disease and that I might have to miss a few
additional days in the future. All of the students, including the few
who were bad actors, were supportive. Many came up to me after
class and asked if there was something which they could do to help.
Throughout my medical ordeal over the next several years, my students provided enormous emotional support.

When I returned to Hopkins on Thursday, the second phase of
the gallium scan procedure was exactly as Dr. Jeffrey had described
it to me. I was surprised, however, by how narrow the table was
that I had to lie on during the scan. What did they have to do for a
genuinely fat person?

While at Hopkins, I also had the slit lamp eye examination. It
was performed in the Wilmer Eye Clinic in one of the older parts of
the facility. The doctor conducting the exam was named Jabs. Although it took considerable restraint on my part, I did not attempt
any "jab-in-the-eye" jokes. It was my guess that this fellow had
probably had it with humor related to his name and line of work.
He probably still carried scars from playground taunting during his
grade school years.

The slit lamp exam was identical to those which I had received in
the Navy. Dr. Jabs explained to me that if sarcoid is present in the
eyes, it can be easily detected by this procedure. He spent considerable time looking, but could find no evidence of the disease in my
eyes. As I was leaving, he recommended that I receive a similar examination every six months by my regular ophthalmologist in Virginia.

I felt reassured by Dr. Jabs' non-findings. If I did have sarcoidosis within me, it had not spread throughout my body. In good spirits, I went to Newport News, Virginia that weekend for the state
high school track championship meet. The temperature was over
100 degrees in the afternoon, but our team did well. Aaron finished
3rd in the mile race and made "all state." He had enjoyed another
successful season and was being actively recruited by several universities.

On June 5 Dr. Baughman called in the evening from Johns
Hopkins to discuss the results of the gallium scan. He said that it

had provided little useful information. There was "no significant accumulation of gallium in my chest or pericardium." He seemed to be disappointed that we had learned so little from the test. I, on the other hand, felt relieved that I was apparently not crawling with sarcoid. Since I had not yet experienced any documented instances of heart problems, I was still hoping that this entire nightmare had all been some type of mistake or misdiagnosis.

Unfortunately such optimistic thinking met a reality check the following evening. At dinner I felt as if my pulse had suddenly gone up. Sharry listened to my heart with the stethoscope which she kept at home. The rate was 160 beats per minute for approximately the next 15 minutes. Then it returned to 80. The same thing happened around midnight. We decided not to call Merlino or Matthews because I had an appointment the next day for an echocardiogram with Bob O'Connell. We did not want to cry wolf too often. In retrospect, I now think that we were still very much in denial.

The echo had essentially the same results as the previous one. There was no degradation. The right side of my heart was still enlarged, but Dr. O'Connell did not seem concerned. I also had blood drawn for a "Chem 6" blood test which Merlino had ordered. The values for glucose, sodium, potassium, chlorides, and carbon dioxide were within normal ranges; the urea level was slightly elevated, but was deemed not to be a problem.

My mother arrived from Kentucky on Saturday. She had come to attend Aaron's high school graduation on June 13. Both as a nurse and as a mother, Mom had been very concerned about the sarcoidosis diagnosis. Although she had no direct experience treating sarcoid patients, she was familiar with the disease and understood the implications. Her attitude had been optimistic from the beginning, but she was clearly worried.

Having Mom and Sharry under the same roof always increased the tension level in the house. Their animosity, based on cultural and personality differences, had remained below the surface for the first several years of our marriage, but, at about the ten year mark, open warfare broke out. They rarely agreed on anything, especially if it was medically related. The fact that both were nurses did little to bridge the chasm. None of us took sides in this conflict. We loved both of them and kept hoping that a miracle would happen and that they would suddenly like, or at least tolerate, each other. It never happened.

On Monday I had an appointment with Bob Matthews. We discussed the gallium results and developed a plan to slowly reduce my daily Prednisone dose. The intention was to gradually wean me from the drug. If it had worked to combat the sarcoid, its effectiveness was now a matter of diminishing returns. Any further good accomplished by the Prednisone would be outweighed by the harmful side effects of extended use. Matthews also touched on the "What next?" issue. He said that I might require a pacemaker or even, eventually, a heart transplant. My interest level in the conversation was so low that I did not ask him about either of these options. That evening I again wore a Holter monitor, but it recorded nothing of interest.

Aaron graduated from West Springfield High on June 13. My best friend, Aaron Spurway, had flown in from his home in Spokane for the occasion. I had difficulty at the graduation ceremony, but it was not medical. Beachballs, noisemakers, inappropriate gestures - you name it - were all part of the proceedings - even during the remarks by the guest speaker. The sad part is that this is a totally avoidable problem. Graduation ceremonies, for example, at Woodbridge High, where I teach, are always a pleasant, civilized experience for both the participants and their guests. The difference is that Woodbridge has stated rules which are consistently enforced.

Mom and Spurway flew to their respective homes following the graduation. With Sharry and Mom now separated by 500 miles, tension around the house decreased immediately. On Tuesday Aaron received a telephone call from the cross country coach at University of North Carolina (UNC) telling him that they "wanted him." There was no money available for scholarship assistance, but they had obtained approval from the admissions office to offer him entry to the university. Aaron had been intending to accept an offer of a partial scholarship at James Madison University, but this development presented a new option. He drove to Chapel Hill, North Carolina the next day to talk with the coach. That evening he called home and told us that he wanted to be a Tar Heel.

The next month was relatively uneventful. I still had not developed symptoms which could be documented. My Prednisone dose was being reduced 5 mg each week. By the end of July, I was down to 20 mg daily.

During the first week of July, I had magnetic resonance imaging (MRI) performed on my chest and abdomen at a local hospital. Although I was placed inside a narrow chamber for the procedure, the experience was not as claustrophobic as I had been led to believe. The results provided no useful information.

On the advice of Bob Matthews, I obtained an appointment to see an arrhythmia specialist, Dr. Ted Friehling. Friehling was a cardiologist, but he concentrated on heart rhythm disturbances. He and his partner, Al Del Negro, had an office close to my home. My first impression of Friehling was surprise at his appearance. He looked young and had curly, black, shoulder-length hair. Was I really about to entrust my life to some hippie-looking character?

Ted's office was, in contrast, furnished in a very Mercedes-like manner. "Even if this guy looks strange, he must be good enough to drag in big bucks from somewhere," I thought. Looking around the examination room, I noticed a photograph of his partner, Al Del Negro, taken while he was running in the New York City Marathon. As a two-time marathoner myself, I felt a kindred relationship to these guys, even before I knew them.

Dr. Friehling immediately put me at ease as we talked. He was friendly and knowledgeable - a combination which I like in a doctor. He examined me carefully and thoroughly but found nothing of concern. At the end of my visit he produced a portable device in a small briefcase for me to carry at all times for the next month. It was called a Cardiocare ECG Recorder. Whenever I felt as if I might be having a cardiac rhythm disturbance, I was to place the circular microphone over my heart and hit the record button on the device. After at least one minute of recording, I would turn the unit off and telephone a toll-free number to receive further directions. Friehling told me that the Cardiocare unit would record an EKG which could be sent over telephone lines for analysis and retransmission back to him. If anything happened in the next month and I were aware of it, we would now have a means to document it.

As I left Dr. Friehling's office with my new electronic companion alongside, I felt as if I were one of the military aides who carries a similar looking briefcase while following a few steps behind the President. That briefcase contains codes and devices to send information to our military forces to authorize release of a retaliatory nuclear attack on our enemies. In the crazy logic of the nuclear age, that briefcase helps to save all of us. Mine was less threatening, but, to me, just as important. It contained a device to record data that might provide the information which could save my life. I found myself gripping the handle on the Cardiocare tightly.

During the week of July 8, I had two appointments with members of my cardiology team. I found it ironic that only two months earlier, I did not know for certain what a cardiologist was, but now I had a "team" of them. I met with Bob Matthews early in the week. He doubted that the intermittent pain in my left upper chest was related to the sarcoid, but he could find no other cause for it. He seemed rather pessimistic about my prognosis, and I left his office feeling helpless and depressed.

On Friday of that week, I drove to Baltimore to see Dr. Baughman again. He stated categorically that the chest pain was not related to my heart and that his primary concern was to wean me from Prednisone as rapidly as possible. If the drug had been effective in neutralizing the sarcoid, its usefulness was now diminishing daily as the negative aspects of the long term side effects were beginning to develop. He also wanted to perform a catheterization of the right side of my heart and concurrently obtain another biopsy of the heart tissue at Johns Hopkins. I replied that I would think about it. Although I did not say anything to Baughman about my real feelings, Sharry and I had discussed various options about Hopkins and had decided that we strongly preferred that any procedures be performed at Fairfax Hospital due to logistical reasons. Why should we opt for my hospitalization so far away when the same results could be obtained locally?

On July 22, I took a cardiac stress test in Dr. Matthews office. I was wired for a continuous EKG and directed to walk, then run, on a treadmill. Matthews increased the speed and the incline of the treadmill as the test progressed. My initial reaction had been, "Piece of cake!" Near the end of the test I found myself looking anxiously at Matthews hoping that he would finish collecting data before I passed out. Just as I was on the verge of crying, "Mercy, Big Bob!!!!", he slowed and lowered the treadmill. I looked at him expecting some form of praise for a fine effort, but all I received was, "OK, Ed."

"OK?" I thought. "How about, 'I have never seen a guy your age do so well' or 'That's a record for this office, Ed.'" or **anything** encouraging.

Dr. Matthews had little else to add based on the stress test. My heart had functioned well and we learned nothing new. Before I left his office, he did discuss some possible options. He again mentioned a heart transplant if my condition worsened. I immediately dismissed this idea, "Bob, I haven't had any symptoms yet! I am still not sure that I have a problem."

"There is another possibility," Mattthews replied. "You can receive a defibrillator. It's a device which is surgically inserted to shock your heart back into a normal rhythm in the event of a problem. It's like those paddles you see on TV shows except that yours would be inside you directly attached to your heart."

"That sounds rather extreme," I answered. "Wouldn't that involve major surgery?" Before Matthews could respond, I added, "I think that I would like to talk to your friend, Dr. Bashore, at Duke before I do anything like that."

Dr. Matthews smiled patiently, "I am not talking about surgery today, Ed. I am trying to let you know what your options may be."

That evening I talked with Sharry about my conversation with Matthews. She agreed that we should not consider any radical steps. Both the heart transplant and the defibrillator options scared us.

The following day I flew to Kentucky with Emily to join my mother for a flight to Arizona to visit her youngest sister, my Aunt Jean. Jean is one of the most colorful and generous individuals I know. Both she and her husband, Tony, are retired from the Chicago area. In her last job, Jean had been a welder, and, by all accounts, a very good one. Having had no personal experience with her work, I would still take Jean over most of the welders I had observed at Navy shipyards. At least, I was confident that Aunt Jean was not on drugs.

My mother's side of our family did have certain rough elements to it. One of her sisters had been murdered with a shotgun by her husband in the front of the family pickup truck. This took place in Kentucky in 1950. The murderer, my uncle, was sentenced to all of 9 months for his act. He did, however, have to sign over title to his two dump trucks to the lawyer who defended him. According to Mom, another of her sisters had been accused by the police of hiring a "torch" to set fire to some run-down housing which she owned so that she could collect the insurance. There was later a mysterious shooting death of this aunt's husband and frequent rumors about her family's involvement with the Mob. I had seen no direct evidence of this other than a large, popular nightclub (with a certain amount of sleazy characters) operated by one of this aunt's sons. For some reason, I had always felt proud of this side of my heritage, particularly whenever I found myself among some of the over-stuffed "blue-blood types" Sharry and I had met while we lived in England.

There were indeed a few unconventional aspects to Mom's family. Aunt Jean fits comfortably in the mold. Two of her favorite things in life are yard sales and slot machines. Shortly before we arrived for our visit, she had borrowed a jack hammer from a neighbor and dug a hole in the concrete slab below her bedroom to place a safe to hide her valuables and slot machine winnings. She had purchased the safe at a yard sale. In fact, much of Jean's house was a testimony to bargains obtained at garage sales. Undoubtedly, her frugality was derived from an exceptionally difficult childhood in the Kentucky minefields during the Depression. Her mother died at an early age, and as the youngest of eight children, she suffered greatly. In addition to continuous financial problems, her father (my grandfather) frequently beat her and ultimately threw her out of the house to fend for herself when she was fifteen. She took a bus to Chicago and not only managed to survive, but flourished due to hard work and ingenuity. Having the same bloodlines, I found that I liked Jean's lifestyle and sense of values. She was a "real" person.

Both Aunt Jean and Uncle Tony had a history of heart problems. As opposed to my situation, the source of their cardiac failure was more definable. In addition to Jean being a heavy smoker, their daily diet had not been heart-friendly, to say the least. Even after both had heart bypass surgeries (they were in the hospital simulta-neously for the operations!), my aunt and uncle were unable to change their lifestyle. Jean stopped smoking for a while, but soon resumed the habit. Although Jean and Tony attempted to alter their diets, few nutritionists would have given approval to their menu choices. They certainly tried, but, as many others with dietary problems have discovered, it is difficult to change life-long patterns in the autumn of your years. But they were happy with themselves and doing better than I in terms of cardiac health.

We had a wonderful time in Arizona. We took day trips from Jean and Tony's home in Mesa to the Apache Trail and spent an afternoon tubing down the Salt River. Jean loaned us her car so that Mom, Emily, and I could take a trip north to the Grand Can-yon. Based on the recommendation of Jean's daughter, Peggy, we had arranged to stay overnight in a small bed and breakfast in Wil-liams, Arizona, about 60 miles from the south rim of Grand Canyon National Park. Peggy owned a very successful consulting firm which did business throughout Arizona. In her travels she had dis-covered our accomodations, the Johnstonian, which was owned and operated by a delightful couple named Bill and Pidge.(Yes, Pidge!). The Johnstonian was clean and cleverly decorated, but was in an older residential part of Williams. Mom and Emily stayed in one room, while I was by myself in an extremely tiny room on the top floor. Just as I was trying to get to sleep, a chorus of wild barking began outside the house. The Johnstonian was sitting in the middle of Junkyard Dog City!!

The dogs continued to bark throughout the night. I could not sleep and, around 2 AM, I noticed that my heart had suddenly started to beat wildly. I became frightened and began to sweat heavily. I foolishly decided, however, not to record the incident on the Cardiocare recorder, which was alongside the bed. My thinking was that I would have to waken Bill and Pidge in order to use their telephone to call the 800 number. Since I did not know which was their bedroom, I rationalized that this was probably not a "real" event and that I should not bother anyone unless I was certain. Of course, I could have easily recorded the event and then telephoned the data to New York in the morning. Maybe the barking dogs affected my thought process. More likely, I was still not ready to accept the fact that my death sentence was real.

In the morning I arose tired, but in a normal heart rhythm. I decided not to tell Mom or Emily. We drove to the south rim of the Canyon and walked part of the Bright Angel Trail before driving back to Mesa. The next day we flew home. When Sharry met us at National Airport, I did not tell her about my apparent tachycardia episode in Arizona. I was now dangerously in denial.

After arriving home, I felt as if I were still on West Coast time. I did not go to bed with Sharry, but stayed up working on bills and other paperwork at the kitchen table. At 2:30 AM I noticed that my heart was again beating rapidly. I went to the family room to lie down on the sofa where I could record the event on the Cardiocare device. After obtaining data for about two minutes, I telephoned the 800 number in New York and began the transfer process.

I was actually surprised that someone quickly answered on the second ring. It was the middle of the night. I explained that I had recorded what I thought had been a heart disturbance of some type. The voice replied, "Rewind the tape, then hit the Play button. After two minutes, hit Stop.

I did as directed. Upon the completion of my part, I wondered what was next. The voice said, "We got it. It looks like you had an episode of supraventricular tachycardia. You are in no immediate danger. We will notify your doctor. It's Friehling, isn't it?"

My voice was not strong and my mind was elsewhere, but I did manage a weak, "Yes. His office is here in Virginia. How can you reach him tonight?"

The voice said that contacting Friehling would not be a problem. I should go to bed and await a call from my doctor. If I had further problems, I should call 911 or go immediately to the hospital.

This got my attention. "911?!!"

After thanking the voice, I went upstairs to wake Sharry to tell her what had taken place. She was again angry that I had not awoken her as soon as I thought that I had a problem. She became really upset with me when I then told her about the incident in Arizona. Through some warped reasoning process, I felt rather pleased that I had cashed two dumb mistakes of omission for the price of just one fit of anger. A great two-for-one deal!

Sharry was too worried to sleep, but I had no trouble dozing off. Dr. Friehling telephoned early in the morning. The Cardiocare people had faxed a copy of the EKG data to his office. He told me that the initial analysis by the technician in New York had understated the problem. Rather than having had an episode of supraventricular tachycardia, I had undergone a dangerous period of sustained "V-Tach" (ventricular tachycardia) and that I should be admitted to the hospital as soon as possible.

Sharry's anger turned into fear. My thoughts drifted between concern and denial. Was I really about to die?

Chapter 5

AMIODARONE

Once again, I chose not to rush to the hospital. I was also angry that my life was being disrupted. I did not have time to be sick. I certainly had done nothing to deserve a death sentence.

These were my thoughts and emotions as I once again packed clothes to be admitted to the hospital. In retrospect, I now understand that I was following the classic sequence of Kübler-Ross' stages of death and dying. The denial which I had been exhibiting during the past three months without confirmed symptoms was now being replaced by anger. "Why me?" was my dominant thought. I was short and uncommunicative with Sharry during the drive to Fairfax Hospital. If I was going to die soon, there was no reason for me to be gracious about it.

Following admission, I was assigned to Room 265 on the second floor. It was the same setup as in May, that is, a roommate, a bathroom, and the cardiac monitoring equipment. Neither the hospital nor the nurses seemed to have changed much in the past three months.

Robin Merlino stopped by my room in the late afternoon to ensure that I had been admitted properly and that I was resting well. The irony was that I now felt fine. The nature of my disease was that either I was totally "normal" or I was on the verge of death. Robin told me that the continuous printout of my heart rate at the nursing station indicated a normal sinus rhythm, that is, a regular heart beat. She examined me and found nothing of significance. She said that she had spoken with the arrhythmia specialist, Ted Friehling. He would be in to see me first thing in the morning.

Sharry and the three children stayed with me during the evening. Aaron and Nelle attempted to cheer us up, but we were all obviously very worried. The uncertainty of my condition was difficult to handle. It was as if we were confronting an unseen enemy in the night.

Dr. Ted Friehling, his partner, Al Del Negro, and their assistant, Kim Hill, came to see me first thing the following morning, Thursday, August 1. Ted introduced Al and Kim to me, since I had never met them. They seemed to be just as likable as Ted. Al was thin, wore black rimmed glasses and had a tired look on his face. Kim was an attractive, young brunette with a pleasant smile.

While Del Negro examined me, Friehling outlined their plan of action. The sarcoidosis, Ted explained, was now causing intermittent ventricular tachycardia, v-tach. As the body's automatic mechanism, the AV (atrioventricular) node, attempted to signal the right ventricle of my heart to squeeze, and thus pump, blood to my lungs, the transmission path for the message was being disrupted by either sarcoid damaged cells or scar tissue resulting from the sarcoidosis. Auxiliary signal sites were being spontaneously established to re-send the message. The result was that the ventricle was receiving numerous conflicting signals. Instead of pumping at an appropriate rate, the heart was beating too rapidly, perhaps 180 beats per minute (bpm) instead of 80. Blood would still flow, but in decreased amounts due to the insufficient time for the chamber to refill between each squeeze.

In the short term, v-tach is not a life-threatening problem. If the heart converts spontaneously, that is, on its own, to the normal rhythm, there is no damage. Prolonged periods of v-tach can be life threatening, because decreased amounts of blood are flowing to the brain and other parts of the body. The real danger is that v-tach will go the other way. If the heart becomes further confused and starts to beat at an extremely rapid rate, called ventricular fibrillation, death may occur instantly because no blood will be pumped. A heart trying to beat at a rate of 300 bpm is essentially worthless as a pump. Before blood can enter the chamber, another squeezing motion takes place. The heart muscle is quivering instead of pumping. Fibrillation, Ted explained, was the death mechanism when a person is electrocuted. The electrical current stimulates the heart into this dangerous rhythm, no blood is pumped, and the person dies.

I understood Ted's explanation. Because of my engineering background, I knew of the same process in centrifugal pumps. If the impeller (a rotating device) in a pump is spun too fast by its motor, fluid cannot be moved because it does not have time to enter the pumping chamber before one of the rotating vanes on the impeller comes around to push it out the other end of the pump. In this situation the pump is said to be "cavitating."

When I gave this explanation to my younger daughter, Emily, she looked confused and then asked me, "You mean like a revolving door which is spinning too fast for someone to enter it?"

"That's exactly it, Emily," I replied, fully aware that my rising eighth-grader had instantly produced a far better analogy than Mr. Engineer.

I responded to Ted, "So my heart is cavitating." Not expecting this doctor guy to be familiar with engineering lingo, I was surprised (and a bit embarrassed) when he quickly replied, "Yes, that's exactly what is happening."

"What doesn't this guy know?" I wondered. "He's one of the top cardiac arrhythmia specialists in the country, he plays lead guitar in a rock band, **and** he knows a lot of engineering! He probably translates ancient Persian sonnets in his spare time."

Having completed his examination of me, Dr. Del Negro now took over the conversation. "What we want to do, Ed, is to conduct an EP study on you."

I interrupted, "What's that?"

Kim answered me, "EP stands for electrophysiology. An EP study is a procedure which allows us to study the electrical conduction system of the heart. The doctors will insert a catheter-type device through a vein or artery into a specific region of your heart. With it, we can electrically stimulate the heart to place it in an increased rate so that we can study the condition."

"So that's why it's called a study," I interjected.

Kim smiled as she continued, "Once we understand what your heart is doing, we can attempt to correct it using various drugs which we give to you intravenously. We may be able to find one that will keep your heart from going into tachycardia. Basically, we give you a medicine, then speed up your heart rhythm to see if the drug keeps you from going into a dangerous rate."

"Am I awake during this?" I asked. "And what happens if my heart goes into tachycardia and you can't get it back to normal?"

Ted broke in, "You will be under light anesthesia. If your heart does not spontaneously convert, we will shock you back to a normal sinus rhythm with electrical paddles. Have you ever seen them used on TV?"

"Sure," I lied, but I got the picture. "Does it hurt?"

"You will be asleep and won't feel it," Al replied.

I did not believe Al.

I also felt that I was the victim of a three-on-one mugging. These guys had all the answers. Nonetheless, I did feel confident that they knew what they were doing. They seemed to be going out of their way to explain what would be going on.

"There is a scheduling problem," Ted said. "Because it is Thursday, we cannot get you on the EP lab schedule until Monday. We want to keep you here on the monitoring system until then. I don't think that it would be safe for you to go home."

Ted's phraseology worried me. "...not safe to go home..." It kept reverberating in my mind as I lie alone in the hospital room. Essentially I was now incarcerated. Although there were no bars over my window, I was now in confinement on Life Row. My only option was to pray and wait.

So I waited. Merlino and Matthews both came to check on me the next day. One thing I quickly learned was the routine of the typical hospital room examination. Nurses, residents, doctors, specialists, - everyone followed the same pattern. After only a few days, I felt that I could do a fairly good impression of a doctor at work during hospital rounds. All I needed was a stethoscope. On the front of the patient move the stethoscope around, pausing for about 5 seconds at various locations on the chest and abdomen. Say, "Uh, huh," at random intervals. Then go to the patient's back and say, "Take a deep breath." Move to a new location on the back and say, "Again." Do this at least 5 times. Then ask, "How are you feeling?" Conduct two additional minutes of small talk. As you leave the room, put a mark on a 3 x 5 card next to the patient's name so that your office personnel can charge $50.00. Go to the next room. My anger was expressing itself in bitter cynicism.

Knowing that each daily visit was costing me, I decided to attempt to get my money's worth. As soon as the doctor entered the room, I would initiate a conversation on some totally medically-unrelated topic. I would continue this dialogue until the doctor figured out how to regain control of the situation. I always enjoyed watching some of the more anal physicians trying to figure out how to return to medical issues so that they could get out of the room in less than 5 minutes. Others seemed to enjoy the break in their routine. For my part, it was pure enjoyment. I was going to be there anyway, so why not pass the time in conversation? Also I felt that I was getting more doctor per dollar. I wondered if Death Row prisoners reacted this way with their attorneys.

That same Friday afternoon I was visited by one of the heart transplant coordinators for the hospital. Her name was Linda Ohler. She was short, well-organized, and pretty. She told me that Dr. Matthews had discussed my case with her and that I might ultimately be a candidate for a heart transplant. After discussing how the transplant program worked at Fairfax, Linda gave me several brochures, and a large, 3-ring notebook to read.

I was polite with Linda, but I was uncertain how to react. In spite of Dr. Matthews earlier suggestions to me, I had never thought of myself as a transplant candidate. It seemed so....final. I was not ready to give up on this heart. Surely Matthews was not ready to throw in the towel. Why was everyone so pessimistic? Maybe I could strike a deal with God. Perhaps if I were a better Christian....?

Unknowingly, I was now in Kübler-Ross' third stage, Bargaining. I wanted to be rewarded for having been a good person. Sure, I had done my share of bad things during my 47 years, but, overall I considered myself to have been a fairly decent person. "Please help me, Lord!" was a frequent thought now. "I promise that I will make it up to you in the future."

Before leaving, Linda said that a cardiologist on the transplant team, Dr. Kevin Rogan, would see me over the weekend for further discussion and questions. I said thanks, but was wondering if my situation was really this bad.

Dr. Rogan arrived on Saturday in the early afternoon. Fortunately Sharry was present because I desperately needed her perspective. She had read all of the literature which Linda had left for us, and she did most of the talking with Rogan. I felt as if I were an invisible bystander listening to two medical professionals talking about someone else.

Dr. Rogan was an extremely young-looking man who spoke in a rapid, New England accent. We decided that he was not nearly as young as he looked. He told us that he had been in Army medicine for 10 years before switching to civilian practice. His office was in the same suite as Matthews, but they were not partners. He was not one of the three heart surgeons who did transplants at Fairfax, but he was a member of the team.

Above all, Rogan was remarkably polite and informative. He explained that I was not yet sufficiently ill to be placed on the heart transplant list, but that we should consider the option if my condition were to deteriorate. He said that we should feel free to contact him or Linda Ohler if we had any questions in the future. As he left the room, I noticed that Kevin walked as quickly as he talked.

Sharry and I talked about the two visits by Linda and Kevin. Neither of us were interested in pursuing additional information on a transplant. We simply did not believe that my situation was that desperate. We were impressed, however, by the attention which we were receiving. This seemed like a good place to be if things did get worse.

On Sunday, a young fellow named Mike came into the room and said, "Mr. Linz?" I said that I was Linz. Mike, it turned out, was a heart transplant recipient. He had been in the hospital for a visit to see a friend and the nurses had told him about my situation. I was struck by how healthy he looked, although I am not sure what I expected to see. I had never knowingly met a transplant recipient, so I did not know exactly what to look for. Mike said that he had received his new heart in April, 1988. Sharry was not in the room at the time, so I was limited in the depth of medical questions which I could ask.

Following his transplant, Mike said, he had encountered no serious complications. As with all transplant recipients, he took medication daily to suppress his immune system so that his body would not reject the new heart. I did not understand all of this, but I smiled a lot and nodded as if I did. Later that evening, when discussing Mike's visit, I told Sharry that I had seen living proof that a transplant was an option. For some reason, we both broke out laughing. If only we knew what lay ahead.

At midnight on Sunday evening I began NPO. Whenever a patient is to receive anesthesia, there is a period prior to the procedure in which no food or drink is taken. This abstinence is designed by cruel, uncaring physicians to put the patient in as foul a mood as possible upon entering the operating room. The "cover story" told to the patient is rather cute: the doctor wants as little as possible in the stomach during anesthesia so that there is less likelihood of throwing up and choking to death. I will let you decide which is closer to the truth. NPO, by the way, stands for the Latin, *nil per os*, which translates "nothing by mouth." A sign saying "NPO" was placed outside my room on the wall beneath my name to fend off any pizza delivery guys who knew Latin.

NPO did not become an issue until everyone else on the floor received breakfast. I certainly did not miss the plastic scrambled eggs or the potholder-tasting pancakes, but some juice would have been nice to take the edge off my nervousness concerning the EP study to be conducted at 10 AM. Dr. Friehling had told me in detail what to expect, but I was still wary. The procedure sounded much the same as the cardiac catheterization which I had received in May, except that my heart would intentionally be placed in a dangerous condition. I regarded the "except" as a big deal.

At 9:45 AM two nurses dressed in blue cotton scrubs came to my room and transferred me to a gurney for the short trip to the EP lab. Sharry kissed me as I left the room and went to a nearby waiting room. She was visibly upset. I did not have time to reflect or worry, because, after leaving Room 265, we took a left, went about 30 yards, hung a right and went through two sets of automatic doors into the EP lab. It was small and cold. Friehling and Del Negro were both there. Ted greeted me as I entered, "Hi, Ed. Let's get this over with."

I was quickly transferred from the gurney to a narrow table surrounded by IV poles and computers. An IV was started. I noticed that there were four nurses in the room to assist the two doctors. Classical music was playing from a boom box near the wall which I was facing. A nurse anesthetist inserted a medication into the IV to put me asleep. My next memories were waking up in something of a daze in the EP lab. Dr. Friehling was gone, but Al Del Negro and Kim Hill were still there. The clock read 12:30 PM. I had been in the lab nearly three hours. I did not feel sore and was in no pain, but there was a huge bandage in my right groin area. I asked, "Am I OK?"

Del Negro answered, "Everything is fine. We will talk to you later in the day."

The next several hours were murky. I remember talking to Sharry as I was taken back to Room 265, but I have no idea what either of us said. At least I was no longer NPO.

Ted Friehling came to see me late in the afternoon. He was in an uncharacteristically somber mood and came directly to the point, "The results of the EP study were not good. We were able to readily induce v-tach in your heart using the pacemaker. We then converted you back to a normal rhythm and tried three different drugs to prevent further initiation. None of them worked."

"I don't understand. What drugs?" I asked.

Before Friehling could answer, I glanced at Sharry. She was pale and obviously understood exactly what the doctor had said.

Ted replied, "We first had to demonstrate that your heart could be placed in and out of VT."

"What's VT?"

"V-tach, ventricular tachycardia. The sarcoid has affected your heart so that it easily goes into VT. That is bad. We then injected you with various anti-arrhythmia drugs, one at a time, to see if they would prevent you from going into VT when we tried again. None of them worked. You went into VT every time. We used the paddles to shock you back to a normal rhythm."

"So that's why I have these burn marks on my chest and back!"

"We had to use a fairly high voltage level. It leaves a mark. It will fade in time. Don't worry about it."

I tried to put the thought that I had been branded out of my mind, but I was unable to do so. Maybe I had watched too many western movies as a kid.

"So what drugs did you try?" I repeated.

"All of the first line types: Lidocaine, Inderal, and Pronestyl. The Lidocaine actually made it worse," Ted responded.

Sharry broke in, "What can be done, Doctor?" There was a tone of desperation in her voice.

"That's what I want to talk to you about," said Ted. His face looked thin and tired. "You have two options. We can put a defibrillator in you. It is called an AICD, automatic implantable cardioverter defibrillator. It monitors your heart rate and shocks you back to a normal rhythm if you go into v-tach. It usually requires open heart surgery. The AICD does nothing to control the sarcoid or the v-tach. It's just there to protect you when it occurs. It's like a safety net."

I had several questions, "Does it hurt? Does it always work? Is it in there forever?"

Friehling was patient with me, "Just having it in you doesn't hurt. If it has to fire, that hurts, but it's a momentary pain - like being shocked. That's what it's doing. It's shocking your heart... Does it always work? Yes, it always shocks you in a dangerous situation. Your heart, however, may not always respond. If the disease reaches a certain point, then nothing can help you. And the AICD itself is a permanent feature. Its batteries are good anywhere from two to five years depending on how often it fires. When the batteries get low, the device can be fairly easily replaced with minor surgery. You see, although there will be leads directly attached to the sides of your heart, the control box is just under your skin in your upper abdomen where it can be easily replaced. It's no big deal."

"What is the other option?" Sharry asked.

"Amiodarone," replied the doctor. "It's a more powerful drug. We do not know if it will prevent VT in you or not. It's very powerful."

I did not like the way Ted was saying "powerful." I was not in the mood to be given two lousy options. The first one required big-time surgery which might not be of any use, and the other involved some dangerous drug. I felt that I was suddenly between the medical equivalent of a rock and a hard place.

Dr. Friehling continued, "Amiodarone works at the cell level. We will have to keep you in the hospital for at least two weeks while we give you a loading dose. The idea is to load you up with the drug, so to speak, and then take you back in for another EP study to see if it will keep you from going into VT."

"Why do I have to stay in the hospital? Is this Amiodarone given intravenously?"

"No. You will receive several pills each day. We have to watch you closely while we are loading you. There have been some instances of bad reactions to the drug. You need to be here in the hospital so that we can act quickly if a problem comes up."

Friehling paused and then added, "There have been some fatalities. It is a powerful drug. We have never had a problem, but it still has to be done in the hospital."

Sharry and I looked at each other. I think that we both felt as if we were suddenly in over our heads. This was serious business.

I was the first to break the silence, "Ted, can we have some time to think this over? Both of these options sound rather drastic. Sharry and I need to talk."

"Sure," he said, "You don't have to decide today. We can get you more information on both the AICD and the Amiodarone. You want to be sure on this. It's a big decision."

"What do you recommend, Ted?" I asked. "What would you do?"

"I'd try the Amiodarone. It may not work, but it's probably worth the risk. We know that the AICD will be only a safety net. The Amiodarone might stop the VT, or at least buy us some time."

I said, "Thanks, Ted. We'll talk, and let you know tomorrow. Thanks for all that you have done. We appreciate it."

As Friehling left the room, Sharry looked at me and visibly gulped. I felt my eyes begin to water. I was scared. Sharry came to my side as I was lying in the bed. She hugged me and said, "Don't worry, Sweetheart, we're going to make it through this."

I asked Sharry what she thought we should do.

"I'm not sure," she replied. "I think that we need to learn more about this drug, Amiodarone. I'm going to go to the nurse's station and borrow their PDR. Let's see what it says."

The "PDR" is the Physicians' Desk Reference. It is a huge (over 2500 pages) manual published annually by Medical Economics Company, Inc. with the cooperation of the major drug manufacturers. Over 3000 pharmaceutical and diagnostic products are listed, complete with color photos of the various pills. The book lists detailed information on each drug, ranging from common over-the-counter products such as Tylenol and Mylanta to the newest and most potent prescription drugs. Each entry contains a general description of the drug, followed by sections discussing its clinical pharmacology, indications and usage, contraindications, warnings, precautions, adverse reactions, overdosage, dosage and administration, and how supplied. An entry for a typical drug is one to four pages in length.

I was familiar with the PDR because we have an old edition of it at home. Most nurses "obtain" a PDR, or its smaller counterpart, the Merck Manual, for their personal use. My mother had procured hers from St. Luke Hospital where she worked. I never asked Sharry how she got hers. Because a new PDR costs around $60, it has a tendency to walk if left unattended.

Fairfax Hospital had attempted to minimize the disappearance of its PDRs by chaining them to the desk at the nurses' station. Sharry and I walked from my room to the chain and began to learn about Amiodarone.

The drug's actual name is Cordarone (cór-duh-rone). It is manufactured by a French firm for Wyeth-Ayerst Laboratories. The chemical name is amiodarone hydrochloride. All of the doctors and nurses at Fairfax referred to it as "Amiodarone," (am-ee-óh-da-rone) although we would occasionally hear "Cordarone." It is a white to cream-colored crystalline powder whose chemical formula is $C_{25}H_{29}I_2NO_3 \cdot HCl$. As a medicine it is packaged as a pink tablet containing 200 mg of the chemical along with several inactive ingredients, including red dye 40. The PDR described Cordarone as "a member of a new class of antiarrhythmic drugs with predominately Class III (Vaughan Williams classification) effects." I had no idea what this meant.

The first thing which I had noticed was the section describing the warnings and side effects. I now understood what Friehling meant when he said it was a "powerful" drug. Cordarone, the PDR stated, is intended for use only in patients with life-threatening arrhythmias because "its use is accompanied by substantial toxicity." Serious lung and liver problems could develop. In fact, some studies had shown that pulmonary (lung) toxicity occurred in 10 to 17 percent of patients given doses of 400 mg/day. Ten percent of these cases were fatal. Amiodarone could also exacerbate the arrhythmia. This had occurred in 2 to 5 percent of the cases studied. There were also other adverse side effects to be expected. Almost all adults on Amiodarone could expect to develop microdeposits on the corneas of the eyes. In many cases there will be extreme sensitivity to the sun, requiring sunscreen and protective clothing. The skin on many patients undergoing long-term treatment develops a blue-gray discoloration. There were many other potential problems mentioned, such as insomnia, thyroid disorders, abnormal taste and smell, nausea and vomiting, and decreased libido. Amiodarone was not a user-friendly drug!

Surprisingly, Sharry and I were not overly alarmed by reading about Amiodarone/Cordarone in the PDR. We both knew, from previous use of the book, that every medicine had side effects and that they were all listed in gruesome detail in the PDR. We had joked that if a person read the PDR, he would never take aspirin.

We did take notice, however, in the section which described how the drug must be administered: "The difficulty of using Cordarone effectively and safely itself poses a significant risk to patients." All of Friehling's remarks were validated. The drug requires a loading dose, because it is slowly absorbed by the body. The patient must be hospitalized during this phase for at least one week, and generally two or more. It is impossible to tell precisely when an effective concentration has been achieved in any given patient. The PDR seemed to be saying, "Load the patient with the drug, watch him closely to see if it is killing him, then take him in for an EP study in a few weeks to see if it works to prevent arrhythmias."

One of the nurses, Teresa, sensed our concern and asked if we would be interested in talking to a patient who was currently on Amiodarone. She said that there was a man in Room 259 who had been on the drug for over a year. He was now hospitalized for a different heart problem.

We thanked Teresa and asked if she could introduce us to this patient. It was still early evening and the man's wife was with him in his room when we entered. He appeared to be in his mid-60's and did not look either blue or gray. His name was Tom.

After exchanging pleasantries, I asked Tom how he felt about Amiodarone. Was it causing him any problems? Did it work?

Tom smiled and said, "Sure, it works, at least for me it does. I've been on it for over a year now. I have this dry cough and I get out of breath easier now, but it ain't too bad."

We talked for a few more minutes, but there were no other medical nuggets to be gleaned. As Sharry and I were leaving the room, Tom called me to his side and whispered, "The real problem with the stuff is that I can't get it up any more. Haven't been able to do it in a year. It makes you limp."

Since Tom's wife was sitting only five feet away, I simply smiled and replied, "Thanks. I hope you get better."

When we returned to my room, I shared Tom's parting shot with Sharry. We laughed and Sharry commented, "I think that Tom's problems may be more related to his age and relationship with his wife than to the Amiodarone." She quickly became serious as she continued, "It's a bad drug, no doubt about it."

"I'm not going to make any decision tonight," I said. "Let's both think about it some more. I certainly do not want surgery if we can avoid it."

Both Sharry and I were accustomed to making difficult decisions and living with the consequences. As we pondered this latest challenge, we discussed some of the "biggies" which we had faced together during my years in the Navy.

In 1974, for example, I had planned to leave the Navy for a career in business. I had submitted a letter of resignation and had been accepted in the MBA programs at both Harvard and MIT. Just prior to my detachment date, I learned that I had also been selected by the Navy as a "CNO Scholar." [The CNO is the Chief of Naval Operations, the senior officer in the Navy.] As a recipient of this scholarship, I would be given two years of shore duty to study anything, anywhere. The payback would be two for one, that is, two additional years of sea duty for each year of study. Since I had completed nine years of service, mostly at sea, at this time, accepting the Navy offer was tantamount to choosing to remain in the service until at least the 20 year retirement point. After considerable debate in which we swayed back and forth several times, we decided to accept the scholarship, attend Oxford University in England, and take our chances in the Navy.

Another major family decision had occurred approximately eight years later when I was in command of the USS KAMEHAMEHA, a ballistic missile nuclear powered submarine. The thrill of command is very individual and is difficult to describe. Having the sole responsibility for a billion dollar ship loaded with 16 ballistic missiles carrying 160 hydrogen bomb warheads, a nuclear reactor and 120 men is humbling. While at sea, we alone knew where we were at any given moment, and the Captain decides where that will be. There is no comparable professional experience in the Navy. Our decision was whether or not to surrender this for the sake of principle.

Although I loved being at sea, the great working relationship with my shipmates and the excitement of submarine operations, my irritation with the manner in which officer and enlisted personnel were treated by the Navy's Nuclear Propulsion Directorate, headed by the legendary Admiral Rickover, was increasing daily. Because of his policy to take whatever measures were deemed necessary to ensure nuclear reactor safety, this organization had long ago dispensed with any concept of fairness or due process. Rickover was truly a total dictator, - and a very senile one at that. Over a thirty year period, the man had cleverly consolidated unassailable power based on a mutually rewarding relationship with key members of Congress. In return for their unwavering support of his program and his policies, Rickover steered a steady stream of government contracts to facilities in the appropriate Congressional districts and states. Due to the unprecedented construction and overhaul requirements associated with the buildup of the nuclear Navy from 1960 to 1980, there was considerable "pork" to distribute.

Because of his solid base of support, no one in the Navy dared to oppose Rickover in any way. The Chief of Naval Operations always deferred to him, as did a succession of Secretaries of the Navy. Within the uniformed ranks, there was total fear. Any action which might jeopardize one's standing with Rickover himself or his Nuclear Propulsion Mafia was avoided.

This paranoia reached ridiculous levels. Whenever Rickover visited a nuclear facility or ship, there were extensive preparations to ensure that he would be pleased. Actually, "pleased" is not the appropriate descriptor. The man was never known to have been pleased. "Not be pissed" would more accurately reflect the goal. Each ship had a "Rig for Rickover Bill," which was a continually expanding multi-page document listing steps to be taken to prepare for a visit by "THE" Admiral. When he visited my first submarine, USS GURNARD, in 1967, the list had reached seven pages. It mandated taking whatever steps were necessary (legal or not) to procure such items as a particular brand of lemon drops from a company in Boston, new Navy uniforms and ship jackets in Rickover's size (he always took these with him at the end of the visit), and whatever equipment and personnel were necessary to mail out over one thousand typed letters to whomever he was trying to woo at the time (generally most US senators and congressmen and a curious collection of dignitaries throughout the world). Since this was before word processors and copying machines, each of these letters had to be proofread by six officers.

Not unlike every Commanding Officer in the nuclear Navy, I had been on the receiving end of Rickover's wrath on several occasions. Whenever your ship was in port, it was not unusual to receive a telephone call at any time, day or night, from his Washington office telling you to standby to talk to THE Admiral. The conversation was always one-sided and consisted of Rickover yelling caustic remarks or questions. He would then hang up. I was generally not bothered by these calls because it was known to be part of the turf. Some of my peers in command actually became sick over these conversations, or, in some cases, worrying about receiving such a call.

My concern was that many sailors and officers were being summarily removed from further assignment in the nuclear Navy due to the whim of Rickover or his underlings. If a sailor made an error in conducting a check of a valve lineup, he could find that his nuclear training designator was removed, that he was disqualified from submarine duty, and that he was re-assigned to an aircraft carrier in the Indian Ocean. These draconian responses to minor cases of human error had major financial and personal implications for the disciplined sailor: the loss of several hundred dollars each month, decreased prospects for promotion, and the disruption of the life of a young, struggling family already under considerable stress.

After approximately 15 months in command of KAME-HAMEHA, I made the decision that I could no longer support and carry out Rickover's personnel policies. I had been sharing my concerns with Sharry over several months, so when I told her of my intention to request to be relieved of command, she was very direct in her response: "Do it."

I wrote two letters. The first was to my immediate superior, an admiral, who was the Submarine Group Commander in Groton, Connecticut. This letter was simply a request to be relieved of command at the earliest opportunity. The other letter was to Rickover. I was polite, but straightforward, in telling him why I could no longer carry out his personnel policies. I also stated that inherent nuclear reactor safety issues mandated an accelerated search for alternate methods of propulsion for submarines.

The Groton Admiral received his letter first. He telephoned me immediately aboard the ship in Portsmouth, New Hampshire, where KAMEHAMEHA was undergoing overhaul. "What the hell is going on?" he roared.

As I explained my rationale, he interrupted and said, "You need to get down here to talk to me." I then told him that I had already mailed a letter to Rickover. The Groton Admiral audibly groaned and said, "Oh, no, why did you do that?" I immediately sensed that he was concerned that my action might adversely affect his career.

Around 11 PM the next night I received a telephone call from Rickover. As usual, he was yelling. His only question was, "Exactly what other (obscenity) forms of propulsion did you have in mind?" He then immediately hung up before I could respond.

The Navy's reaction was swift and predictable. As requested, I received orders to be relieved of command. Much to the chagrin of the Nuclear Mafia, there were no discrepancies noted by the relieving officer. Our reenlistment rate was among the highest in the Atlantic Fleet, there were no material or equipment problems, and the enormous quantities of paperwork were all in order. There were no grounds for an ex-post-facto tarring.

Upon completion of the change of command, I was temporarily assigned to the Groton admiral's staff. Because Sharry's mother was hospitalized in nearby Mystic, Connecticut, I requested that my new assignment be "anywhere on the East Coast." As we waited for the Navy's response, we learned that we had become "Typhoid Marys." Sharry had received a reminder in the mail to attend the monthly CO Wive's Club meeting, but suddenly there was a phone call from the admiral's aide uninviting her. I think that her exact words to this obviously embarrassed young officer were, "And just what made you think that I had **any** intention of coming?" Considering the circumstances, I would have probably worked a few obscenities into the reply. Most of my colleagues, on the other hand, were very understanding and supportive. A few who were currently on the receiving end of Rickover's wrath were openly jealous.

Two weeks later I received message orders to report to a Battle Group Commander's staff assigned to the aircraft carrier, USS CONSTELLATION, headed to the Indian Ocean. Apparently it had taken several working days and phone conferences between Washington and Groton to find an assignment for me exactly the opposite of "anywhere on the East Coast." The Nuclear Mafia had exacted their revenge.

I immediately attempted to appeal my new orders via letters to Senators and Congressmen. From my own experience answering such letters, I knew that this effort was going to be a total waste of time. In fact, I knew of no instance in which the complaining sailor or officer ever received any satisfaction. Still, I felt obliged to go through the motions in my own case. Maybe lightning would strike.

We gave away our dog, sold our house, packed our possessions, and drove two cars with three kids across the country to San Diego. There we stayed in a Navy motel for four weeks while I attended a course on aircraft carrier group operations. The fact that I had never set foot on a carrier in my life did not seem to be a factor in the Navy assigning me to provide advice to the admiral who would be in charge of the aircraft carrier and the ten or more ships operating in conjunction with its Battle Group.

Joan Metz is one of Sharry's cousins. She and her husband, Peter, live in the Boston area. They had attended the change of command ceremony when I had taken command of KAMEHAMEHA. When Peter learned that I was about to be exiled to the Indian Ocean by a vindictive Navy, he called a former colleague who was then a "high ranking official" in the new Reagan administration. This political appointee telephoned the Secretary of the Navy, John Lehman, to ask that he look into the matter. Lehman's personal attorney happened to be Spike Karalekas, a Naval Academy classmate of mine, whom I had known at Annapolis. Lehman asked Spike to get together with me and Sharry to hear an unabridged version of our case. We met with Spike at a hotel in Los Angeles the following week while he was there on business. We were enroute from the school in San Diego to the admiral's staff in San Francisco, so it was a mutually convenient location to meet. Over a two hour period we explained to Spike exactly what had taken place. He was very receptive and promised to prepare a detailed report for Lehman.

One week later, just as I was preparing to depart for the Indian Ocean and CONSTELLATION, Spike telephoned me to tell us that Lehman was sympathetic to my cause, but that the "Navy brass" were really against me. He (Lehman) wanted me to come to Washington as soon as possible to resolve the matter. I told the admiral to whom I was assigned about Lehman's request. He was absolutely gleeful in his cooperation. He hated Rickover's guts, as did most non-nuclear flag officers at the time. Within two days I flew back to D.C. to meet Lehman.

Our meeting in the Secretary's office was private. Lehman asked his aides to leave. He then said to me, "I have read Spike's report. Tell me exactly what happened."

After I gave the Secretary a brief synopsis, he responded, "Rickover and his nucs have definitely screwed you. I am going to overrule them. Would you like to have an assignment here in Washington?"

"Yes," I replied, "as long as the job is on the East Coast, we will be happy."

Lehman then added, "I am probably going to fire Rickover shortly. Whom do you think I should replace him with?"

With little hesitation I said, "Mr. Secretary, I'm too far down in the trenches to tell you whom to select, but I will tell you whom **not** to select." I then listed four senior nuclear submarine admirals, including the one in Groton, whom I had long-standing professional and/or personal reasons to dislike.

As it turned out, none of these four were selected. I suspect that each of them had probably ruined their chances many times over on their own. Nonetheless, I still felt buoyed by the fact that I had been asked for my opinion.

I returned to the West Coast with new orders in hand. I related what had happened in Washington to my admiral friend on the CONSTELLATION. I told him that my intentions were to complete the initial phase of our deployment with him so that he would have time to obtain a replacement for me. He roared with laughter, "Ed, maybe Secretary Lehman will send ole Rickover himself out to the Indian Ocean to relieve you. That old bastard has shipped enough sailors out there over the years. Maybe he should see it for himself! It would do him good." Now this was an admiral that I could like.

Three months later I was in my new assignment in Washington advising the Chief of Naval Operations on arms control matters. We had moved to Springfield, Virginia and life was again sweet.

Sharry and I reflected on these two major decisions as we sat in adjoining chairs in my hospital room. It seemed as if the Lord had been in our corner in several previous rounds. We prayed that He was still with us in our current time of need.

The following morning, August 6, 1991, was typical for a summer day in Washington. By 9 AM the humidity was already unbearable and the temperature was headed to 100 degrees Fahrenheit. In my hospital room the weather was not a factor. It was almost uncomfortably cool. I was sitting up in the bed with a blanket over me when Dr. Friehling came in just before noon. Sharry and I had talked on the phone for over 30 minutes earlier in morning and had finally reached our decision. Before Friehling could say hello, I said, "Let's do it. Let's start the Amiodarone. I'm ready."

Friehling smiled. He then explained to me what to expect over the next several days. I would begin taking the medication immediately after lunch. The dose would be heavy: 1800 mg/day. I would receive nine tablets a day, three separate sets of three 200 mg tablets. "The nurses will be watching you closely," Ted assured me. "We will also be conducting several tests to determine baseline levels for kidneys, liver and blood. You will have to have a new chest x-ray so that we can keep an eye on your lungs. Get yourself some good books, because you are going to get bored in here. Al Del Negro or I will see you daily. After a week or so we will decide when to conduct an EP study to see if this stuff works for you."

We then talked about guitars and music for the next 15 minutes. Ted, I learned, not only is a rock musician and singer, but also has a world-class collection of guitars of famous performers. For a brief period, I forgot about my medical problems and enjoyed the conversation.

Dr. Friehling was correct about becoming bored. During the next week I spent most of the time walking in the hallway and talking to whoever might listen. I had no immediate noticeable side effects or toxicity problems from the Amiodarone. The monitoring system indicated that I had no instances of arrhythmia during this period. The question which no one could answer was, "Is it working?"

My girls cross country team began practice on Monday, August 12, without me. I had discussed my situation with the boys team coach, Vic Kelbaugh. We had developed a plan in which my two co-captains would conduct the practice following the instructions which I had given. Vic would be there as a safety monitor and to take care of administrative problems. It never occurred to me that I might have to give up coaching due to my condition. I felt fine and was back in full-scale denial.

One week after beginning the Amiodarone therapy, Friehling surprised us by walking in to my room and saying, "I am going to let you go home for a few days. You have been entirely stable since we began the loading. Just take it easy and be back here Friday for an EP study. We'll do it first thing in the morning. If you have any problems at home, call 911."

I did not ask Friehling to explain. I felt as if the warden had just given me a weekend pass! Soon I would be "outta here." Sharry was in the room with me during Friehling's visit, and, upon hearing that I could be released, left immediately to pick up our car. While she was gone, one of the nurses, Kathleen, gave me detailed discharge instructions. Basically my duties were simple: take three Amiodarone tablets three times each day. Return for an EP study on Friday. Don't die.

I was happy to be home because Aaron was leaving for college on Friday. We discussed how to handle this in view of my returning to the hospital the same day. Previously we had planned on all of us driving to Chapel Hill with him to help transport his belongings and move into the dorm. Nelle was elected to represent us. Although she was only 16 at the time, we had no problem with her driving our pickup truck to North Carolina and back by herself. Nelle was a rather independent operator.

The EP study on Friday lasted less than two hours. The results were great. The Amiodarone had successfully prevented all attempts by Ted and Al to induce arrhythmia. By evening I was home and feeling elated. Friehling had placed no restrictions on my activities. I could resume coaching immediately and begin the new school year on August 27.

Life was once again sweet.

Chapter 6

ON THE PILL

Amiodarone was not a big deal. The maintenance dose after I was discharged from Fairfax Hospital in August 1991 was initially 400 mg daily. Dr. Friehling reduced the dose to 300 mg/day two months later. I remained at that level for the next three years. There were no immediately apparent side effects. Over the next several months, however, I did begin to develop an increasing sensitivity to sunlight. As the drug reached equilibrium levels throughout my body, it became necessary to wear long sleeve shirts and a large brim hat in order to prevent sunburn. This condition became progressively worse in subsequent summers. By 1994, I had to coat my exposed skin with heavy duty sunblock in order to be protected. I often joked with my friends that "heavy duty" in my case meant at least SPF 5000!

Sharry noticed that my face was developing a blue-gray pallor as the months on Amiodarone continued. Frankly, I was unaware of this discoloration, but for years I had also managed to find ways to overlook the obvious fact that my hair was turning gray. It is difficult to give aging a hearty hello as one looks into the mirror each morning.

What no one could see on the surface was the damage being done to some of my internal organs by the Amiodarone. Dr. Merlino conducted periodic blood tests to monitor the condition of my liver, kidneys, and thyroid. The results indicated that these organs were being adversely affected, but that the damage was acceptably low. Because the Amiodarone was successfully preventing further arrhythmias of my heart, the trade-off was one which we had to accept.

Within a year, I learned during a visit to my ophthalmologist, Dr. Leonard Barmack, that tiny microdeposits had started to form on the cornea of my eyes. These were known side effects of Amiodarone. They did not adversely affect my vision. Leonard, whose life was eyes, seemed to be highly intrigued by this discovery. I was his first Amiodarone patient, and he now had data to share with his eye doctor friends at the next ophthalmology convention. He even arranged for me to have the interior of my eyes photographed by a cornea specialist using a customized Polaroid camera. Sure enough, there were swirls of tiny black dots, resembling a constellation in space, on the photo which was taken. Dr. Barmack kept the photograph in my records to use as a baseline for future reference in case there was a deterioration.

Dr. Friehling had not placed any serious restrictions on my activities. He told me to resume a "normal life" of teaching and coaching. He recommended that I not participate in any marathons, but I was allowed to run shorter distances and exert myself moderately. One day every other month I wore a Holter Monitor for 24 hours to monitor my heart rate. Of course, nothing of significance heart-wise was recorded during any of these wearings. Much to my disappointment, I still was unable to convince Sharry to conduct "scientific experiments" in bed while I was wired.

Teaching had become a significant part of my life. I had begun this second career at Woodbridge Senior High School in the fall of 1985 immediately upon retiring from the Navy. I approached the first day of class with considerable apprehension. Sharry had been more than a little skeptical of my choice for a second career, because, she was quick to point out, "you have never been in a public high school in your life."

Her facts were correct. All of my grade school and high school education had been in Catholic schools where discipline and learning were inseparable. My 1959 high school graduating class at Covington Latin School had just 31 students, none of which were minorities or females. Now I was about to teach in a 3000 student school in the metropolitan Washington, D.C. area with a strong racial and ethnic mix. Presumably half the students on any given day would be girls. Would I be out of my league?

I did have some preparation. The teacher certification courses which I had taken during the past two years at George Mason University involved observing classes at local high schools. It was an eye-opener. Some of the teachers were highly skilled and effective. Others were content to make it through the day in one piece.

One mathematics teacher whom I observed had obviously established an unwritten contract with her students: don't give me any trouble, and I will make this course as easy as possible for you. She would begin class by taking roll for the first five minutes. Then she would go over the previous day's homework assignment by asking the student in the front seat to her left to put the first problem on the blackboard. The student behind the first would take the next problem, and so on, until all of the homework was covered. This process took about twenty minutes. Then the teacher would spend five minutes covering new material. As soon as this was over, she would write the assignment for that night on the board and tell the students that they could begin to work on it until the end of class. She followed this exact process for all five days during which I observed her. In one week I saw her actually teach for less than 30 minutes total.

During another of my observation sessions, I was sitting in the back of a "Consumer Math" class when a girl, who had been quietly filing her nails, suddenly stood and yelled at the boy across from her, "You miserable fag! Quit bothering me!"

The teacher, who had been using an overhead projector trying to explain how to write a personal check, did not have much of a reaction to this incident. In fact, he apparently did not regard it as an "incident." His only response was, "Tina, sit down." The student answered his request with a stream of shouts justifying her claim regarding the boy's sexual inclination. Of course, he responded in detail with comments about her rather extensive social life. All of the other students found this quite entertaining. I then knew where the daytime television talk shows developed their format. What I found most interesting was that the teacher did not say anything to me about this outburst during our discussion after the class. "What am I getting into?" I asked myself.

I also observed several inspirational teachers in action. An older man named David taught calculus with an absolute passion. His students were attentive, busy and quiet. They seemed to genuinely enjoy being in the class. Even with this group, I noticed that a boy and a girl sitting near me in the back of the room were able to caress each other's thighs while taking what appeared to be perfect notes. Young love will find a way!

I learned that good teaching is not restricted to the college prep type of courses, such as calculus. I watched a "general math" class composed of 10th graders in which the material was on the 5th grade level. The teacher, a woman in her late 20's, was incredibly well organized and in total control. She was determined that her students would learn something, and I think that they did.

With this limited background, I confronted my first group of students at Woodbridge. I had been assigned a teaching schedule of five geometry classes, all in different rooms. As a new teacher in a crowded building, I did not have the luxury of my own room. My desk was a cardboard box containing all materials, papers, etc. which I carried from classroom to classroom.

The irony was that I had never taken a geometry course in my life. Covington Latin was strictly a college preparatory institution. We covered the 7th through 12th grades in four years. In order to do this and to include religion classes and a heavy dose of the classics, it was necessary to gloss over some of the more traditional subject areas, such as geometry. I had not shared my mathematics "black hole" with the principal when he hired me. Based on the total number of **college** credits which I had obtained in mathematics over twenty years ago, I had been certified by the Commonwealth of Virginia to teach any **high school** mathematics course. The fact that my knowledge of geometry consisted primarily of knowing how to spell it was not an issue. I was certified.

In fact, I was certified to teach mathematics, chemistry and physics. Based on my actual educational background, my real expertise was in economics. I had obtained an M.A. in economics from Oxford during the mid 1970's when I had attended Christ Church College on a Navy sponsored fellowship between submarine assignments. I had also recently completed doctoral level economics courses taught by the Nobel Laureate, James Buchanan and the conservative columnist, Walter Williams, at George Mason University.

In spite of my questionable math background, the initial challenge for me in teaching was not the mathematics, but the presentation. How does one motivate teenage students to listen, to study, to learn? I did have considerable classroom teaching experience from my days in the Navy. There I had taught both officer and enlisted personnel, many of whom were tired, disinterested, and non-motivated. The classroom scenario aboard the submarines had often been cramped and uncomfortable with few, if any, audiovisual aids. These circumstances had led me to develop an active, "in-your-face," teaching style. I had never taught from behind a desk or in a static manner. My style involved movement, props, and frequent interaction with my students. It worked well with sailors, and, fortunately, also with my new charges.

I quickly developed a reputation as "that new weird math teacher." I was loud and outrageous. We laughed a lot. On some days, we would do constructions of geometric figures in chalk on the ceiling using a meter stick and a large wooden compass. The rectangular tiles up there were great for illustrating various types of angles when a transversal (a line intersecting two or more lines) was drawn across them. We went on "field trips" around the school building and the parking lot looking for examples of geometric principles. By Thanksgiving of my first year of teaching, I knew that I had made the correct decision for a second career. I really enjoyed going to work each day, and I was good at it. Most of my students were putting forth considerable effort, and there were no discipline problems.

For me, each class day was similar to putting on a one act play five times. The first period was sometimes shaky, but by afternoon I was always on a roll. The jokes which did not work in the morning had been discarded and replaced with new ones. If the first period students did not understand my explanation of a concept, I would keep adjusting in subsequent classes until an approach clicked. I never felt badly about the first period being Mr. Linz's "geometry guinea pigs" - everybody had a first period class in which much the same was taking place - and most also had afternoon classes which were better presented. It all tended to balance.

Most of my colleagues were excellent teachers, both in the classroom and as leaders of extracurricular activities. I soon realized, however, that an outstanding high school does not necessarily have a teaching staff composed exclusively of geniuses. A principal attempting to assemble an optimum staff for a large school cannot hire only those who are talented as classroom teachers. It is equally important to have a solid coaching staff for sports, enthusiastic sponsors for extracurricular activities, and a few really BIG bodies to break up fights. There are also requirements to have role models representing different races and cultures. When a school, such as Woodbridge, has an Hispanic population approaching 15 percent, it is imperative to have several Spanish speaking staff in the building.

In order to achieve this mix of talent and interest, a good principal will often sacrifice teaching skills for some other needed attribute, for example, a willingness to devote the extra hours required to be the sponsor of the Science Club, or the JV basketball coach, or the faculty representative for the Vikettes (our kick-line dancers).

One of our most effective faculty members did not teach. Haig was the school's audio-visual expert. His stated duties involved movie projectors, VCRs, computers, and a variety of equipment, but his real value to the school was the deterrent threat which he created for unruly students. Haig's office is in the library which is located in the middle of the school. Any student creating a disturbance could look forward to having to confront Haig, all 6 ft 8 in, 280 lb of him. He had several posters of The Terminator, Arnold Schwarzenegger, in his office and had the type of deep voice which itself generates nightmares in most teenagers. His body was as well toned as Arnold's. **No one** wanted to mess with Haig.

Because our administrative staff at Woodbridge understood this important trade-off, they had assembled a well-balanced staff. Discipline throughout the school was excellent. I recall less than five fights per year anywhere on school grounds. Our athletic teams were also the envy of the area. Academically we could compete with any of the top schools in the region. It was a superb situation for me as a new teacher.

After teaching geometry for three years, I was approached by the principal to teach physics. I jumped at the offer. Although mathematics had been a great way for me to begin as a teacher, physics was directly aligned with my personality - and based on my nuclear engineering training in the Navy, I actually knew the material!

On day one of the course, I informed my students that we were about to embark on a study of LIFE - physics was simply the vehicle which we would be using on our journey. Each of the areas of physics involved countless opportunities to explore the world around us: forces, motion, collisions, gravity, electricity, magnetism, light, sound, optics, nuclear reactors, atomic energy, lasers. Our lab experiments always involved hands-on procedures and data gathering. We fired bottle rockets, designed, built and tested "egg delivery vehicles," and used Geiger Counters to measure actual radioactive material. My classes would run up stairwells in the back of the building to estimate human horsepower.

In addition to these "fun" learning experiences, I also demanded considerable problem solving by my students. There was written homework every night, except on weekends (as a student I had always hated weekend assignments). Much to the disappointment of most of my students, I also required that they complete a four month long science project. Most initially hated this aspect of the course because they had to prepare a detailed written report of at least 10 pages in a specific format detailing their findings. By the time that the students presented their report in February, many had decided that this was the most enjoyable and rewarding part of the course. I personally had mixed feelings. The projects were excellent learning experiences for many because it was usually the first time that most students had studied a physical phenomenon in detail and presented the results in a well-written report. When the students stood in front of their classmates to present their findings, I always shared their excitement and felt that the project assignment had been worthwhile. On the other hand, reading and critically evaluating over 125 reports was an incredibly time-consuming task for me. Since I read the reports four separate times as they were being prepared from October to February, it was difficult to be enthusiastic knowing that several weekends and nights at home would be consumed in the evaluation process. When the final student report was completed at the end of February, I always felt physically exhausted.

My quizzes and tests were notoriously "challenging." Students were required to show all of their work. Although many students hated the fact that Mr. Linz **never** gave multiple choice tests, by the end of the first semester they loved the idea because they could receive partial credit on a problem or essay even if they were unable to present the "correct" answer.

How any educator can evaluate students using multiple choice quizzes, tests and exams is beyond me. I have heard all the arguments why "properly constructed" multiple choice tests are valid - blah, blah, blah. In truth, the **only** rationale for using multiple choice instruments (educator jargon) is expediency, that is, ease of grading. Faced with a requirement to obtain frequent grades, many teachers simply give "A,B,C,D or E" tests in which the answers are penciled in on a machine-graded Scantron sheet using the famous #2 pencil. The fact that the student who guesses the correct answer, D, receives the same credit as the student who has studied and diligently works out the same answer is scandalous. Even worse is the situation where a student knows 90 % of a problem, but is unable to do the final 10 % and receives zero credit by a programmed grading machine for penciling in answer C instead of D. Showing one's work eliminates this injustice and also allows me as a teacher to understand exactly what students do not understand about a problem or a concept. My first directive as a principal would be to throw out every Scantron machine in the building. I assure you that this alone would make me a very unpopular principal with many teachers.

Many of the physics problems which I assigned to students involved hamsters. "I hate hamsters," I would say early in the course. Terrible things happen to hamsters in my class, at least theoretically. They fall off cliffs into "Lake Jake" far below, they are shot out of cannons into walls, they are electrocuted, and they receive enormous quantities of ionizing radiation. Actually, I am totally neutral on hamsters, but I have found that typical high school students seem to understand theoretical concepts such as impulse and momentum better if they can relate the idea to some semi-outrageous situation with a tinge of humor. Naturally there have been some students who, as animal rights advocates, have been offended by perceived images of smashed and maimed hamster carcasses, but their complaints never went far with the administrators.

After watching many teachers in action, I came to the conclusion that the good ones are often controversial. Challenging students to reach their potential necessarily involves mentally prodding, pushing, praising - an entire range of *action* verbs. What works to help one student sometimes offends another. Working with a class of 25 to 30 students, the teacher does not have the luxury of one-on-one motivation. An effective teacher is one who is continuously throwing off intellectual sparks, much as a grinding wheel spinning against a metal blade. Hopefully the sparks land on the innate curiosity of individual students who then ignite their own imagination and skill. Sometimes the sparks land in unintended areas creating controversy. It is tempting for school administrators to solve problems and complaints about such teachers by simply extinguishing the source. Fortunately, the principal and assistant principals at Woodbridge did not routinely take this easy route, but worked to protect and encourage those teachers who were taking chances by throwing off sparks.

During my first year of teaching physics, I was involved in one incident in which I was definitely on the receiving end of spark-throwing. It was not a happy experience. We were in the midst of a lesson on electrical charges. One of the classic physics demonstrations involves the use of a large piece of equipment called a Van de Graaff generator. The Van de Graaff uses a motor-driven leather belt to transfer electric charges from the air to a metal sphere located at the top of the belt. As the charges reach the sphere, they spread uniformly over the surface. Since there is nowhere for the charges to go (the sphere is not grounded), they build up, producing an extremely high potential (voltage) on the surface of the metal.

I usually place the Van de Graaff on a table in the front of the classroom. I then ask for a student volunteer to stand on a wooden chair behind the table with arms extended over the sphere. Before turning on the generator, I direct the student, "Put your hands firmly on the sphere. Don't worry, this can't hurt you." (I always crossed my fingers as I said this!)

We then turn the Van de Graaff on. Initially nothing seems to happen. Soon, however, the student's hair starts to stand straight up. Everyone laughs, we take a photo of the student, the machine is turned off, the student quickly pulls her hands away from surface of the sphere, and the generator is then grounded to remove the charge. Then another student volunteer repeats the process. I generally have a contest to select who had the most outrageous "bad hair day." (The hair stands up because the student's body simply becomes an extension of the sphere. Since there is no path to ground for the charges to escape, they proceed to the surface of the person. Because the charges are of the same polarity, they attempt to repel each other. This action causes individual hairs to try to get as far away from each other as possible. The resultant effect is a porcupine look). I have to be careful which student volunteers to choose when doing this, because I learned, much to the delight of my male students, that light-weight skirts do the same thing as hair.

After conducting this procedure during my first year of teaching physics, I planned to show the class a short experiment involving the Van de Graaff. I left the machine running as I prepared some materials about three feet away. I should have sensed impending trouble when my eyebrows started to rise, literally! Before I realized what was about to happen, the center of my forehead was struck by a bolt of electrical charge that knocked me unconscious. When I awoke, I was lying on the floor near the Van de Graaff. Several students were hovering over me, but the first thing that I noticed was the loud, unmistakable laugh of Toni, one of my favorite students. She thought that I was acting. Never before had one of her teachers pretended that he had been killed in class. As soon as I assured myself that I was alive, I tried to save face by declaring, "See, I told you that it can't hurt you."

For the next several weeks, I had to endure several versions of, "Hey, Mr. Linz, seen any good charges lately?"

When Toni learned that I had not been acting, she apologized. I laughed and replied, "Toni, it was a good deal. Now I am eligible for workman's compensation." The experience must have been a positive one for Toni. She recently completed teacher education training at Grambling University, although I do not think that she will ever go near a Van de Graaff generator again.

At least 95 percent of my teaching experiences were positive. I thoroughly enjoyed the daily interaction with my students. Many have remained in contact with me after they have left Woodbridge. I have been to their weddings and college graduations, and have even held their babies. I do not remember all the names, but most of the faces will stay with me forever.

My health while teaching at Woodbridge was excellent until the first symptoms of sarcoidosis appeared in the summer of 1991. I ran daily and prided myself on being able to outsprint any of my students on a steep downhill course behind the science department. I would bait the class for most of the winter and then, in late spring, we would take a "field trip" outside on a nice day for the challenge run. I never lost a race until 1990, when age caught up with me. I popped the gastrocnemius muscle in my left calf in a race against my 4th period physics class. My sprinting days were over.

I loved coaching even more than teaching. Perhaps I enjoyed the instant gratification which came from watching our athletes do well in competition. Success is easier to measure on the track than in the classroom, and there were frequent articles featuring our athletes in the local papers. In truth, what I really liked was the fact that there were no homework papers to grade.

I myself had not run competitively in high school. Covington Latin had only two sports, basketball and baseball. I had played both - neither particularly well in terms of current standards. At the Naval Academy, I tried out for the plebe cross country team. I had never run over two miles at one time in my life. When the team went for a 10 mile training run the first day of practice, I knew that I was in over my head. I managed to hang on for the next two weeks, but I was then cut. The remainder of my running in college was at the intramural level. I had won most of those races, but the competition was not world class. Most of my competitors were running only because some upperclassman had told them they had to run that day. So the sport of cross country was not entirely new to me. When I watched someone running, I could echo the words of one of my more famous fellow Oxonians, "I feel your pain."

Working with athletes seemed to be a natural extension of teaching. I had coached youth soccer and baseball for several seasons, so I did have experience in coaching. What I did not have was any expertise in the theory of running or how to coach someone to run well. But there are books on the subject. I also watched other track coaches and asked many questions. I found that several physics and mathematics principles were directly related to track. To my surprise, for example, I noticed that many high school runners were inadvertently running well over 1600 meters in a 1600 meter race because they did not remain in the inside lane. We also had sessions on how to use centripetal force to advantage when trying to pass a runner on a track.

Coaching cross country was even more personally rewarding than working as an assistant in track. I ran with the girls every day rain or shine. We essentially formed a social club revolving around running. When I took over as head coach, we had nine girls on the team, and some intensely disliked each other. Within two years we had over 40 teammates who seemed to genuinely enjoy one another. The key to coaching girls, I found, is to make the activity "fun" for them. The two co-captains arranged frequent parties, organized a system of "secret pals," and treated everyone the same regardless of their running skills.

The friendships which I formed during these years of coaching remain today. Many of the girls have now completed college and are confronting the real world. One of my former captains, Meredith Carter, is midway through medical school. The two co-captains of one of my recent cross country teams, Julie Vance and Emily Linnemeier, went on to become varsity runners at separate universities in North Carolina. During college, they continued to ask for advice on the same things which we discussed at West Springfield: their academics and their love lives. Coaching is more than sports.

Based upon Dr. Friehling's recommendations, I decided to resume a relatively normal routine in the classroom. I would no longer challenge my students to races or compete with them running up stairs, but I was determined that an observer on any given day would be unable to recognize that I had any health problem, much less a fatal heart disease. As a coach, I had to make some adjustments. Instead of going daily with the girls on 4 to 10 mile training runs, I planned their route so that I could meet them at prearranged locations with water and encouragement. I drove my pickup truck from one location to the next with a large Igloo cooler full of ice water. This arrangement actually worked better than running with the team, because, in addition to the "mobile water cooler" aspect, I was able to provide a ride back to the school if one of the runners became sick or injured.

On August 27, 1991 I reported to Woodbridge High to begin the 1991-92 school year. This would be my first experience teaching while on Amiodarone, on the pill, so to speak. The initial days are always teacher work days in which we prepare rosters, obtain textbooks, set up classrooms, and perform whatever else is necessary to greet 150 new smiling faces the following week. I did not inform most of my colleagues about my recent hospitalization, nor the arrhythmia problems over the summer. I was feeling fine, and I did not want my health to be a gossip item in the teacher's lounge areas. (Actually this was not a possibility at Woodbridge because we were so overcrowded that teacher's lounges had long ago been converted to additional classroom space).

By Friday of that first week, I was ready, and even anxious, to begin classes the following Tuesday, when the students returned. Once again, fate intervened to complicate matters. I was on the south side of the house mowing the lawn on Saturday morning around 11 AM. Suddenly Nelle came running from the house screaming and waving her arms. I turned off the mower so that I could hear her. She yelled, "Dad, come quick. Grandma has been injured in a serious car accident. A doctor in Cincinnati is on the phone!"

Mom had been driving four of her friends to a picnic about 30 miles from her home in Kentucky when the car went out of control. Apparently, based on what could later be re-constructed, her right front tire had gone off the road into some fresh deep gravel alongside the highway, which had just been opened for traffic. When she turned the steering wheel to bring the car back onto the road surface, the tire dug into the gravel, causing the car to flip over several times as it rolled down an embankment.

Mom was seriously injured. She was removed from the crushed car by "jaws of life" equipment and flown in an emergency helicopter to University Hospital in Cincinnati. Her injuries were massive. The emergency room physician told me, "We don't know if she will make it. She has a serious skull fracture and undetermined internal injuries. The prognosis is poor."

I was in shock. Mom had not been hospitalized since my birth. I regarded her as immortal.

I flew to Kentucky on the first flight the following morning. Sharry had argued that she should come with me, but I insisted that she remain with the children. We had telephoned the bad news to

Aaron in Chapel Hill. His exact words were, "Oh my God, not Grandma!" Nelle and Emily were also distraught. Emily was particularly close to her grandmother; during our recent trip together to the Grand Canyon the two of them had been inseparable. I promised to assess the situation so that we could decide what to do next.

Sharry's concerns were considerable. We had no track record of how my heart would respond during a severe emotional crisis. I did not think of this aspect of her worry until several months later. All of my thoughts were focused on my mother.

Although I was expecting the worst, I was still unprepared for the first glimpse of Mom as she lie in Intensive Care. Her head was shaved, exposing extensive bruises and sutures. Her left arm was fractured, her face was ashen, and she was unconscious. She was on a ventilator to assist her breathing. Her official condition was listed as critical.

The doctors treating Mom were very candid. If she were able to make it through the first 48 hours, her chances would be better. The swelling from the skull fracture was creating a dangerous condition. She could die.

I stayed with Mom throughout the day and early evening. Her condition did not improve. I telephoned Sharry to discuss what we should do. Having no brothers or sisters, I was the sole decision maker. I needed Sharry's advice. Classes were to begin at Woodbridge two days later. It would be very difficult to have a substitute perform all of the administrative chores associated with the first day of the school year. On the other hand, I did not want to leave my mother in such a tenuous condition. Sharry recommended that I stay in Kentucky and that she fly there to join me. I did not like that approach - what about Nelle and Emily? Who would be with them? They were both beginning school also. They needed a parent at home to help them through this difficult period. They were both terribly worried about their grandmother. One of us needed to be there.

After considerable discussion, we decided that I would remain in Kentucky until at least the next afternoon. If Mom's condition was stable, I could catch a late flight to D.C. If things worsened, I would stay.

Early the next morning I spoke with Bob and Mary Leurck. They were life-long friends of Mom. At the time of my birth, Mom and Pop had been living in a two bedroom apartment above Bob's parents, Ray and Dorothy Leurck. Bob was two years older than I. His dad owned a Pure Oil gasoline station, which ultimately became a very profitable operation. The Leurcks are one of the hardest working families I have encountered. Although neither Bob nor his older brother, Ray, attended college, they both became successful entrepreneurs. Bob invested in local properties and was one of the most highly respected building contractors in the northern Kentucky/Greater Cincinnati area. His projects (mostly apartment complexes and commercial buildings) were solidly built and attractive additions to their neighborhoods. Even after acquiring considerable wealth, Bob and Mary lived very unpretentious lives. When I left the area to attend the Naval Academy, Bob became Mom's "local son." They saw each other several times weekly and shared many social activities. He even took her with them on their vacations, including a lengthy trip to Alaska in their Bluebird motor home.

I had always been grateful to Bob and Mary for the attention and love which they had shown Mom over the years. When I was away at sea, I felt better knowing that she had such good friends watching over her. Because Mom was active in several organizations and clubs, she did not have a shortage of friends in the area, but the Leurcks were special.

After telling Bob and Mary everything I knew about Mom's condition, I asked, "How are the girls?"

"The girls" were the four ladies in the car with Mom. They had been close friends for over half a century. In the spring of 1938, twelve nurses who were recent graduates of Speers Nursing School in Dayton, Kentucky had formed a social group, which they called the '38 Club. These ladies had met monthly since then for evenings of card playing and gossip. Most married, raised families, and worked as nurses, but, as far as I know, they **never** missed holding the monthly meeting for over 50 years! I knew all of these ladies and their families well - everyone referred to them as "the girls." Although I had initially learned from the emergency room doctor that no one else had been killed in the accident, I knew that there had been other injuries.

Mary answered my inquiry, "Ophelia, Ida Lee, and Mary have relatively minor injuries. They are all going to be OK. Ophelia had a collapsed lung, Ida Lee has some broken ribs and bruises, and Mary has a bruised heart."

"What about Esther Lou? I asked.

"She's not doing too well, Edwin," Bob interjected. (All of Mom's friends called me Edwin. They also referred to Mom as "Hogan," her maiden name). "She has a broken back and is paralyzed. They don't know if she is going to make it."

"Oh, no!" I was for the first time becoming nauseous. These ladies were like aunts to me. They were all over 75 years old, they did not deserve this.

"I talked to the state policeman who was at the scene," Bob continued. "Hogan lost control somehow or other. She and Ophelia were in the front seats and had their seat belts on. Ida Lee, Mary, and Esther Lou were all in back. They weren't wearing seat belts. As the car rolled over going down the hill, the roof caved in on your Mom's side. Her head kept getting smashed each time the car flipped over. Esther Lou was behind her. She apparently hit the roof because she wasn't restrained. They think that's what broke her neck. You should see the car. It's really smashed."

"What can we do to help, Edwin?" Mary asked.

"I am going to see how Mom is doing this afternoon. If she is pretty much the same, I think that I may fly back to Virginia until Friday. If you could keep close track of Mom's condition and let me know if anything worsens or if she becomes conscious, I would really appreciate it."

The Leurcks said that they were happy to help us. I spoke with the doctors at noon and again, around 4 PM. Nothing had changed. I decided to fly home. It was an extremely difficult decision, perhaps the most anguishing I had to make up to that point in my life. I did not know if I was doing the right thing. I had been submerged in the Pacific on GURNARD when Pop passed away. I did not want to be away if Mom were to die.

Sharry and the two girls met me at the airport. We exchanged long hugs. I am certain that Nelle and Emily felt that the world was against them. Within the space of a few months, they had been hit initially with news that their father had a fatal disease and now their only living grandparent had been seriously injured in a car accident. We did not speak much during the ride home from the airport.

I went through the opening day motions at school, but my thoughts were elsewhere. I telephoned the Leurcks each evening to receive an update. On Thursday the news was good. Mom had come out of the coma. Her prognosis for recovery was better. Immediately after classes ended on Friday, I flew to Kentucky to be with Mom.

She was still in Intensive Care, but was conscious and aware of my presence. I cried when I saw her. She looked as if she were in terrible pain, but there was obviously a strong fighting spirit within her determined to overcome the adversity. She had to struggle to speak, and her voice was feeble. Her first words to me were, "How are the girls?"

I lied to her, "They're all fine. Esther Lou is still here in the hospital, but everyone else is already home. You are going to be OK soon yourself."

I could tell that Mom knew that I was not being straightforward about Esther Lou. She forced a smile (which caused my eyes to water) as she said, "I know Esther Lou was hurt pretty bad. I was awake for a while after we rolled down the hill. They couldn't get us out of the car for a long time. I don't remember much else. I hope that the girls are OK." I was holding her hand. As she spoke, Mom would lightly squeeze my index and middle fingers. I wanted very much for her to live.

The Leurcks and other close friends visited Mom each day. We all agreed that if willpower were a factor, Mom had an excellent chance. She was a fighter.

On Sunday evening I again flew back to Virginia. I had an appointment with my cardiologist, Dr. Matthews, the following afternoon after school. Everything went well; there was no evidence of further arrhythmias. I was now down to a dose of 15 mg Prednisone daily. Surprisingly, I felt well in spite of the emotional trauma and a lack of sleep worrying about Mom.

While in Kentucky over the weekend, I had met on Saturday with a local attorney to assist me in case of legal action against

Mom. Although no other vehicles were involved, Bob Leurck had recommended to me that a lawyer friend of his look after Mom's interests. Although all of the ladies in the car were life-long friends, there were going to be considerable medical bills all around, especially for Mom and Esther Lou. Bob's advice proved to be particularly sage.

When I returned to Kentucky on Saturday morning, Mom's condition was considerably improved. She had been transferred to a "step down unit" where she was closely monitored by hospital staff. Although she was in a two bed room, there was no roommate. We had a wonderful afternoon together. We talked about how much she had improved and began to make plans for her transfer to a rehabilitation hospital near her home in northern Kentucky. It was now clear that she had lost vision in her right eye and hearing in her left ear due to the head injuries, but her arm was healing well and she was very alert. Despite the devices strapped around both her legs, which inflated automatically every few minutes and squeezed gently to help prevent the formation of blood clots, she seemed remarkably normal.

I left the hospital at 3 PM to visit the rehabilitation hospital which had been recommended to us by hospital discharge planning personnel. The facility was new and impressive. I felt comfortable knowing that Mom would be well cared for there. The staff came across as enthusiastic and competent. Their tentative rehab plan for Mom seemed realistic. I returned to the hospital in an ebullient mood. I was anxious to share my findings with Mom. The doctors had told us that she could be transferred at the end of the coming week. I felt as if our prayers had been answered with a miracle.

As I rounded the corner to Mom's hospital room, I saw two nurses run out the doorway of her room. They both yelled, "Call a code!"

I ran the last few feet to the door, but a man in a white coat restrained me from entering. I assumed that he was a resident. As I looked over his shoulder, I saw Mom lying face up on the floor. There were several medical personnel desperately working on her. They were apparently in the midst of CPR.

The man in the white coat pulled me by arm to a nearby room. He asked, "Are you a relative?"

I nodded, "Her son."

He looked me in the eye and said, "Your mother collapsed while we were walking her to the bathroom. We are trying to revive her."

The word "revive" hit me as if I had been rammed in the stomach. Before I could say anything, I heard "Clear!" followed shortly by "Again!" from Mom's room. The white coated man left before I could ask any questions. I never saw him again. I was in total shock.

As minutes passed without information from the room, I knew that Mom had died. I kept praying that I was wrong. "Please, God, let her live!" I repeated over and over.

After perhaps 20 minutes, a doctor entered the room where I was waiting. His face was somber. I knew that my prayers had not been answered. He reached for my arm as he said, "Mr. Linz, we were unable to save your mother. We tried everything, but she has passed away. I'm sorry."

I sat and cried for at least 10 minutes. I was alone and angry.

The cause of death was bilateral pulmonary emboli. As Mom had walked with the assistance of a nurse to the bathroom, two blood clots had broken loose from veins deep in her legs and become lodged in her lungs. Death had been essentially instantaneous.

I telephoned Sharry and the Leurcks. It had been a cruel twist. Mom had fought her incredible injuries so successfully, only to have a bolt out of the blue take her from us. We decided that it was God's plan that she join Him at this time. It certainly did not make us feel much better, but this faith did provide the framework for constructive grief and acceptance.

Sharry, Nelle and Emily flew to Kentucky on Monday. Aaron arrived from North Carolina that evening. Mom's remaining sister, my Aunt Jean, arrived from Arizona on Tuesday morning. Mom's niece, Carole Ulmer, drove from her home in northern Indiana with her daughter, Natalie, and two grandchildren, Anna and Katherine. There was a well-attended viewing at a funeral home in Fort Thomas, Kentucky on Tuesday evening. We buried Mom next to Pop the next morning after an emotional church service. It was Wednesday, September 18, 1991, my 48th birthday, and I had lost my best friend.

The next two months were a stressful blur. I had to return to Kentucky several times to attend to legal matters. Fortunately, my attorney was both competent and well-connected locally. I had learned from my father at an early age that the latter attribute was supremely important in Kentucky.

There were indeed several pressing legal matters. One of the insurance companies attempted to avoid payment by claiming that Mom had not been wearing her seat belt at the time of the accident. Since the sheriff's accident report was woefully brief, the only evidence was the hospital report which mentioned bruises inflicted by the seat belt. It did not take long for my attorney, Kurt, to have a very straightforward conversation with the insurance outfit. Kurt told me that their attempt to cheat us was not unusual. Their bluff was, as he put it, "worth a try" because several thousand dollars were involved. I wonder how many accident victims have been robbed by insurance companies using this ploy. My experience in dealing with medical insurance companies had already taught me to be extremely wary of every move by these people. They are definitely not on your side. Being "in good hands" may not be such a favorable location.

The other legal matter involved a suit against Mom's estate. It was ultimately settled out of court. I felt as if she had been robbed. We decided to settle in order to avoid protracted litigation which might require my presence in Kentucky. Sharry was very firm in her advice. She warned that we should consider my own health problem and the uncertainty associated with it. I was being kept alive only by taking a pill with dangerous side effects. The added stress of legal proceedings would not be helpful, she argued.

The other continuing reminder of Mom's death was the problem of disposing of her furniture and personal effects. As a product of the Great Depression, Mom did not throw anything away. Her house was jammed with belongings, often three or four of each. The basement was stocked with sufficient food and supplies for a lengthy nuclear war. During some of my trips to Kentucky to confer with Kurt, I spent most of the time making runs to a local homeless shelter with Mom's clothing and furniture. On one weekend when Aaron joined me, we used Bob Leurck's pickup truck to "donate" twelve full loads of junk and trash to a dumpster behind the local K-Mart. There was a definite sense of adventure in sneaking tons of garbage into someone else's dumpster. Since Mom had purchased so many things from K-Mart over the years, I saw a certain justice in our actions.

The fall of 1991 was hectic. I had little time to worry about my sarcoidosis. In addition to the frequent trips to Kentucky, I still went about the duties of teaching and coaching. Since these responsibilities were at different high schools located 12 miles from each other, I seemed to always be rushing about. Classes at Woodbridge began at 7:30 AM and ended at 2:05 PM. Because I usually remained in my classroom after school to provide tutoring for students requiring assistance, I did not leave Woodbridge until 2:45 PM. Then I would speed in my truck to Springfield for cross country practice. The co-captains led the team through stretching and warm-up exercises until my arrival. I always spoke to the team for at least 15 minutes before they left on a training run. Usually I would have them meet me at a local junior high school where we conducted various training drills until 5:00 PM. On Tuesdays we would participate in a local meet against another high school. This involved riding a "cheese box" (the girls' term for a school bus) to and from the meet. Most evenings I arrived home around 6:00 PM, just in time to fix dinner. Sharry's job usually kept her at work until later, so I was generally the designated chef. I liked this arrangement, because I enjoy cooking and none of us wanted to wait much later to eat.

On most weekends, the cross country team traveled to an invitational meet, frequently outside the immediate area. This meant that we had to leave early Saturday morning to drive to the location. Since these were typically all-day affairs, I would not return home until evening. Sundays, therefore, were my only day for rest and relaxation - unless I had lab reports or tests to grade from physics. I did not allow myself sufficient time to sleep. Five hours per night was not an uncommon occurrence. In retrospect, this was not an enlightened life style in view of my medical condition. I did not, however, have any further instances of arrhythmia of which I was aware. The pill seemed to be working.

In mid-December, after the cross country season had concluded, I arranged for a substitute to teach my classes, and drove with

Sharry to North Carolina to see Dr. Thomas Bashore at the Duke University Medical Center. From the time of his initial diagnosis of the sarcoid in May, Bob Matthews had wanted his friend, Bashore, to examine me. The Heart Center at Duke had a long history of treating patients with cardiac sarcoidosis due to the relatively high incidence of the disease in the Carolinas. We would have gone sooner, but the opportunity had not presented itself due to my hospitalization in August followed immediately by Mom's accident and death.

The Duke Medical Center is a huge complex comprised of many buildings located over a several block area in downtown Durham. After the long drive, we were anxious to see the doctor. There were no parking spaces available on the street, so I pulled into an open spot in a parking lot belonging to the Cricket Inn directly across the street from the North Hospital section of the medical center. I could have paid to use the hospital parking garage, but I have always been philosophically opposed to spending money to park. (Sharry asserts, probably correctly, that my core philosophy is *"CHEAP"*, and that the parking thing is only a minor subset of this religion). At any rate, I decided to chance being towed or ticketed rather than paying a few bucks to the Duke parking garage. As a UNC Tar Heel fan, I found a degree of pleasure in ripping off any aspect of a Duke Blue Devils' operation.

Sharry and I were both somewhat apprehensive as we walked to our appointment with Dr. Bashore. We had developed a certain comfort level with the Amiodarone therapy. It seemed to be working, and I was able to lead a relatively normal lifestyle. Neither of us wanted more bad news. We were not sure what could be gained from a visit to Bashore. Still, we had decided to do it, in the hope that he might have some insight into treatment for the sarcoid. When you are living on Life Row with a diagnosis of a fatal disease, there is a real urge to try anything. Maybe someone would tell us that there was a cure or a treatment or ....anything!

Dr. Bashore's office was on the 7th floor. The building was very new and was actually a large hospital divided into "zones." There was even a subway system, the "PRT" (Patient Rapid Transit), in the basement connecting this hospital to the older buildings on the university grounds. Large groups of medical students in short white coats seemed to be everywhere. This was a very busy place.

My first indication of trouble came as I left the elevator on the 7th floor. The water fountain did not work. "Was this an omen?" I thought.

We did not have to wait long to see Dr. Bashore. He was a short man, approximately my age, with a thin face. He was pleasant, but serious.

"I have read your file," he said. "Your case is highly unusual. It is difficult to believe that you have sarcoid. In fact, I have never seen anything quite like this. We'll do a few more tests on you here today and I will get back to you. Tell Bob Matthews that I said hello."

He then examined me, finding nothing remarkable in the process. We took the PRT to the South Hospital for the blood tests, x-rays and echocardiogram which Bashore had ordered. Within two hours we left Durham for the short drive to Chapel Hill to see Aaron. We did not receive a parking ticket while at Duke, so I considered the visit successful.

Just before Christmas, Dr. Bashore telephoned Matthews with his analysis. He concurred that the biopsy presented unmistakable evidence of cardiac sarcoidosis. He agreed with the steady reduction in Prednisone (I was now down to 7.5 mg/daily). I did not, of course, know exactly what else Bashore said to Mattthews, nor did I particularly care once I learned that he had nothing new to offer.

Aaron came home for the holidays. Christmas, 1991, was not a very joyous season. I had a fatal disease, and Mom was no longer with us.

Chapter 7

NEARLY BEYOND

The new year, 1992, started out well. My students returned from the holidays refreshed. We spent the next three weeks preparing for the semester examinations. All went well. No one failed the first semester.

There were no classes on January 27 and 28 so that the teachers could calculate grades for submission and prepare plans for the second semester. During these "teacher work days" I had a relaxed routine. Since I kept student grades on my computer throughout the school year, I did not have to spend much additional time preparing final grades. Consequently, I was usually able to have free time to socialize with my colleagues - something which few of us had the opportunity to do during normal school days.

On Tuesday, January 28, I left Woodbridge around 2 PM and met Greg, the father of one of my cross country runners, for some racquetball near my home at South Run Recreation Center. Greg was retiring from the Navy soon and was interested in becoming a high school teacher. I had invited him to visit Woodbridge to see first hand what may lie ahead. He had taken up my offer and had spent two weeks observing classes (both mine and others).

I had not played racquetball with Greg previously, and we were unaware of each other's skill level. Shortly after play began, I noticed that I was becoming fatigued. Greg was a good player, and we were having some lengthy rallies for each point. At the end of the first game, I asked that we take a short break. During this intermission, I was breathing heavily and sweating profusely. I had always been a heavy sweater, so I did not regard this as an unusual situation. After approximately five minutes, I said, "OK, let's get back to it. Your serve."

Greg gave me a long look and asked, "Are you sure you're OK? We can quit now if you want."

"No way," I responded. "I'm fine. I'm just not in good racquet-ball shape."

Although the second game was going in my favor score-wise, I was having to stop to get my breath after each point. I was worried that Greg was thinking that I was using this as a ploy to gain an advantage. With the score at 11 - 8 in my favor, I stopped playing and asked Greg, "Do you mind if we quit? I'm not feeling well. I think that I'd better go home."

In fact, I was feeling exhausted. I was gasping for each breath. My gym clothes were soaked with sweat. I had to sit immediately.

Greg replied, "Sure. No problem. Do you want me to stay here with you? I'm not doing anything."

"I'll be OK. I just need to get my breath. I'm going to sit here for a few minutes, then take a shower, and go home. There's no need for you to stay."

Greg rather reluctantly went along with my request. He did not know me that well and did not want to offend me by being pushy. He left.

I remained sitting outside the racquetball court for ten minutes, then slowly shuffled to the locker room. With considerable effort, I took off my soaked clothes and lay naked on a narrow wooden bench between lockers. I had a towel draped over my groin area. I do not know how long I remained there, but I do remember a tall, older man coming over to me and saying, "Hey, buddy, are you OK?"

"I'm fine," I snapped.

He persisted, "If you're not OK, I can get you some help. I can have the front desk call 911."

"Thanks, but I'm fine. I just want to get some rest before I shower. Thanks for asking."

"Now go away and leave me alone," I thought. In retrospect, I imagine that my condition must have looked rather serious to that fellow. Most men simply do not talk to naked strangers in locker rooms.

After the man left, I struggled to my feet and inched toward the shower. I had to stop every 10 feet to get my breath. I did not realize that I was in big trouble. It did not occur to me that I might be having arrhythmia. The pill had fixed that problem, I thought.

The shower took over 15 minutes because I was having diffi-culty moving. Somehow or other, I inched back the length of the slippery walk from the shower to the bench in front of my locker. I sat exhausted for several minutes to regain sufficient energy to dress myself. When I reached the stairs from the locker room to the lobby, the height of the steps looked insurmountable. I thought of calling for help, but foolishly decided to soldier on. It must have taken me ten minutes to climb that one flight of steps. Fortunately, my truck was parked near the entrance. The sun had set and it was bitterly cold. Each breath left a plume of vapor in front of me as I shuffled slowly to my truck for the short drive home. When I walked into the family room from the garage, Sharry was taking off her coat after just arriving from work. I gasped, "I'm going to lie down. I don't feel very well."

I fell backwards onto the sofa in the family room. Sharry rushed to me and grabbed my wrist to obtain a pulse. She felt nothing.

"I'm calling 911," she said.

As she went to the phone, I protested, "You don't need to do that. I'll be OK."

Sharry ignored me. She spoke directly to Nelle, "Go outside and look for the ambulance. Turn on the light outside the garage so that they can find us easily."

As soon as Sharry finished providing information to the 911 op-erator, she brought her stethoscope to my side to try to obtain a pulse directly from my chest. The heart beats were too fast to count. "Emily, get me my blood pressure cuff. It's on the front seat of the Nissan," Sharry directed.

Unable to hear a reliable pulse to obtain a blood pressure read-ing, Sharry was beginning to lose her relatively calm demeanor. "Where **is** that ambulance?" she worried aloud.

I was conscious, but very tired. I was not certain what was hap-pening to me.

Sharry held my hand while we waited for the ambulance. We did not speak. After approximately five minutes, we heard a siren.

A fire truck arrived shortly. Nelle directed two young EMTs through the garage into the family room. As one medic interviewed Sharry, the other prepared to start an IV in my right arm.

"I cannot feel a radial pulse. He's in VT. The apical pulse is too fast to count. He's on Amiodarone. Friehling's his doctor. He has cardiac sarcoidosis," said Sharry, all in one breath.

"Slow down," urged the young medic. "Talk to me plain and slowly."

The EMT working on me attached EKG leads and obtained a reading. He did not comment on the results, but folded the strip of paper and put it in his pocket. He then drew several blood samples.

Three additional medics entered the family room. From my prone position they all looked alike - young, obviously fit men operating in a very business-like manner. They exuded confidence.

Our neighbor, Hugh Boyd, came to the door and asked how he could help. Sharry requested that he and his wife, Sandy, take care of Nelle and Emily while we were at the hospital.

I do not recall how I got there, but the next thing I knew was that I was in the back of an emergency vehicle. I remember being disappointed that it was a truck instead of a traditional ambulance. I wondered if the driver would use the siren.

He did, but only at some intersections.

I know, because I was conscious throughout the drive to the hospital. Sharry was riding in the front with the driver. The two medics with me in the back did not speak to me. They were in radio communication with the emergency room; I was cargo.

I remember being able to follow our progress toward the hospital. As we made each turn, I mentally charted our route. It was now past 6:30 PM, but rush hour traffic was still heavy. As we reached Braddock Road, about three miles from Fairfax Hospital, one of the medics reported to the ER, "His pulse is still real high. What should we do? He doesn't look too good."

"Push 500 units of Lidocaine," came the reply.

"No, not Lidocaine. It makes me worse!" I yelled.

The EMTs ignored my scream and quickly injected the Lidocaine through the IV.

I was now worried - very worried.

"He's getting worse," yelled the EMT into the radio. "What do you want us to do?"

"Where are you?" came the response.

I could have answered. I knew that the truck had just rounded the cloverleaf onto the Beltway. We were less than two miles away. "If these guys don't kill me with the Lidocaine, I might make it," I thought.

"We're on the Beltway. ETA less than five minutes."

"Push another 500 units of Lidocaine," came the reply from the ER.

"No!!!" I yelled, "You're killing me. **Please** don't do it! Wait until we get to the hospital. Get hold of Friehling. He knows what works."

My protests fell on deaf ears. I watched in horror as another 500 units of Lidocaine was injected through the IV line. I started to feel woozy.

Maybe this was the end.

As the vehicle pulled into the emergency room entrance to the hospital, I quietly thanked God that I was still alive. I remember feeling the cold January air as I was moved from the truck into the ER. "Now I will be safe," I thought.

Sharry did not share my optimism. While I was being transferred from the emergency vehicle to a room in the ER, she was directed to wait in a small conference room. In reality, the room was more suitable for mop and supply storage than as a waiting room for a frantic relative of someone close to death. There were no windows or reading material. As opposed to all of the other hospital waiting rooms, there was not even the ubiquitous television to numb the mind. "I felt as if I had been put into a closet and told to wait until I was allowed to come out," Sharry later recounted. "I never felt more alone. My only companion was fear."

In contrast, I had considerable company. I was now lying on a narrow table in a small room filled with medical personnel, who all seemed to be flitting about me like gnats around a sweaty body. I was conscious and intelligible, if not lucid. The emergency room doctor, a young woman, was speaking to me, "How do you feel, Mr. Linz?"

"I am in v-tach. I've been this way since just after four. They gave me Lidocaine in the ambulance. I told them not to. It makes me worse. Is Dr. Friehling here? He is my doctor. He knows how to handle this. I think that I am dying. I can talk, but it is hard to breathe. I will tell you everything that I feel. My toes are tingling. Where is Friehling?"

"OK," she replied quietly. "We are going to help you. Dr. Friehling is in-house. He should be here shortly. Stay calm."

"I think that I am losing feeling in my feet!" I did not shout, but my anxiety was increasing. I tried to wiggle my toes, but I could feel nothing in response.

"Now I can't feel anything below my knees. I can't feel my legs!" For the first time in my life, I started to worry about dying. The end seemed to be approaching rapidly. I would never see Sharry or our children again. I started to pray intently to myself, "Oh, God, please take care of my family. Please help them. Please!"

"I can't feel any of my legs! I'm dying. Where is Friehling?!"

"You are not going to die, Mr. Linz," assured the doctor. She was shouting orders to the cloud of gnats around me. I have no idea what she said or what procedures and medications were being tried. It seemed to me as if there were at least twenty faces hovering over me. I was beginning to detect a collective sense of panic.

My own terror increased as I now began to lose feeling in both hands. "My hands! I can't feel them any more. Do something! Please do something!" I yelled.

No one responded to my shouts. For some reason, I then began to calm down. I decided to use all of my energy to pray for life. I would continue to report symptoms as they developed, but my mind was repeating to itself, "I am going to live. Help me, Lord. I am going to live."

The loss of feeling had now spread upwards throughout the length of both arms. "My arms are gone," I stated calmly. I was struggling to breathe, but my concern was that the only parts of my body left with feeling were the trunk, face and mind.

A tingle began in my chin. "My face. It's beginning in my face. It's spreading up. My cheeks. I'm dying. I'm dying, aren't I? I'm dying," I sobbed.

To my horror, my tongue now started to curl upwards from the tip. My speech became slurred, as I reported this development to the doctor, "I don't think that I can talk much longer. My tongue is curling up."

It was at this moment that I became resigned to death. I attempted to yell out, "Good-bye, cruel world!" but no intelligible sounds came from my mouth. My mind was still alert, and I felt cheated that I had been denied final words. I remember trying to conjure up something more appropriate than "Good-bye, cruel world," in the event that my speech returned, but nothing seemed appropriate other than prayer. Soon I regained focus and began repeating to myself, "Help me, Lord." I continued this three word request for the next several minutes, or so it seemed. My eyes remained open and I was able to watch the continuing despair on the faces around me. I was determined to fight death with every ounce of remaining energy. I would not give up.

As I hung on the edge of death, I did not see angels, saints, or any of the other heavenly creatures which the nuns had promised during grade school. But, as I stared at the ceiling, unable to move anything except my eyes, I began to experience a warm glow of acceptance. It was as if I had entered a calm from the storm of activity raging around me. Suddenly, I felt as if a large hand was pushing gently on my forehead to prevent me from falling over a cliff into darkness below. I was certain that I heard a quiet voice saying, "Not yet."

At that moment I knew that I was being given a reprieve. The Lord wanted me to remain on Life Row.

Suddenly I felt my tongue begin to uncurl. It had been in a tight ball against the roof of my mouth. As soon as I could speak, I gasped, "I can talk! My tongue is back to normal. I can feel my cheeks!"

The loss of feeling process slowly reversed itself in an exactly opposite order. Once my face was returned, my arms began to develop feeling from the shoulders down to the fingertips. I chronicled these gains to the doctor who had remained at my side during the entire experience.

Within five minutes I could feel my entire body. I felt as if a miracle had taken place. My eyes were running with tears as I mumbled, "Thank you, Lord." I heard no reply, nor did I have any vision of a celestial being. I was certain, however, that God had been with me.

My heart rate, as reported by one of the gnats in the room (someone had been calling out blood pressure and pulse readings every 30 seconds, or so) was still consistently over 180 bpm. Medically I was not out of the woods. I remained in ventricular tachycardia. Although I could die at any minute, I knew that I would not.

The mood among the ER personnel changed noticeably as Dr. Friehling came into the room. The young doctor who had been re-assuring me looked particularly relieved. "We're going to get you out of this right now," Friehling announced as he smiled at me. "You won't feel the shock. We will put you asleep for a moment before we put the paddles on you. You're going to be OK."

I wondered if I would have burns again from the paddles. Before I could dwell on this thought, I passed out from the narcotic which had been injected into the IV line.

Ted Friehling was correct. I did not feel the shock. In fact, I did not know exactly how many shocks were required to return my heart to a normal rhythm. Nor do I remember how long I remained in the ER. When I awoke, I was by myself in a small hospital room with no windows. I felt fine, but I did have the tell-tale burn marks on my chest and back.

Sharry was unaware of the developments in the ER until Ted came to see her. She had been, in effect, in isolation and was on the verge of a breakdown. Apparently, Ted asked if Sharry was present as soon as he entered the ER.

"You did all the right things," he assured her. "I ordered them not to shock Ed until I got down here from upstairs. I was hoping that he would convert on his own. When do you think he began v-tach?"

"Probably just after four when he was playing racquetball," Sharry replied. "He was definitely in it when I first saw him just after six."

"A couple of hours in v-tach. Amazing! He went through a tough period a few minutes ago, but I'm sure he will be OK," Ted smiled assuredly. "I'll be right back."

In less than five minutes, Friehling returned to Sharry, "He converted right away. He's fine now. Normal sinus rhythm. He went right back in one shock. I'm going to send him to the CCU tonight.

We'll see how he is and talk more tomorrow. You can go in and see him now."

"Thanks, Doctor. I'm so glad that they did not try to convert him in the emergency truck. Thank God that you were here."

"I'm always here," joked Friehling as he left Sharry to return to the second floor to complete an EP study on another patient. It was after 8 PM. He had been in the hospital since 7 in the morning. I later learned that this was a rather routine day for Ted.

Sharry spoke with me in the ER before I was taken to the Cardiac Care Unit (CCU), also on the second floor of the hospital. I do not recall the conversation or even seeing her. Apparently she told me that she had called Nelle and Emily at the Boyd's to tell them that I was OK. Nelle had then relayed the news to Aaron in Chapel Hill.

When I awoke the following morning, it was now Wednesday, January 29. As soon as I saw that the clock was indicating 6:45 AM, I worried about who was going to teach my classes. It was the first day of the new semester. There were no lesson plans, of course, because I had not anticipated almost dying and ending up in a room somewhere in Fairfax Hospital.

Before I could dwell on the teaching problem, a technician entered the room. He was pushing a large machine in front of him. His way of saying "Good morning" was to announce, "Chest x-ray."

"Why?" I asked.

"The doctor ordered it," he replied. He was obviously annoyed that I asked.

"Which doctor? All of mine know how I feel about x-rays. Which one ordered it?"

The technician was really angry now. "Are you refusing doctor's orders?"

"Well, I'm not getting any x-ray until I know who ordered it. Tell the nurse. If this is refusing doctor's orders, then, yeah, I'm refusing doctor's orders. You can log it however you want."

The technician, who was a thin, young male, mumbled something unintelligible under his breath and departed the room. He left the x-ray machine near the bed. A nurse soon arrived to defuse the situation. "I'm Janet, your nurse. Welcome to the CCU. What's the problem on the x-ray?"

"I try to minimize my exposure to x-rays. All of my doctors support this. I cannot imagine any of them ordering a chest x-ray without first discussing it with me."

"No problem," replied Janet. "Dr. Merlino will be in to see you later this morning. I will ask her about it when she comes in. Do you feel like eating breakfast?"

"Yes, thanks. Is there a phone here? I need to call my wife about my job."

I talked with Sharry for several minutes. We agreed that she should go to work. Nelle and Emily would be in school. I asked Sharry to call Pam White at Woodbridge to tell her about my hospitalization. "Tell her that I will give some lesson plans to Cecil Jarman over the phone later today. We'll let her know when I will be back after I talk to the doctors today."

"Don't worry about Woodbridge. They'll survive without you for a few days," Sharry responded.

I ate everything on the breakfast tray. I felt pretty good about myself. In the past 24 hours, I had dodged a deadly sarcoid bullet and successfully eluded an x-ray. I did not want to address the question, "What next?"

Before I could refine these reality avoidance maneuvers, Robin Merlino came into the room. She smiled as she took my hand, "I am glad that you are OK, Ed. That was a close call. Has Ted Friehling talked to you about options?"

"Options? What do you mean? What options?"

"The Amiodarone isn't reliable. You almost died. You shouldn't try to walk out of here just on Amiodarone. Next time you may not be as lucky. You need to talk to Friehling about getting a defibrillator. You need more protection. He can tell you what will be involved."

"That's open heart surgery, isn't it?" I asked. "I'm not sure that we are at that point yet."

"Probably, but you cannot go on safely like this. The medicines are not totally effective. Talk to Bob Matthews also. No one knows for sure, but the sarcoid may be getting worse. In my opinion, you are in considerable danger without a defibrillator."

Dr. Merlino then examined me. As she was leaving the room, she turned and smiled, "By the way, Ed, I talked to the nurse about the x-ray. Some intern ordered it. I have taken care of the situation. You will not be receiving any more x-rays unless Matthews, Friehling, or I order them. They can't believe you out there at the nurse's station. They have never seen anyone refuse an x-ray before. I'll see you this afternoon."

Just before noon, I was transferred from the CCU to a bed on the second floor. It was the same unit that I had been in during the Amiodarone load-up phase the previous August. I was happy to see that my nurse friends, Kathleen, Jennifer, Mark and Donna, were still assigned there.

The hardware sales pitch began in earnest shortly after lunch. Ted Friehling, Al Del Negro and Kim Hill - the arrhythmia specialists, or, as I preferred to call them, my "rhythm and blues team" - came to see me. Al did not beat around the bush, "Ed, we think that your only choice now is to have a defibrillator. The Amiodarone has worked as well as can be expected, but, as this incident indicates, it is not foolproof. You need the protection of an AICD."

"Tell me everything about it again," I requested. Ted had spent nearly 30 minutes explaining the AICD to Sharry and me in August. I had forgotten most of the details, except that AICD stood for Automatic Implantable Cardioverter Defibrillator. I did remember the basic premise of the device: it would shock my heart back to a normal rhythm in the event of tachycardia. [The terminology for defibrillators seems to be constantly changing. In 1992, AICD was used by all of my doctors. By 1994, most were referring to the same device as an "ICD."]

Al answered me, "Kim brought one with her. Take a look at it while I talk to you about it."

Kim produced a metallic box approximately the size of a wallet. As she handed it to me, I noticed that it was considerably heavier than I expected - at least a pound, I estimated. One end was flat and was covered in soft plastic. The other was rounded and smooth to touch. Three wires were attached to the plastic end via sealed connectors. Two of these had a clear plastic coating which gave them the thickness and pliability of spaghetti (after it has been cooked). The wire itself, inside its covering, was thin and gray and was just under two feet in length. These wires were connected to two identical mesh rectangular "paddles" containing 20 small squares approximately 1/2 inch on a side. One side of the paddle was covered by a thin plastic coating, but on the other side, the small squares had exposed metal screening. The paddles resembled the business end of a small fly swatter.

As I ran my fingers over the mesh paddles, Al explained, "Those get sewn onto the sides of your heart. When the computer circuitry inside the box senses a dangerous arrhythmia, a switch closes and the batteries inside charge up a capacitor. If the condition is still there after the capacitors are fully charged, another switch closes and an electrical charge is sent through the wires to the paddles. Your heart gets shocked, but we don't need as much charge as the external paddles use, because it is directly against the tissue. It doesn't have to travel through all that skin and muscle. It's already there."

"How much of a shock is it? Will I feel it?"

"You'll feel it," laughed Ted. "It's not that bad. We can adjust the level based on how much it takes to convert you. We will test it several times after it is installed to ensure that it is working and that we have set a good level for it to operate reliably."

"That middle wire, see how it divides into two other wires?" asked Kim. "Those are the sensing leads. The ends of those two are connected to small screws which will be inserted into your heart tissue. They detect the continuous electrical activity of the heart, like an EKG. That's how the box knows when to start charging the capacitors. There is also a pacing capability with those same sensing wires. We can program the computer to try to pace your heart out of a dangerous rhythm before it tries to shock you. There is a lot of versatility."

"Screws go into my heart? Paddles get sewn onto the sides? Where does the box go?" I asked.

"We make an incision just below your ribs on the left side. The surgeon will then create a small pocket in that fleshy area. There is a lot of muscle there to hold it in place. The box fits right into that pocket."

"Doesn't it stick out? Will I have a big lump in my stomach? Can you see it?"

I had several other questions, but Ted interrupted, "Sure, you can see a lump if you are naked. If you are wearing a shirt, no one will probably notice. You can move around without it bothering you. After a month or so, you probably won't even know that it's there."

The engineer in me then came out, "What kind of metal is this box made of? I assume that it has to be something which will not react with my body tissue. Do you know what it is?"

Al took this one. "I think that it is titanium or some stainless steel alloy. I'm not one hundred percent certain. You're right. It has to be non-reactive. It's going to be in there for a while. We don't want an infection. That's why there is also so much plastic. Obtaining materials which can be safely used in the human body for extended periods of time is a real technical challenge."

"How dangerous is all of this?" I asked. "Am I going to get shocked often?"

Al looked at Ted before he responded. His tone was serious. "Let's not kid ourselves, Ed. You are already in a dangerous condition. No one knows the status of your sarcoidosis. Maybe it's getting worse, maybe not. It really doesn't matter, because the damage has already been done. We know that your heart will go into tachycardia even with the Amiodarone. Next time you might die. The AICD gives you protection. The surgery to implant it has all the risks of a normal open heart operation. We have never lost anyone putting in an AICD."

"OK, but what about the shocks? How often?"

"There is no way of telling," said Ted. "It depends on your body. Maybe once a month. I don't know. Maybe less often. It varies from patient to patient. Al didn't mention this, but you might get more than one shock at a time. If the first shock doesn't convert you, the AICD will re-charge and fire again. It keeps doing this until you convert or, uh, you won't convert."

"I suppose that you can program it to play 'Taps' when that happens," I wise-cracked. "With all of this shocking going on, how long do the batteries last in this thing?"

"It depends on how often it fires. Generally, at least two years. Sometimes they go five years. You will have to come to our office every two months to let us check it."

"How do you check it?"

"It's easy," interjected Kim. "We put a radio transmitting device on your skin directly over the box and interrogate it with a lap top computer type device. We get a read-out which tells us everything about your heart and the AICD during the preceding two months. We can look at every unusual rhythm which occurs. It gives us a print-out and also tells us how much battery life is remaining."

"All of that from this little box?" I asked.

"If you knew what it costs, you would understand."

"How much does it cost?"

"About thirty thousand. But it has a two year warranty," replied Ted, sounding somewhat like a used car salesman.

"I need to talk this over with Sharry. This is pretty heavy stuff. I don't know what to do. Do you have these things lying around ready to install?"

"The ones we use are 'investigational devices.' They don't have full FDA approval yet, but we can get one for you, - at least, I think so. I will check tomorrow. We will probably use a model made by Telectronics. Talk to Sharry. Make sure that you both want to do this. I really do not know of any other viable option," concluded Al.

As they turned to leave the room, Ted gave me an encouraging smile, "Hang in there. If you have any other questions, have the nurse get us. We are here every day." Kim squeezed my leg and smiled also. I really liked these folks. What I did not like was their message.

Shortly after my "rhythm and blues" team left the room, I realized that I had not asked them if the costs of the AICD and the surgery to implant it would be covered by my insurance. When Sharry arrived after her work that afternoon, we discussed the insurance problem and all of the pros and cons associated with the AICD. We came to no decision that evening. We did decide that Sharry would call our insurance company the next day to inquire about our coverage, and, if necessary, to plead. We had been very fortunate so far in the first year of our medical ordeal, because our two insurance plans had paid most of the expenses. We were now, however, headed into deeper financial waters. I did not want to impoverish my family due to my medical problems. Whether or not we could afford this proposed treatment was a factor in my decision process. Sharry's approach was different: we would do whatever was necessary to obtain the appropriate medical treatment.

Kim Hill had left us a video on AICDs. It had been prepared by the manufacturer, Telectronics, and was essentially sales propaganda for the device. To view the video, we walked down the hallway to a small room containing a TV and VCR used by the nurses for training during day shift. It had a happy ending, in fact, several of them. Everyone lived happily ever after. My main reaction to the film, now that I knew the price of the device, was that I wanted to buy some Telectronics stock.

By morning I had come to a decision. I would not have the defibrillator implanted. I would go home and take my chances. I had gone nearly six months on Amiodarone with only one incident. For all I knew, it may have been a one time event due only to playing racquetball. The surgery and the shocking seemed too extreme.

When Robin Merlino came to my room early that morning, I informed her of my decision. "Have you told Sharry yet?" she asked.

"No. I will talk to her later this morning. I'm going to tell Friehling when he comes in. You look like you don't approve."

"You know how I feel, Ed. You are making a big mistake."

Dr. Merlino did not debate me. She completed her usual physical examination and left without further comment. I was somewhat disappointed because I knew from my experience on the debate team at the Naval Academy that I needed an opponent to enable me to hone my arguments before I attempted to convince Sharry that I was making the correct decision. It was going to be a tough sell.

I later learned that as soon as she left, Merlino telephoned Sharry at home. "We need you to be here at noon today. Ed tells me that he is going to go home without the AICD. We are going to hit him then with all three of us at once, Bob Matthews, Ted Friehling and myself. If you can help us, we might be able to turn him around on this. He **has** to have the AICD to have a chance."

Sharry thanked Merlino for the invitation and for her strong interest in my case. "This is why I wanted a civilian doctor," Sharry thought to herself as she hung up the phone. "I cannot imagine this type of follow-through in military medicine or even in an HMO. God, we are lucky to have Merlino."

I was unaware, of course, that a scheme to manipulate me was underway. Sharry arrived just before lunch with the good news that our insurance companies would cover the AICD expenses. She had telephoned Blue Cross/Blue Shield, and with little argument, had been granted approval for the implantation. Dr. Friehling's office had also spoken with Blue Cross that morning, and everything was set.

I responded to Sharry's insurance news in a soft voice, "Thanks for making all the calls and getting their approval, but I'm not going to do it. There's just too much risk and too many unanswered questions. I'm going to go home. I'm being monitored here continuously and my heart is working fine. I think that it was an isolated incident. I won't play any more racquetball."

I was expecting a big argument, but Sharry was relatively low key. "I think that we would be making a huge mistake," she replied firmly. There were tears forming in her eyes. "This really is a family decision. Have you thought about us?"

A hospital worker came into the room with my food tray. "Let's talk about this after lunch," I requested. "Of course, I have thought about our family."

Ten minutes later Robin Merlino walked into the room. She looked very sad. "Ed, let me tell you why I feel so strongly about this. You see, I lost one of my patients last year due to an arrhythmia like yours. It wasn't sarcoid related, but I had a chance to save him if I would have insisted on an AICD. I didn't, and he is dead today. I do not want that to happen to you and Sharry. The AICD can save you. You need to have it."

I did not argue with her. I could tell that she was very upset with me. I appreciated her advice and friendship, but I was not yet ready to change my mind. "Thanks, Robin. Thanks for being so straight. I'm scared by all of this. I just can't do it now. I think that I will be safe at home. As long as I don't do anything stupid, I'll be OK. No more racquetball!"

Robin talked with Sharry outside the room for a few additional minutes. I could not hear their conversation. I was now more confused than before. I did not know what to do.

Before I could sort out these thoughts, Dr. Matthews came into the room. As always, he walked briskly to the large chair near the wall, sat down, and crossed his legs. He always seemed to be wearing the same type of socks. "I understand that you don't want the AICD, Ed. Why not?"

We then engaged in a lengthy debate. Matthews spoke quietly and softly as if he were lecturing a small group of medical students. He answered each of my objections with facts. He was, in Sharry's words, "eloquent and brilliant," while I had been "petty and stupid." After about fifteen minutes, my thought process had been exposed as irrational, and I knew it. I was still not prepared, however, to cave.

I maintained my position for the next two hours. Sharry and I talked little. I could sense her frustration with me. I sensed, however, that she knew that they had me on the ropes. Friehling provided the knock-out blow as he entered the room. Instead of his usual smile, he sternly demanded, "Well, what have you decided?"

I looked over to Sharry and then back to Friehling. "OK, let's do it," I mumbled, closing my eyes in the process.

Friehling simply nodded and said quietly, "I think that you are making the correct decision. We haven't located a device yet, but I still think that we can get one by next week. First we have to do an EP study on you. I will try to get you on the schedule for tomorrow afternoon."

Sharry smiled as Friehling left the room. She did not tell me until two years later how I had been set up by Merlino.

The EP study provided generally good news. Although Al and Ted were able to put me into v-tach rather easily, they were also able to control it by pacing. I could be returned to a normal rhythm without a shock being required. The AICD would be set to try to pace me several times, before it would shock.

The weekend passed quickly. I had telephoned Pam White at Woodbridge on Friday morning before the EP study and brought her up to date on my situation. We agreed that she should attempt to obtain a long term substitute teacher who knew some physics to take my classes while I would be recovering from the surgery. I told her to expect me to be gone at least a month. The science department chairman, Cecil Jarman, called me on Saturday to tell me that they had located a recently retired Air Force general who was willing to teach for me. Cecil gave me the general's name and phone number so that I could contact him with instructions. On Sunday I telephoned him and talked for nearly an hour. I felt comfortable with him. He was enthusiastic and relatively knowledgeable about physics. I tried to be encouraging, but I did not envy his assignment. He had never taught before, so he was about to enter a minefield. I knew that my classes would be cooperative with him, but walking into a high school classroom in the middle of the school year as a rookie teacher would be challenging. As it turned out, he did very well.

Once the teaching issue was settled, my thoughts focused on my medical problem. I was still uncomfortable with the decision to have the AICD installed, but I did not tell anyone, including Sharry. How do you admit that you are afraid to die? I had been "nearly beyond" only a few days earlier. Now I was about to have patches sewn onto, and screws inserted into, my heart. Things did not look good.

I had been in dangerous situations many times during my years in the submarine force. As a junior officer aboard my first submarine, USS GURNARD, we had hit the bottom of the ocean off the California coast while we were cruising at a high speed submerged at a deep depth. The only reason we survived was that the bottom was sand, instead of rock or coral. On numerous other occasions I had been involved in submerged operations locating and trailing Soviet submarines, similar to those described by Tom Clancy in his book, *The Hunt for Red October*. On more than one occasion I was convinced that we were going to die during these submerged games of chicken. But none of these situations had the psychological impact of my stay on Life Row. I felt as if I were now a target directly in the cross-hairs with a steadily decreasing amount of wiggle room to avoid the next shot.

As I tried to fall asleep that evening, I was trying more than ever to bargain with God. "Please help me," I begged. "I'll do anything..."

For the first time since being placed on Life Row, I was crying. I was now fully aware of my mortality. I began to wonder if I would be able to locate Mom and Pop in heaven. I do not know when these thoughts ended and my dreams began that night.

Chapter 8

HARDWARE

An AICD was located on Monday, February 4, 1992. Surgery was scheduled early the following morning. The surgeon, Paul Massimiano, had gone over the implantation procedure with me the night before. I liked Massimiano. He was tall with slightly drooping shoulders. His hair was gray, going on white, although he appeared to be younger than I. Overall, he reminded me of some of the tall officers I had served with on submarines who had developed a semi-permanent stoop from the restricted head room aboard ship.

Dr. Massimiano's soft-spoken approach was straightforward, "This is not going to be difficult. First we are going to try a transvenous placement of the AICD. That doesn't require open heart and is the easier way to do this. The AICD itself will go into a pocket which we create down here in your abdomen." He rubbed his hand over that area of his stomach. As I nodded he continued, "The wires to and from the AICD will be threaded into veins into the right side of your heart. The problem is, due to your sarcoid, it may not work. We may not be able to establish reliable electrical continuity. If that's the case, then we will have to do a thoracotomy. That's an incision just under your left breast." He drew an imaginary line in a concave arc under his left nipple. I got the idea.

When I nodded again, Massimiano continued, "We will then spread your ribs to gain access to the heart. I will sew the defibrillator leads onto the side of your heart. The sensing leads will be screwed into heart tissue. The box itself goes into the same pocket whether we do transvenous or open heart."

"If you have to use open heart, how do you get the wires from the heart to the box?" I asked.

"First I create a passage under the skin with my finger. I know, it sounds terrible, but it's really simple. Once I have a tunnel, I just push the wires through it from below the heart to the location of the AICD. It's about five inches or so."

"I should never have asked," I thought to myself. The image of someone poking their fingers through various parts of my body was not particularly uplifting. I tried, of course, to maintain a brave front, "Yeah, that sounds pretty simple. Will I be able to feel those wires after this is all over?"

"I doubt it. You will be able to feel the box. It's big. But the wires are very fine and are far enough under the skin that you won't know they are there."

"So, are you doing the whole thing? What do the arrhythmia doctors, Friehling and Del Negro, do? Just watch you?"

"One of them, Ted Friehling, I think, will be there, along with a tech rep from the AICD manufacturer. Ted will not be doing the actual surgery tomorrow, I will. But he will be there to test the device before we close you up. The AICD will not be permanently turned on until later in the week. You need to talk to him about that. I am just the plumber to get the thing in."

I thanked my plumber for taking the time to explain the procedure. As he left, I yelled to him, "Don't stay up late tonight. Get plenty of sleep."

Massimiano turned and smiled. I am sure that he had heard the same thing hundreds of times from patients.

Sharry was with me when the gurney arrived to transport me to the operating room. We kissed good-bye. In spite of Massimiano's assurances that this was no big deal, we both knew that I was about to undergo a potentially dangerous procedure. If the transvenous procedure did not work, my chest was going to be cut open and my heart would be handled and sewn. This was a big deal.

Sharry smiled and waved as I began the trip to the elevator. I thought that I saw her starting to cry.

My next memory was waking with a terrible pain in my throat. I had a tube there which was apparently helping me to breathe. I felt as if I had been hit by a very large truck, which had then backed over me several times. Everything on my body from my shoulders to my belly button hurt. None of my doctor friends had discussed this aspect of the procedure.

Overall, however, I was very happy. I was alive. I kept repeating to myself, "Thank you, Lord."

Sharry was near the bed. I assumed that I was in the Intensive Care Unit (ICU) because Dr. Massimiano had told me that I would be taken there following the surgery. I wanted to talk to her, but the tube in my throat, the respirator, made this impossible. I kept falling in and out of sleep. Everything was a fog, but I knew that I had survived. I was still on Life Row.

The following morning I was conscious and was taken to the third floor to recuperate. It was a difficult day. My body still hurt tremendously. Every time I attempted to move, I winced in pain. I was receiving medication for relief, but the only effect that I could notice was a dramatic intensification of nightmares when I would fall asleep. The images during those dreams were vivid and frightening. I had not had nightmares since I was a teenager, so I was unaccustomed to this agony. Several times during the day I woke up terrified and sweating profusely. I became angry that I had not mentally prepared myself for the realities associated with a major surgery.

Sharry was also not having a good day. She had left work at the Health Department just before noon in order to arrive at the hospital shortly after I was transferred to the third floor. When she first saw me, I was tossing and turning in a fitful sleep. The ventilator had been removed before I was transferred from the ICU, and I was yelling incoherently. As I woke with a start, I began to scream requests for water. Sharry was annoyed that no nursing staff had apparently been in the room since my arrival. She went to the nursing station to obtain a pitcher of water.

Once I settled down, we talked. My throat was still extremely sore, but I could carry on a limited conversation. Most of my comments revolved around the pain I was encountering. Sharry told me that both Massimiano and Friehling had spoken to her immediately following the surgery. As Massimiano had predicted, the attempt to use the transvenous placement method had been unsuccessful. The sarcoidosis had created too much damage in the right ventricular area of my heart. Friehling kept repeating, "We couldn't get good thresholds." He did not explain, Sharry said, exactly what this meant, and she did not ask. The bottom line was that the easier method would not work, and that open heart surgery was required. I had been cut open, patches were sewn onto the sides of my heart, screws were inserted into the heart tissue, and wires were run back and forth under my skin from the heart to the AICD now bulging from my left stomach area. I was now full of hardware.

Approximately two hours later, a nurse, an older Hispanic lady whom we did not know, came into the room and took my vital signs. I had been tossing and turning following another nightmare. The nurse spoke harshly to Sharry, "Why don't you go home? You are upsetting him."

"I beg your pardon?" Sharry was shocked. "What was he like this morning?"

"He was much better. He's only been bad since you've been here."

As a nurse, Sharry was very offended. She could not believe the insensitivity of this nurse. Instead of providing support in this difficult time, the lady was laying a guilt trip on her. Sharry responded, "Thanks for your opinion. I'm his wife, and I'm staying."

The nightmares continued through the next afternoon. I decided to ask that the pain medication be discontinued to see if that was the cause of the horrific dreams. To my delight, the nightmares went away. I was able to tolerate the pain by taking Tylenol 3 (Tylenol containing 30 mg of codeine). Maybe I was going to survive this ordeal after all.

The AICD had not yet been turned on. On the next morning, Friday, February 7, 1992, I was taken to the EP lab. As I was wheeled into the room on a gurney, Friehling and Del Negro waved hello, but offered no verbal encouragement. Both seemed more tense than usual. Working together closely with their team of nurses and a Telectronics tech rep, they used a magnet to place the AICD in an operating mode. Over the next two hours they installed set-points and took readings as the device was thoroughly tested. The bad news was that its pacing function would not convert me successfully to a normal rhythm. Each time that my heart was externally stimulated by the doctors into tachycardia, the AICD sensed the dangerous condition and attempted to pace me to a lower heart rate. Unfortunately, my heart would not cooperate, and did the exact opposite by speeding up to an even more danger-ous condition. When this happened, the only route back to a nor-mal sinus rhythm was via a shock, which the device delivered suc-cessfully on each occasion. I did not feel the shock because I was under a mild anesthesia during the entire EP study. Although this was certainly a disappointing and sub-optimal situation, the AICD was definitely performing its primary mission of shocking me when-ever I went into v-tach.

Dr. Friehling gave us the bad news when I was returned from the EP lab around noon. Sharry and I were very disappointed because the pacing had been successful only a week earlier during the EP study prior to the AICD implantation. Friehling told us that, based upon the unsuccessful tests, he had decided to turn off the pacing function, so that it would not exacerbate an arrhythmia when it oc-curred. He also told us that both he and Massimiano were sur-prised at the appearance of my heart during the surgery. Appar-ently it was white and enlarged and rather sickly looking, compared to a healthy heart. There was an obvious line of demarcation of disease at the septum, the tissue dividing the right and left sides of the heart. "The sarcoidosis is definitely there on the right side of your heart," Friehling said grimly. "It is really strange how it seems totally limited to the right side. The left side looks fine. There is a clear break at the septum."

"When do you think that the AICD is going to fire, Doctor? How long before I get shocked?" I asked.

"Who knows? It could be later today, next week or maybe never. It depends on whether or not you have v-tach. If you do, we know that it will fire. When you get out of here, you will have to come to our office every two months for us to check the unit."

I found Ted's comments grim. I began to wonder what it would feel like when I was shocked. Each time that the external paddles had been used on me, I was anesthetized so that I would not feel the shock. What might happen if the device fired while I was driving? I decided to ask. "Ted, can I drive with this thing in me?"

"I wouldn't recommend it," was all that Ted would say. I read his body language to say, "It's up to you. Just don't say that I said it was OK."

I paused for a moment and then said, "I see." I was angry at myself for not discussing this subject prior to the AICD installation. I decided to adopt a "wait and see" approach. If the device did not fire in the next few weeks, maybe I would drive. I also wanted to experience the magnitude of the shock before making a decision. Driving was an important part of my life. I was not about to surrender that nugget without data obtained first-hand.

With so many thoughts racing through my mind, I did not sleep well that night. A hospital room is a terrible place to recuperate from surgery. Doctors understand this fact and attempt to get their patients home as soon as possible. The nightmares were no longer a problem, but I was still very restless and sore. I wanted to return home, recover and proceed on with my life.

Ted gave me the good news on Saturday that I could go home the following morning. The surgeons were satisfied that I was healing sufficiently well from the surgery. The chest tubes had been removed, and my vital signs were stable. The continuous monitoring had indicated no further instances of arrhythmia. I was able to spend several hours on Saturday in a bedside chair. I had not yet walked more than a few steps in the room, but, at ten on Sunday morning, I was discharged from the hospital.

Seeing our home as we approached on Huntsman Boulevard in Springfield was a total thrill. I was smiling broadly as Sharry helped me into the house. I was incredibly weak, but I could move. It was taxing to walk the short distance from one side of the living room to the other. After a few steps, I was completely winded. But I was **not** in the hospital, and I was **not** dying, and I **did** have new hardware protecting me.

The next three weeks were encouraging. Sharry stayed home from work only the first three days. Although I had considerable difficulty sleeping for over two hours at a time, I could see immediate progress in my overall condition. I forced myself to walk further and further each day. I spent considerable time listening to some very funny audio tapes by Garrison Keillor. Several times I had to turn off the tapes because I was laughing so hard that my incisions hurt. I soon learned to hold a pillow in my lap as I listened to the tapes so that I could clutch it firmly against my midsection whenever I began to double over in laughter. After one really painful laughing episode, Nelle said, "Hey, Dad. Remember how you sometimes say, 'I thought I would bust a gut laughing?' Well, it looks to me like you just might do it!"

Nelle's note of caution was valid, but I had become convinced that laughter was therapeutic for me both mentally and physically. The tapes kept me from lying around feeling sorry for myself, and I believed that the shaking of my stomach muscles was speeding the healing process.

I gained strength with each passing day. On February 19, Sharry drove me to Massimiano's office for an examination of the surgical site. All was well. I was healing fine at both incisions. The following Tuesday we saw Friehling for an appointment at his office. He placed a circular metal device, about the size of a hockey puck, on my stomach directly over the AICD. "I'm using this to interrogate the device," he explained. "It uses radio signals to query the computer in the AICD. The box inside you sends information back to my laptop computer to tell me exactly what has happened to your heart since we turned the defibrillator on two weeks ago. I can even get a printout on this strip of paper."

I watched in amazement as Ted typed instructions on his keyboard. I was lying flat on an examining table while this computer in my stomach was talking to my doctor. They appeared to be having a great conversation, because Ted would periodically mumble, "How about that!"

"Is everything OK?" I asked.

"Sure. No arrhythmias. No incidents. It looks great. I am going to change a few settings, but you're fine."

Ted and Sharry exchanged some pleasantries while I dressed. "He really is a genuinely nice person," Sharry remarked as we reached the car.

"Yes," I replied, "but I wonder what he and the computer were talking about."

I felt well enough to return to work the following Monday. I was able to walk slowly, but without much pain. The first few days back were demanding. I had been away from the classroom for four weeks, and there were numerous administrative details to tend to. Because my sub had done a great job covering the material, none of the classes were too far behind the syllabus. We would be able to catch up rather easily. My students were happy to see me, because, as one of my favorites, Jessica, put it, "The general was a nice guy, Mr. Linz, but we missed you a lot because you tell better jokes." That certainly made me feel like a top notch educator. "Maybe I should go into stand-up comedy," I thought.

Spring passed by rapidly. I continued to regain strength and was able to resume my normal routine at work and at home. I had frequent doctor appointments with Merlino, Matthews and Friehling, but there was no bad news from these visits. April 22 was the last day on which I took Prednisone. Matthews had been slowly weaning me from this steroid. If it had helped to counter or slow the sarcoid (there was no way to determine if it had), its effect would be complete by this time. The consensus among my doctors was that it would be counter-productive to continue further doses of the drug. I was still taking Amiodarone daily. It seemed to be working to prevent arrhythmia, although I was now careful not to overexert myself physically. I had no intention of playing racquetball or running in any 10 K races. Going to the brink once, and living to tell about it, had been enough for me. I was not going to do anything stupid.

In late May, I had a scheduled EP study done by Al Del Negro at Fairfax Hospital. The procedure was conducted on an outpatient basis, and I was home by evening. This time Al was able to use the pacing function of the AICD to override and control the arrhythmia which he induced. Since it now appeared to be of some benefit, he decided to leave it turned on. The advantage was that I might be successfully paced out of v-tach rather than having to endure the painful shock. The really good news was that the computer inside the AICD had indicated that there had been no instances of sustained v-tach during the past two months. Maybe the Amiodarone was working!

At home that evening, Sharry and I had a lengthy discussion concerning our future. We recalled Dr. Matthews' prediction that we might have two years before the sarcoid took me. Now that I had spent one year of that on Life Row, we had only one year remaining. "Maybe a miracle will happen, maybe the Amiodarone will buy us more time, maybe..." We went through many "maybe's" that night. Finally, we decided to use part of our remaining time together, however long, to do something special. After I had brought up a few ideas to consider, Sharry looked at me and said, "How about Alaska?"

I thought that her suggestion was superb. We had not been able to go on our annual visit to Ocean Isle Beach, North Carolina the previous year due to my hospitalization in August. I was reluctant to head to the beach because of the extreme sensitivity to the sun that I had developed from the Amiodarone. Alaska sounded like an intriguing alternative, because I could wear long sleeve outfits and still be comfortable.

Within the next week, we decided to take a cruise from Vancouver, British Columbia to Juneau, Alaska and then spend the next week or so traveling around other parts of Alaska. We scheduled the trip so that Nelle and Emily would be at Camp Varsity during the period in which we were gone from home. Both girls had been to this summer camp in previous years and were in love with it. Nelle was a counselor now, while Emily was just your basic happy camper.

I wrote a letter to Telectronics, the maker of my AICD, to ask what precautions, if any, I should follow at the airport security checkpoint. They replied that I must not pass through the metal detectors (because my device is turned off and on by means of a magnetic field). The preferred method of passing airport security, they said, was to present my laminated card indicating that I had an AICD and to be hand-frisked by security personnel.

Although we were somewhat apprehensive about traveling so far from immediate medical help, we boarded the flight to Vancouver in great spirits. It was now late June, 1992, and we had experienced no sarcoid-related problems since the AICD had been installed in February. After a day touring Vancouver, we boarded the cruise ship, Westerdam, to begin our cruise along the coast of British Columbia to Alaska.

As the ship was pulling away from the pier in Vancouver, I noticed that the Captain did not sound the ship's whistle, which other cruise ships, merchant vessels, and warships routinely use when backing from a pier with an obstructed view. We did not hit anything, but I remarked to Sharry, "If I see the Captain, I'm going to ask him about this." Two nights later, during the Captain's reception, I was introduced to the Captain, a Dutch officer who appeared to be in his mid-50's.

"Captain, I'm Ed Linz. I used to drive submarines around. I am curious why the ship did not sound a prolonged blast as we backed away from the pier in Vancouver. I realize that it is not technically required under the International Rules of the Road, but the other cruise ships seemed to be doing it. Is there some special rule in Vancouver?"

The Captain stared at me as if I had smacked him. Reception lines in cruise ships are all smiles and pleasantries, so I was surprised by his attitude and response. "There's never anything back there anyway," he growled. His glare at the aide on his right seemed to demand, "Get this guy out of here before I kill him." Sharry and I were quickly moved along in the line, so that other passengers might have the opportunity to meet Captain Personality.

Having been on several cruises prior to this Alaskan experience, I was taken aback by the Captain's remarks. Did he have a similarly cavalier attitude toward other aspects of seamanship and navigation? Later that evening, Sharry raised an interesting point, "Aren't we headed into iceberg waters?"

Knowing that this captain might regard the possibility of icebergs with the same "there's never anything there anyway" approach, we completed the remainder of our cruise as unpaid lookouts. I later wrote a letter about this incident to the president of the cruise line, but I received no response. Based upon our experiences during other cruises, we concluded that there are a lot of other ships out there without Captain "What, me worry?" types in command and that we would stick with them for future vacations at sea. In view of my deteriorating medical condition at that time and Dr. Matthew's grim prediction, it now seems rather remarkable that I was still thinking of future cruises. Actually, there were no activities that I was willing to concede to my disease until they became physically impossible. I believe that this defiant attitude was an important aspect of my mental approach to Life Row.

There was a doctor on board Westerdam, so I did not feel totally unprotected if I developed arrhythmia. I am not certain what he could have done other than to send an SOS, but, nonetheless, there was that warm fuzzy feeling knowing that a doctor was "in house."

When we debarked to begin the land portion of our trip through Alaska, this was not the case, but I did not initially worry.

We flew from Juneau to Fairbanks and then took the Alaskan Railroad to Denali Park, the home of Mt. McKinley. Early the next day on a tour bus deep into the park, I suddenly realized that I would be in a rather precarious situation if the AICD started to fire. We saw lots of grizzly bears and moose, but no cardiologists or EP specialists. Apparently, the latter two are not native to the park.

After spending several days in Anchorage (which we both loved), we decided to fly to Kotzebue, a small Eskimo village north of the Arctic Circle, just so we could say that we had been north of the Arctic Circle. This was a big mistake. BIG mistake.

We arrived at the Kotzebue airport in mid-afternoon. Our first indication of trouble was that it was incredibly hot - nearly 90 degrees! Unfortunately we were dressed for 50 degrees. Our accommodations for the evening were at the only lodging in town, a two story Motel 6 type of place. It was sparsely appointed. Of course, there was no air conditioning, but neither were there screens on the windows. By early evening we had recognized the dilemma: either sweat to death in our room, which was at least 100 degrees, or open the window and be invaded by swarms of the largest, most aggressive mosquitoes we had ever encountered.

After considerable debate, we decided to follow Sharry's plan. We stripped off all our clothes and opened the window. As the mosquitoes invaded, one of us sitting at the window smashed the insects as they attempted to enter. The other would be trying to get some sleep on the bed. We did this in two hour shifts through the night. During my shifts at the window I kept thinking about how I should have been worrying about mosquito repellent instead of the AICD when we planned the trip. As we boarded the plane the next day to fly south to Nome, we did not wave a fond farewell to Kotzebue.

The remainder of our Alaskan adventure was very pleasant. At the conclusion we flew from Anchorage to Seattle to rendezvous with my life-long friend, Aaron Spurway. He and his wife, Coco, had driven over from their home in Spokane. I had become friends with Spurway during our first class (senior) year at the Naval Academy in 1965. He was an outrageous, and truly eccentric, character. We spent much of our free time together getting drunk at sleazy bars in and around Annapolis. These "social skills," initially developed following Navy football games and at Officer Clubs while on midshipman summer cruises, were an unfortunate legacy which plagued me for many years following graduation.

By the time we rendezvoused in Seattle, both Spurway and I had long since given up alcohol. Although our initial years following the Academy had been characterized by a succession of alcohol-related adventures and near-disasters, we were both fortunate to survive without permanently injuring ourselves or others. I had been thrown into jail several times, Spurway had been kicked out of the Navy's nuclear program, and his first marriage had failed. Neither of us were proud of our indiscretions, but there was a definite bond which had developed. After our time together in California, our paths diverged. I remained in the Navy and ultimately received command of a submarine. Spurway returned to his roots in the Pacific Northwest, did surveying work in the national forests, and then became a successful newspaper publisher in Spokane.

Throughout our ordeals and occasional triumphs, Spurway and I had corresponded almost daily. He was my best man when Sharry and I married in 1970. Our son, Aaron, born in 1973, was named after him. My last marathon prior to being placed on Life Row had been run with Spurway at my side. Next to Sharry, he was my best friend. It was particularly difficult, therefore, for me to enjoy myself in Seattle with him. I found myself continuously wondering if I would ever have another opportunity to see my best friend. We had been through many challenges together, but our current opponent, sarcoid, seemed to be far ahead at the moment. Neither of us addressed the issue, but as I boarded the plane for our return flight to Virginia, I felt as if it was a final good-bye.

Shortly after arriving home, I had a bi-monthly AICD checkup. When Dr. Friehling finished he said, "There's a lot of apparent arrhythmia on the trace for the last month. There is so much that it is difficult to believe. Have you felt anything funny?"

"No," I replied. "We went to Alaska, but, other than a shortness of breath when I exerted myself, I felt nothing unusual. Does that thing record mosquito bites?"

Ted ignored my sarcasm. "OK. We'll have to watch this. Telectronics has been having some trouble with some of their units. Don't worry. You're still protected. The device will work if you have an event."

We worried, at least initially. Both Sharry and I had the same paranoia. It was as if someone was out to get us: first an unknown, usually fatal, disease hits us, and now the protective device which required open heart surgery to install may be developing a problem. When were we going to receive good news?

We decided to adopt a positive attitude and proceed on with our lives. Things could be far worse. I was still alive, our family was intact and our finances were still sound. If new problems arose, we would confront them at that time. We had learned not to waste our brain cells worrying about things which we could not control.

In late August, I returned to teaching and coaching. I was happy to see both my students and my athletes. By this time the Amiodarone had created such a level of sensitivity to the sun that I had to use sunscreen on exposed portions of my skin whenever I went into sunlight. This was not a problem as I was teaching, but it did necessitate some adjustments to my coaching routine. I began to wear long sleeve shirts and a broad rimmed hat to every cross country practice. The girls on the team knew of my medical situation and were always very cooperative and understanding. I had at least two incidents of apparent arrhythmia in the early fall. During these episodes I "felt funny" and had a pulse in the 120 bpm range for several hours. Since the AICD was set to act only at higher pulse rates, the device did not fire. Whenever I wore a Holter monitor to attempt to record these events, nothing, of course, happened.

The AICD checkup in mid-September was uneventful. The device continued to show what Friehling described as "excessive noise." Because there had been no degradation since July, we decided to do nothing and hope that it did not get worse.

The week of October 19-26, 1992 was not a good one for me. As the school bus carrying our cross country team returned to the West Springfield High School following a meet at another school, I scanned the lot for my car. Not seeing it, I yelled out, "Someone has stolen my Volvo!"

The girls immediately assured me, "No way, Coach. Who would want to steal a Volvo **station wagon**?"

They definitely had a point. Not only was it an unglamorous station wagon, it was an old, unglamorous station wagon.

The girls were wrong. I called Nelle at home and she came immediately to help me search. After looking around the school grounds for nearly an hour, I reported the theft to the police. It was now 6:30 PM. At 7:15 PM, we received a phone call from an excited policeman.

"Mr. Linz, we found your car. It was abandoned over near Hidden Pond. Unfortunately, it's on fire!"

"On fire?!! Are you sure?" I asked.

"It's license number CGL 703 and it's a yellow Volvo wagon. That's your car, isn't it?"

Watching one's car burn is not a pleasant experience. It had been stolen from in front of the school while I was at the meet. The firemen recovered some textbooks left in the back seat by the thieving vandals. Unfortunately, the books were also stolen, and the crime was never solved. We later purchased a van to replace the Volvo, but it was a $15,000 net loss.

The week got worse.

As I was filling a large Igloo cooler with ice water on our front porch before heading to cross country practice on Thursday, I suddenly felt my knees begin to buckle. As I started to collapse to the concrete, I grabbed at the column near the step. Just as my hand touched it, I felt an incredible punch in my chest. Wham! It was as if I had been hit by a railroad tie, end on. The force instantaneously straightened me upright.

I did not immediately realize what had happened. My chest was sore and I was dazed. I stood motionless holding on to the column. I did not know what to expect next. The afternoon was mild, and I noticed that several birds were chirping nearby. Suddenly I understood that I now knew what it feels like to be on the receiving end of an AICD firing.

As I regained composure, I decided to try to reach Friehling or Del Negro to ask what to do now. Fortunately, their assistant, Kim was in the office to take my telephone call. When I told her what I thought had happened, she asked, "Where are you now?"

"At home. I'm OK, I think. I'm lying on the couch."

"Ted's here, but he's with a patient. I know that he will want to talk to you. I'll get him."

After a short pause, Dr. Friehling came on the line, "Tell me what happened."

I explained to him everything that I could remember. I expected him to order me to go to the emergency room immediately.

"Sounds like the device did just what it's supposed to do, Ed. How do you feel now?"

"Fine, I guess. I don't feel any arrhythmia. Everything seems normal now."

"Relax for the next several hours," cautioned Ted. "I don't have to see you. You're safe. The device is working to protect you. That is why you have it. If it fires again in the next 24 hours, call me and then go to the ER. When are you scheduled to see me next?"

"In two or three weeks, I think."

"That's fine. We will check the device then to get a readout. It's been over six months since we installed it, so I doubt that you will have a reoccurrence in the near future. Sooner or later, though, it's going to happen again, and probably when you least expect it. It's doing just what it's supposed to do."

"Thanks, Ted," I said glumly as I slowly put down the phone. Although I was relieved that I did not have to go into the hospital, I suddenly felt very vulnerable. Several questions raced through my mind. What would have happened if I had fallen when the device fired? Would I have hit my head on the concrete? Who would have been there to help me? What might have happened if this had taken place while I was driving?

Not only did I not attempt to answer these questions, I went immediately to my truck to drive to cross country practice at West Springfield. I was worried that no one would be there to tell the girls what to do. The district championship was to be held the following Wednesday, and, in my rather curious thought process, nothing else was more important. (Actually, I suspect that there are many coaches who would understand this reasoning).

I found the team just where they were supposed to be, doing just what they were supposed to be doing. The captains had them stretching in front of the school. Without getting out of my truck, I spoke to two of the runners, Julie Vance and Emily Linnemeier. I told them that "something had come up" and I would be unable to stay with the team that afternoon. I told them where the girls should run. Julie smiled, probably guessing that I had some type of medical problem which I did not care to discuss. I drove directly home and returned to the couch in the family room.

I decided not to tell Sharry until she came home from work. She was upset that I had not telephoned her as soon as the device had fired. Dinner was tense. I think that we all knew that I was headed downhill. The only question was the severity of the slope.

I saw Al Del Negro and Kim Hill for the scheduled AICD checkup on November 10. He confirmed that I had been in v-tach prior to the firing on October 22 and that the device had operated correctly. Unfortunately, the electrical noise in the device had worsened. Because of her concern over the apparent malfunctioning, Kim had contacted the manufacturer. She learned that there was a history of problems with the model which had been implanted in me. Some of the solder joints on the electrical connections inside the box had failed in approximately one percent of the units. Kim showed me a fax which the manufacturer had sent to her. It was actually a form for me to sign indicating that I had been informed of the potential problem. It stated that 7 of 1099 model 4202 devices had failed and that 4 of 520 model 4210 devices had encountered the same type of solder joint failure. The next paragraph was not encouraging:

"Susceptibility to failure arises from possible variations in the welding process. The gas pressure inside the can may vary, and if low, abdominal forces against the can may result in solder joint failure. Also the activity of the patient and the length of time since the implant can play a part in the solder joint failure."

Al explained that I had two options: (1) Continue with the existing device with the current bi-monthly checkup supplemented by the use of a "Guardimate" - a device to be used at home daily to interrogate the defibrillator to see if it was still working, or (2) Replace the AICD with a re-engineered model or a totally different device.

Kim handed me a "Guardimate." It was the approximate size of a Walkman and had a few buttons and lights. "Just place it directly over your AICD each morning, push the button and see if the green light comes on. If it does, it is OK."

"What about the replacement option?" I asked.

Al drew a sketch of the AICD hookup inside my body as he responded, "That might be a problem. We can't be certain that the noise is coming from this known solder problem in the box. There are two other possibilities. The screws which hold the leads onto your heart may be loose, or the connectors between the leads and the box may be the problem. There is no way to determine which of the three possibilities is the culprit without having surgery."

"Another open heart surgery?" I asked.

Dr. Del Negro's face was very grim. "Not necessarily. We would open up the abdominal cavity first to examine the box. If it or the connectors are the problem, we can replace them without further surgery. If they are OK, then, yes, we would have to work on the leads on your heart."

I remained silent for at least a minute while I pondered the options.

"Al, are you sure that I am safe now? Is the device still protecting me?" I asked.

"Currently, yes. In the future, I don't know. It's a difficult situation."

I noticed that I was beginning to sweat. I did not want to be in this high stakes poker game. The card playing analogy influenced my answer, "I'm going to stay with this hand for now. I'll use the Guardimate and see what happens. I need to talk this over with Sharry. We haven't rushed into any major decision so far. I'll get back to you if we decide to do the surgery."

Kim demonstrated how to use the Guardimate. The green light flashed on indicating that all was well with my AICD, at least for the moment.

Dinner that evening was not a joyous event. We discussed the options, but kept returning to our bad luck. 1 out of 100 units had this solder problem. We were apparently the 1. Sharry concurred with my view that we should not have the surgery now, but it was obvious that she was under no illusions about the long term. Sooner or later, we were going to have to face the issue again.

My blood pressure had been rising steadily over the past several months. Dr. Merlino was closely following the problem. I had been on Dyazide, but it was not achieving as much of a reduction as hoped for. On November 20, she stopped the Dyazide and had me begin a different type of blood pressure medication, an "ace inhibitor" two days later. The second day after beginning the new drug, I began to develop severe stomach cramps, but I did not tell anyone because we were scheduled to go to the beach in North Carolina for our annual Thanksgiving day family reunion with Sharry's four sisters and their families. This decision to grin and bear it was stupid, but I had a fairly consistent track record in that regard.

I was miserable the entire time at the beach. I had difficulty walking along the ocean, and I spent most of the time sitting or lying down. Although I ate little, my stomach felt bloated - as if it had been inflated with an air pump. As soon as we returned home, Sharry insisted that I call Merlino's answering service to tell her that I was having problems.

I saw Merlino after school on both Monday and Wednesday. She immediately stopped the ace inhibitor and placed me on a different blood pressure medication, Capoten. By this time my legs were also starting to swell. "Ed, you have all the classic symptoms of right-side heart failure. The sarcoid has obviously progressed to the point where the heart is simply not pumping well. You are having a consistent fluid build-up in your extremities. We need to put you on a diuretic to help eliminate those fluids. I'm going to start you on Lasix twice a day. It will diminish the fluid retention."

"Failure? What do you mean by failure?" I asked in an incredulous tone.

"It's a technical term. We have known for over a year that the right side of your heart is enlarged. It is now obviously not functioning as it should. Blood is flowing, but the rate and pressure are inappropriate. This causes a buildup of fluid in cells throughout your body. That's why you felt bloated and why your legs are swollen. This is called edema. I cannot give you anything to help the underlying condition. The heart failure is here to stay. What we can do is to help your body to remove the excess fluids. That is what the Lasix will do."

By the end of the week I felt much better. What Robin did not tell me was just how well Lasix did work. After taking the pill at 7 AM, within 45 minutes, I had an unbelievable urge to urinate. Then, at almost exactly one hour intervals for the remainder of the morning, I would find myself dancing on my toes with the same problem. Fortunately, my classes were only 45 minutes long. I soon learned never to put myself in a situation where I could not visit a friendly urinal at short notice. In one of my daily letters to Spurway I wrote, "This is ridiculous. I've never met a urinal that I didn't like." He had the good taste not to comment.

Our Christmas in 1992 was restrained. Our son, Aaron, had come north from Chapel Hill for the holidays, but we all knew that my health was headed south. I was no longer able to exercise due to a shortness of breath, my blood pressure remained high, the AICD was probably going to have to be replaced, and I frequently felt lousy. Still, we managed to count our blessings and thank the Lord for what we did have. Maybe a miracle would happen.

Unfortunately the meter was running on Dr. Matthews' initial prediction concerning my longevity. I was now three-fourths of the way through the time which had been given to me. My initial optimism was being eroded by the reality of my worsening condition. I was no longer able to smile off my illness. It was beginning to seriously affect important parts of my life. I found myself frequently in Kübler-Ross' fourth stage of death and dying: depression. I did not like my situation, but there was little I could do about it as I waited on Life Row. We definitely needed a miracle.

Chapter 9

DOWNHILL

The new year, 1993, began on an ominous note. During my bi-monthly checkup of the AICD with Dr. Friehling, he determined that the electrical noise in the unit had now reached the point where the unit must be replaced. I relayed the news to Sharry, and we decided to go ahead with the surgery at the end of the month when the first semester examinations at school would be over. If complications did arise (for example, the need to have open heart surgery to repair the leads on the heart), it would be a more convenient time for me to be out of school for a month. We conveyed our decision to Friehling and he agreed with our reasoning. He told us that Telectronics now had a new AICD model which was designed to eliminate the solder joint problem. He would be able to obtain one by the end of the month.

I continued to be examined by Dr. Merlino at regular intervals. In addition to taking 300 mg of Amiodarone daily, I was also on 100 mg of Capoten and 60 mg of Lasix. She took frequent blood tests to follow the condition of my liver and kidneys. Some of the liver parameters were outside the normal range, but this was consistent with the right side heart failure.

I went to Fairfax Hospital on the morning of January 28 to go through the required tests prior to the surgery scheduled for the following morning. Before the surgery, I drew a line across my upper stomach region with a black felt tip marker. Below the line, I wrote "OK." Above the line, on my chest, I wrote "NOT OK." I had given Ted and the surgeon, Dr. Albus, a cardiac surgeon, specific instructions. "You can open me up to check out the box and its connectors. You can replace the box if it is the problem. Basically you can do whatever is necessary as long as it does not involve my heart. You do **not** have my permission to do open heart surgery at this time. If you find that it is required, sew me up and then we will talk about it. I am not going through another open heart until we think about it a lot more."

They agreed. Fortunately, the issue became moot. Once my abdomen was opened, Friehling and the Telectronics tech rep quickly determined that the AICD box was the problem. It was replaced rather easily with the new, improved model. I was home the following day with a new device and a very sore mid-section.

I remained at home for one week before returning to work. An EP study of the new unit indicated that it was working well. This device could be programmed to deliver variable energy level shocks in a sequenced manner. Based on results obtained during the EP study, Friehling set the AICD to attempt first to pace me out of the dangerous rhythm, then, if unsuccessful, to implement a shock using a low energy level, then an intermediate level, then maximum. Remembering the incredible bolt delivered by the old unit when it fired back in October, I was happy that technology was marching forward to provide some more palatable options. Still, I was not looking forward to the next shock.

Dr. Merlino continued to try various medications to reduce my blood pressure, which remained higher than desired. She directed me to discontinue Capoten and to start taking 20 mg/daily of Zestril (Lisinopril). We achieved slightly better results with this approach, but the high blood pressure was a continuing problem.

The next month, March 1993, I was feeling sufficiently well to take our older daughter, Nelle, on a brief trip to England to see her roots. It was a spur of the moment thing. I had seen an advertisement for a very low air fare to London. Without asking Sharry or Nelle, I purchased two tickets and arranged for a rental car at Heathrow airport. I knew that Sharry would successfully talk me out of such risky business if I sought her approval, so I decided to go with the non-refundable ticket ploy. There was some heated discussion, but Nelle and I left the U.S. on March 11.

We had a great time in Britain. Nelle was born in Oxford eighteen years earlier during my studies at Christ Church College, so our visit was a homecoming, of sorts. Although Nelle did not remember our small duplex in the Summertown section where we were living at the time of her birth, she enjoyed hearing me recount for her the stories of our life in Oxford during the mid-1970's. Her delivery in a "birthing room" at the Radcliffe Hospital was attended by a student midwife and myself. We used the LaMaze techniques which Sharry and I had learned in anticipation of Aaron's birth a year and a half earlier. (Unfortunately I had been at sea during his birth and Sharry had to enlist a friend to be my surrogate). As we walked through the small villages outside of Oxford, I told Nelle my memories of her and Aaron riding side-by-side in a double stroller as Sharry made her daily visits to the fishmonger, butcher, bank and greengrocer's.

"I notice that there seems to be a betting shop in each of these towns," remarked Nelle.

"The British seem to like to bet on everything," I replied, wondering what odds they might post on my chances of living beyond the two years predicted by Matthews. "I remember going into one of those places only once while we were here. I bet five pounds that Miss Germany would win the Miss Universe contest that year."

"Did you win?"

"She wasn't even fourth runner-up."

I changed the subject to tell her about my studies. Since Nelle was about to head off to Indiana University in the fall, I thought that she might like to hear about the British system of higher education.

"I really liked it here. It was as if I were on an intellectual sabbatical. I would go to school for eight weeks, have the next six weeks off, then eight more weeks of studies, six weeks off, then a final eight weeks in school before a 16 week summer break. We always traveled. You don't remember it, but we spent one summer in Bavaria in Germany studying German and another camping our way through Scandinavia."

"Cool! I wish that I could do that."

"It was not as easy as it sounds," I cautioned. "The studies were based on the tutorial system which is centered around a 'don.' I went to some lectures and participated in some seminars, but most of the learning comes from your interaction with the don."

"What's a don?"

"A professor who has his offices in one of the colleges which make up the university. He assigns the student a topic, like, 'The British are primarily responsible for the problems in the Sudan.'

Then he would give me a list of books and journal articles to read. I would then go to the Bodleian Library to read as much as possible over the next two days. On the third day I would 'go to press.' That is, I would hand write about 20 pages either pro or con - it didn't matter which - and then take it in to read to him the following week. I could spend only three days on each of these papers because I usually had to do two a week. After I read the paper to him, he would then grill me for the remainder of the hour making me justify my conclusions. By the end of the eight weeks, I had pulled a lot of all-nighters and was exhausted. It wasn't that easy. Fortunately you and Aaron were great babies. Basically we had a great time here."

"Didn't President Clinton, go to Oxford too?" asked Nelle.

"Yeah, he was a Rhodes Scholar, but he never finished his studies. He didn't get his degree. Maybe he got distracted. I don't know. No one seems to ever raise the issue with him. I saw several young Americans when I was here that had other priorities than studying. I hope that he does a better job as President than he did here and ..."

"He invites us to the White House!" interrupted Nelle.

"Fat chance," I muttered as I changed the subject. I was silently hoping that I would live long enough to vote against him if he did not invite us. Thoughts about just how long I was going to live were becoming not only more frequent, but also less rational. "Am I turning into a bitter, old man?" I wondered to myself.

Throughout our trip, Nelle did all of the driving. Apparently driving on the left side comes naturally to someone born in England. We stayed at bed and breakfasts and ate most of our other meals in pubs. She carried our suitcases and was very protective. I felt at times as if we had reversed parent-child roles. She kept asking me, "Are you OK?" In Oxford I had some difficulty in walking from college to college (there are over 30 in the university) due to my worsening condition. I was intensely aware of my disability because I kept thinking of the ease with which I had traversed these short distances just 16 years earlier during my student days in these same streets. When we toured Warwick Castle, I had to sit frequently to catch my breath. I was unable to climb the stairs to the top of the castle walls. I realized that the sarcoid was winning.

The remainder of the spring of 1993 was relatively uneventful. My medical condition continued to slowly degrade, but it was nearly imperceptible to those around me on a daily basis. Although I could now walk up only one flight of stairs until I had to stop to get my breath, I learned to adjust. We had two healthy teenagers at home to mow the lawn and to do other physically oriented chores. Nelle became very good at changing the oil in all of our cars, and Emily learned to split wood (although she did not like it!). In retrospect, this forced labor may have been a blessing for both of the girls, because they learned several skills to bolster their confidence for "the real world."

Late in the spring, I became suspicious that the replacement cost of my new AICD had not been covered under the two year warranty of the original unit. We had sent a copy of the warranty to both the hospital and Blue Cross/Blue Shield immediately after the surgery in February. Since we had heard nothing from anyone on the subject, I decided to investigate. When I telephoned Fairfax Hospital, a clerk said that she would "look into it." As I suspected at the time of her promise, we never heard from this clerk again. Two weeks later we received a statement from Blue Cross informing us that they had paid over $23,000 to Fairfax Hospital for the AICD. Sensing that Blue Cross had been ripped off, I called Telectronics to ask why they had not stood by their warranty on the AICD. A very pleasant person at the firm informed me that he had mailed a check several weeks ago to Fairfax Hospital for "23-something." I then called Fairfax back to check out their version. A voice, identified only as Sally, answered.

"Telectronics tells me that they have sent you a check to cover the cost of the new AICD which was implanted in me on January 29th. Can you please check your records to see if this money has arrived?" I asked.

After being placed on hold for at least 10 minutes, Sally told me that the check had been received.

"But I have a statement indicating that Blue Cross/Blue Shield has also sent you money for the same unit."

There was a long pause and then the confession, "That's right. They did. We got it about two weeks ago."

"It sounds to me as if you have been paid twice."

"Well, that's one way to look at it."

"Why haven't you returned the check to Blue Cross/Blue Shield?" I asked incredulously.

"They haven't asked us for it," came the reply.

"But they don't know about the other money that Telectronics has sent to you."

"What's your point?" asked Sally. Her tone indicated that she was becoming impatient.

I took a deep breath. "The point is that you have been paid twenty three thousand dollars twice for the same AICD. That's a problem. What are **you** going to do about it?"

"I told you," Sally retorted. "**We're** not doing anything unless Blue Cross/Blue Shield asks us for it."

Sensing that the conversation had become circular, I concluded the call, "Thanks. I'll see what Blue Cross wants to do with this."

I immediately dialed Blue Cross/Blue Shield of Virginia at their toll free number in Richmond. Incredibly, this conversation went no better than the last.

After being shuffled from one clerk to another through several iterations, I was finally connected to a woman who acted as if she had lost the draw and had to take my call. I explained the two check, double payment situation as slowly and carefully as possible.

"So what do you want me to do?" was her response.

"You could begin by contacting Fairfax Hospital to check this out. There is twenty three thousand dollars of your money involved."

"That's not how we do it," she explained. "We are not allowed to ask them about stuff like this."

"Wait a minute," I yelled. "Are you telling me that, even though you now know that Fairfax Hospital is stealing over twenty thousand dollars from your company, you are not going to do anything about this?"

"Look, if this is so important to you, why don't you write us a letter telling us all about it? Maybe we can look at it then."

"Before I hang up, let me make sure that I have this correct." I was speaking very slowly. "I've told you how you can get twenty three thousand dollars back for your company which was paid incorrectly for a piece of medical equipment which was covered by a manufacturer's warranty. And you're telling me that I have to write you a letter. I don't think so. Maybe this is why you guys have to keep raising your rates all the time. You are giving away all our money!"

I hung up in disgust.

I called Sharry at the Health Department to share my morning telephone conversations with her. From her tone alone, I knew that someone at Blue Cross/Blue Shield was about to have a very bad day.

That evening Sharry received three calls at home from various levels of Blue Cross/Blue Shield of Virginia management hierarchy. Judging from Sharry's responses, each caller was begging her understanding and forgiveness. "It had all been a terrible mistake, please forgive us, I have no idea how this could happen, thank you for your interest, please forgive us, we are reviewing all of our internal procedures, please forgive us, blah, blah blah..." was the general theme.

"Just what did you say to them today after I spoke with you?" I asked.

Sharry smiled, "I spoke with a few people down there. I told them that if they didn't have this straightened out by tomorrow morning I was going to call a friend at the *Washington Post* and see if she was interested in how Blue Cross of Virginia is in collusion with Fairfax Hospital to steal the public's money. I yelled a little."

Knowing Sharry's temper, I winced in sympathy for the poor souls who had been on the receiving end of her calls.

The following day, we received several additional phone messages from various management levels of both Blue Cross and Fairfax Hospital. The debate on a national health care plan was a hot topic in the Washington, D.C. area and no health provider organization wanted to be in an expose on the front page of the *Post* or any other newspaper.

I am convinced that neither the hospital nor the insurance company was actively attempting to steal or give away the $23,000. Both, however, are massive bureaucracies with many employees who recognize no connection between their daily work and the corporate well-being. It is not their personal money, so why worry?

During May of 1993, I took two field trips with my physics students. The first was to Virginia Power's nuclear electrical generating plant on Lake Anna, which is a two hour school bus ride from the high school. I had conducted this trip for several years, so that my Advanced Placement physics students could see a practical application of the theoretical material which we had been studying. Now, because of the effects of the Lasix which I was taking, I had to schedule a pitstop enroute so that I could relieve myself.

During our trip to Lake Anna the previous spring, I had learned that anything over one hour in a bouncing school bus puts the average Lasix taker in an incredible zone of pain. This Lasix lesson was dramatically reinforced later that fall. I was driving by myself to a cross country meet north of Baltimore when the effects of the diuretic suddenly "kicked in." There were four cars of cross country runners and their parents following me as we drove north on the Baltimore-Washington Parkway. As I continued to look for **any** pit stop, the pain in my groin began to become unbearable. I yearned to urinate - anywhere, anyhow!! Because of the manner in which the Parkway had been constructed, there were no restroom facilities or even any convenient places to pull over and run to the woods. I decided to empty the remaining apple juice from a bottle which I had been drinking and to use the bottle as an emergency urinal. This was a bad idea. After determining that I had to pull my pants down in order to have a clear shot at the bottle, I paused at the thought of being pulled over for exposing myself. This concern was only fleeting, because, by then, I was almost in tears from pain. While driving 50 miles per hour, I wriggled free of the top of my pants, and fired away. It felt wonderful, until I noticed the unmistakably warm and wet sensation of urine all over my lower extremities. I had missed the bottle.

The lesson from these experiences was that I could not allow myself to be far from restroom facilities at any time, particularly in the morning immediately after I had taken the Lasix. So we now visited a friendly McDonalds going and coming from Lake Anna. One of the students yelled from the back of the school bus, "Mr. Linz, why are we stopping so soon?" I did not answer as I ran from the bus to the restroom.

Our other annual class trip was to Busch Gardens, a theme park in Williamsburg, for Physics Day. Although the stated purpose of this outing was to participate in various physics-related activities on the roller coasters and other thrill rides, I made no secret of the fact that we were there to enjoy ourselves. The students brought home-made accelerometers, and I provided stop watches to gather data. Because it was now difficult for me to walk the hills in the park, I planned my day so that I could take the train and the gondola from one sector of the park to another. I did make one colossal error in judgment when I foolishly went on a roller coaster. Everything was fine until the bottom of the first hill. As the car in which I was riding followed the tracks and started up the second hill, my AICD felt as if it was going to continue downwards to China. I felt particularly stupid as I realized that I was trying to violate Newton's First Law of Motion. I did not have much time to reflect on the irony of this, because we soon entered a loop-de-loop, followed by a series of sharp turns. This was **not** a ride for a passenger to have a free floating metal box inside of him. But I survived, and it did make a great discussion point in class the next day.

Following Nelle's graduation from high school in June, we drove to the midwest to see her new home at Indiana University. When we returned, the east coast was in a very intense heat wave. I had been elected to take our dog, Sydney, to obedience school classes each Tuesday evening so that she might develop improved manners. Sydney was less than a year old, and was rather "headstrong." Obedience school would be the cure, or so we thought.

The lady who taught the class was rather headstrong herself - in fact, she would have made a wonderful drill sergeant. Although it was an early evening class, the temperature was still over 100 degrees. The humidity was suffocating. After putting us through one hour of rigorous training in a field just outside the same South Run Recreation Center where I had almost died during the racquetball adventure, our not-so-friendly instructor lined Sydney and me up with our fellow students to receive a dog biscuit, presumably for the dog. Just as she handed me the biscuit to give to Sydney, my AICD fired. I doubled over in shock and yelled, "Wow!!"

As I tried to straighten up, I noticed that the instructor had a very perplexed look on her face. Was I some type of weirdo? After a brief pause, she asked, "Are you OK?"

"No. I am **not** OK. I am going to sit down for a few minutes. Can you take the dog?" Without waiting for a reply, I handed her Sydney's leash and went immediately to the shade. She followed me. After regaining my composure, I explained what had happened. The expression on her face seemed to say, "Buddy, I don't know who you are and I don't like your dog, but you had better not die on me." I am certain that a fatality, dog or master, would have involved a lot of paperwork for her. Once the lady sensed that I was going to live, her interest evaporated. She left, and I was alone with Sydney.

I remained sitting for the next twenty minutes until I was certain that I was able to drive home. I found my pulse on my wrist. It was steady at 76. When I arrived home, I telephoned Friehling's answering service to ask that he call me. Within 10 minutes, Ted was on the phone.

"I would not recommend strenuous exercise, Ed, in this heat and humidity. You just cannot do this type of stuff anymore. Cool it, or the device is going to fire again. You can still do moderate exercise. In fact, I want you to. But don't overdo it. When do I see you next?"

"In two weeks, I think."

"Fine. Call me right away if it fires again. And get Sharry or someone else to take the dog to obedience school."

I thanked Ted and then reflected on my condition. Things could be much worse. I was now past the two year estimate which Dr. Matthews had given me to live. I was still able to teach and coach, although with some adjustments in each. I was able to drive and enjoy a relatively normal lifestyle. In the 18 months since the AICD had been installed, it had fired only twice. Things could be **much** worse.

Throughout the fall of that year, my stamina continued to decline. At cross country meets, I now had to watch the races from one or two locations rather than the four or five that I had previously been able to run between as the races developed. As I grasped the reality that this would probably be my last year of coaching, I became very depressed. In the classroom, I was forced to develop a teaching style which required less movement and more sitting. At home, Emily and Sharry began to do more and more for me. I was slowing becoming an invalid. Stairs were now a major challenge. Although I could walk a few steps at a time, I now had to stop for almost a minute to regain my breath before continuing. I was fully aware of what was now happening on Life Row, and I was frightened.

I was also having more frequent appointments with Dr. Merlino. She was following my blood tests closely because of her concern over the long term effects of Amiodarone on my liver, lungs and kidneys. Some test results were slightly out of specification, but, surprisingly, there were no serious outliers. The heart remained the major problem. The last echocardiogram had shown that the right side was continuing to enlarge. How much longer it would last as an effective pump was unclear.

On Monday, February 7, 1994, I felt terrible at school. I was completely exhausted by the end of classes at 2 PM. I decided to drive directly to Merlino's office, which was about 45 minutes away. I had a scheduled appointment the following day, but I needed immediate help. As soon as I entered the doctor's office, Donna, the receptionist, took one look at me and said, "I think that Dr. Merlino will see you right away."

Robin's first words to me were, "Ed, you look terrible. Let me check your vitals."

Dr. Merlino was now looking very pregnant. She was expecting twins in July. I felt sorry that she was having to work so much during the final months of her pregnancy. I asked, "Robin, how are you feeling? Are you taking any time off?"

She did not answer my questions. "Your pulse is under 50. You are in complete heart block. How did you manage to get here?"

"I drove. What's 'complete heart block'?"

"The heart's natural pacemaker is not working properly. The normal conduction path is blocked. The sarcoid has probably affected it. This is not a surprise. Do you know if your AICD has a pacemaker in it?"

"The way I understand it, the unit has two pacing functions," I replied. "One is set to protect me in the event of tachycardia. I forget exactly where it is set at now, but somewhere around 130. If my heart rate goes above that, it energizes at a slightly higher rate to try to gain control so that it can pace me back down to a normal sinus rhythm. That way I don't get shocked right away, if the pacemaker function can handle the problem. But there is also a pacemaker function on the lower end. I don't think that it is turned on. Its use shortens battery life of the AICD, and I haven't needed it up to this point, so Ted has left it turned off."

"Well, you may need it now. I'm going to take an EKG and call Friehling's office for advice. They will know just what kind of hardware you really have."

Dr. Merlino ran the EKG herself. I sensed that she did not want to leave me. As I dressed, she telephoned Friehling's office.

"Ted is on his way out of town to attend some conference. His receptionist said that if you can get to his office in five minutes, he will still be there. He is flying out of Dulles. Do you think that you can get over there by yourself?"

"Sure," I said. "His office is just three blocks away. I made it here from school in heart block. I can drive there in heart block. I can be there in a few minutes."

"Take this EKG printout with you. And tell his receptionist to call me when you arrive so that I know that you made it OK."

"Thanks, Robin. Take care of those twins."

I was at Friehling's office within ten minutes. It took me longer than I anticipated because I could walk only very slowly to and from my truck. I felt exhausted when I reached the door to his office.

"Go directly to the examining room," the receptionist ordered. Merlino had obviously called ahead.

Although Dr. Friehling was supposed to be on an airplane leaving for Dallas in just over an hour, he was the picture of calm. Kim Hill was with him, and, as usual, they worked together quickly and effectively. As Kim placed the radio transmitter over the AICD, Ted started typing on the laptop. In less than a minute, he said, "There. It's on now. I have it set at 80 beats a minute. You should feel better shortly."

In fact, I felt better instantly. I sat up, stretched my arms above my head, and said, "Thanks, Ted. Now what?"

"We need to insert a pacemaker in you. This one in the AICD is very primitive. It paces you at a set rate and it eats up the battery for the other AICD functions. However, it will protect you until we can put a separate pacemaker in sometime next week. We can get one of those new ones, can't we, Kim?"

"I'm sure we can. I'll take care of it. You need to get to the airport. All of your papers for the conference are in your car. Call me on the way to the airport if you need me to Fed-Ex anything else to you in Dallas. Now get going so that you don't miss your plane. I will finish up with Ed."

Less than ten minutes later, I was driving home. I felt fine. I had been repaired by a laptop!

Sharry was not elated by my news when she arrived home. I had called her on the car phone during the short trip from Merlino's to Friehling's office to tell her that I was in heart block and would keep her updated after my visit with Friehling. Unfortunately, I forgot to do so. She had spent the next hour and a half worrying about me. She finally called Friehling's office, but they had closed at five. "Is he in the emergency room again?" she wondered. No, I had stopped at a 7-11 to get a Slurpee.

The pacemaker was implanted by Dr. Del Negro on February 17, 1994. It was a straightforward procedure performed in the EP lab at Fairfax Hospital. I was placed under local anesthesia while Al made an incision just below my left collarbone. He then inserted two screw-in, transvenous pacing leads into my heart through the subclavian vein using the fluoroscope to achieve accurate placement. One lead was screwed into the wall of the right atrium, the other was positioned in the right ventricle.

Al then tested the leads for electrical continuity before connecting them to the pacemaker, a Synchrony III rate-modulated, dual chamber, manufactured by Siemens, Inc. It was a totally state-of-the-art device about the size of a book of matches. Just like the AICD, the electronics are enclosed in a hermetically sealed, bio-compatible titanium case to guard against adverse reaction with the body. The tech manual for the pacemaker bragged that the same case also serves to block the intrusion of "body fluids" and to reduce the level of outside electromagnetic interference (emf) which could interfere with pacemaker operation.

Dr. Del Negro created a subcutaneous pocket in the fleshy area beneath my left collarbone. After testing the device and checking the leads to the pacemaker, he stitched it into position and closed the incision. In addition to being fully programmable with bi-directional telemetry, my new hardware contained a small piezo-electric crystal designed to sense my level of activity and adjust the pacing accordingly. As opposed to first generation pacemakers which could deliver only a set pulse rate, this high-tech model had all the latest bells and whistles. If I started to walk, the "pizza" crystal (as Emily called it) would sense the motion and increase the pulsing signal. When I lay asleep, it would return to a low rate. It could do nothing to help in the event of tachycardia - that was still the responsibility of the AICD.

As I was being taken to a recovery room following the pacemaker implantation procedure, the manufacturer's rep handed me an 82 page tech manual on the device. He was sincere, but I could not help thinking, "As if this is going to help me if this sucker goes bad? I am at the mercy of God and his electrons!"

I was out of the EP lab by noon and home the same evening. I now had two metal encased computer systems inside my body keeping me alive. "What next?" I thought.

Chapter 10

THE CRASH

As the spring of 1994 brought new life to the flowers, grass and trees in Northern Virginia, I began to accept the fact that I was slowly, but surely, dying. The sarcoidosis was an unrelenting foe. Each card which we had played to counter its latest thrust was only a delaying action. The drugs and the devices inside me were stop-gap measures to slow the inevitable. There were no other defensive measures available. I would have to play the hand which was dealt me.

My realization that I was approaching the end of Life Row did not send me into a state of constant melancholy or bitterness. By now I had rationalized my condition and was mentally prepared for the conclusion. I had slipped quietly into Kübler-Ross' fifth, and final, stage of death and dying, acceptance.

My daily routine did not change. I continued to teach at Woodbridge High School. I did make adjustments when necessary if I found myself in a situation requiring more physical stamina than I possessed. Most of those around me, except Sharry and Emily, probably did not notice a change. We made plans for a family vacation at the beach in North Carolina during the first week in August and a short get-away for Sharry and me at a bed and breakfast in Michigan near the end of June. We were not planning on trouble.

I was continuing to see Merlino, Matthews and Friehling on a regular basis. Friehling and his group concentrated on my arrhythmia problem and the operation of the AICD and the pacemaker. Matthews restricted his observations to cardiac problems other than the rhythm disturbances, and Merlino looked after everything else. It was a nice division of labor. During one of my visits with Matthews following the pacemaker implantation, he said, "Ed, I want you to get a mugga."

"What's a mugga?" I asked, wondering if I could get one free on some dark alley in D.C..

"It is a test to measure how much your heart is pumping each stroke. It's official name is 'multi-gated acquisition study' and it is abbreviated MUGA. That's why it is called 'mug-ga.' Actually it will be a resting MUGA."

"Where do I get this mugga? And what all is involved?"

"You can have it done at Fairfax Hospital. It is a nuclear test. A technician down in Nuclear Medicine will inject about 3 cc of sodium pyrophosphate into your blood stream to tag the red blood cells. By 'tag' I mean 'bond.' Then you will wait, maybe 20 minutes or so, for this process to take place. The technician will then inject a small amount, 25 millicuries, I believe, of a radioactive isotope into your blood. It attaches itself to the sodium pyrophosphate. You will then be placed on a table so that a machine can measure the radiation from the isotope in your blood as it passes through your heart. A computer analyzes the results and computes a number which reflects the percentage of blood being pumped out of your left ventricle compared to the total volume in it. For a normal heart the percentage is 45 to 65 percent. I need to know what yours is now. It will undoubtedly be lower. It is a good way to follow the pumping effectiveness of your heart. This will give us a baseline to determine quantitatively how much the sarcoid is affecting you."

I interrupted, "What isotope is this? How long of a half life does it have? I assume that it is a gamma emitter, isn't it?"

By now, Dr. Matthews had become accustomed to my physics teacher questions. He smiled as he patiently answered, "It's technetium-99. It is one of those artificially-made isotopes used in medicine. I don't know its half life, off hand - ask them when you have the test. It's a gamma emitter - most of them are, because the radiation has to pass through the tissue of your body to the detector, and betas and alphas can't make it that far."

I nodded as he continued, "There is some other useful information which we can get from the mugga, such as a check of the wall motion of your heart, but the ejection fraction is our main concern. The whole thing will take about two hours."

Dr. Matthews' estimate was a good one. When I received the MUGA the following week, I learned that the half life of the isotope was 6 hours. I once again took the opportunity to get my physics classes involved. The following morning at school during first period I went to the teacher's restroom to obtain a urine sample in a beaker. As I was racing back to my classroom with the sample, I literally bumped into the principal, Pam White, as I rounded a corner. Somehow or other, I managed not to spill the radioactive urine on her, or the floor.

"My God, Ed! What is that?" she reacted.

"It's hot pee. We're counting it in class today to determine its half life. Want to watch?"

Pam had the good taste not to ask anything else. "Uh, no thanks. I think that I'll pass on this one. Let me know how it turns out."

Upon my return to the classroom, we used a Geiger counter to measure the number of counts per minute of gamma radiation being given off by the isotope in the urine sample. Although nearly 24 hours had passed since I had been injected with the technetium, the count rate was still high. The students recorded the count and the time of day. As the day progressed, each class took a reading of the same sample. By the end of the day, we had gathered nearly 8 hours of data. The following day we measured the sample again in each class and then calculated the actual half life. The students were surprised by the consistency of the results and how closely their answers for the half life came to the stated value of 6 hours. Surprisingly, no one seemed to be offended by our lesson involving my urine, but we were, by then, nearly 3/4 through the school year. My students (and presumably their parents) were accustomed to strange happenings in Mr. Linz' physics class. I was hoping that someone would call Pam White to complain, so that she could respond, "What are **you** so upset about? He nearly spilled the stuff all over me."

When I saw Dr. Matthews for an appointment in mid-March, he had the MUGA results. "Your ejection fraction was 38 percent. That's less than the normal range, but not as bad as I expected. Things could be a lot worse. How are you feeling?"

"Not so hot. I get winded quite easily now. I have to stop to get my breath frequently whenever I go up stairs. I also can't walk very fast. The good news, I guess, is that the AICD has not fired since last summer. I certainly don't need that."

"Your breathing is probably not going to get any better, Ed. The pulmonary function tests which you have had indicate declining capacity, but the real problem is your heart. I would be lying to say that things are improving."

I knew exactly what Matthews meant. I think that both of us were recalling his estimate three years earlier that I might have just two years to live. We both understood that I was now on borrowed time.

Merlino continued to monitor the condition of my liver and kidneys through frequent blood tests. The results indicated that all was not well with my liver. Because three of the parameters were out of the normal range, Merlino ordered an ultrasound test of the liver. The test was conducted in much the same manner as the echocardiograms which I had received at routine intervals since 1991 - a sonic probe rubbed over the skin in the area of the target organ. Nothing unusual was noted. We knew that the combined effects of the Amiodarone and the right heart failure were creating increasing damage to the liver, but nothing could be done.

May brought the annual Busch Gardens Physics Fair field trip and the Advanced Placement physics test for my seniors. The school year was almost over. I was looking forward to our planned family trips.

Aunt Jean and Uncle Tony arrived for a visit on Memorial Day. They were in the final stages of a cross country vacation from their home in Arizona. I was happy to see them. I had an appointment with Merlino on that Friday morning, so I took off work for the day so that I could give Jean and Tony a quickie tour of Washington after seeing Robin. All had been reasonably well at 9 AM during my doctor's appointment. Shortly after we arrived in D.C., however, I began to feel very tired. We drove around the Capitol area and then parked in the Union Station lot for a walking tour of the revitalized train station and its shops. By noon, I was feeling exhausted. I apologized to my aunt and uncle for cutting the tour short, but I had to get home. I was not certain that I could drive home safely. I said nothing about just how ill I felt to Jean and Tony.

I did not mention my problem to Sharry that evening, because I had promised Aunt Jean that I would take her to Annapolis to see the Naval Academy the next day. I knew that if I told Sharry how terrible I felt she would insist that I see a doctor immediately.

The trip to Annapolis was a nightmare. I could barely walk. I felt as if I would not be able to drive the 50 miles back to Springfield. My chest hurt, I was out of breath, and I wanted to be in bed.

As soon as I walked in the door at home, I told Sharry what had happened. We telephoned Friehling's answering service, but both he and Del Negro were not on call. We soon received a return phone call from a doctor who was covering for them that weekend. He was not familiar with my history, and the sound of his voice suggested that he was young. After I explained what had happened during the past two days and how I was now feeling, he said, "Sounds like you're probably in 'a-fib,' that's atrial fibrillation. It's not that bad if you can still get around OK. Go to Friehing's office first thing Monday morning and have them take a look at you."

"Monday morning?" Sharry yelled, when I explained this new doctor's advice. "I'm calling Dr. Merlino. I think that someone needs to see you **now**."

I did not protest. I was hurting.

Sharry telephoned Merlino's answering service immediately. Although it was now nearly 7 PM on a Saturday evening, Robin returned our call within ten minutes.

"What's up, Ed?" she asked.

"I'm feeling real bad, Robin. My pulse is all over the place. It is really erratic. We just talked to some new arrhythmia doctor who is covering for Dr. Friehling this weekend. He thinks that it is a-fib. He wants me to wait until Monday to see someone."

"No way!" exclaimed Merlino. "We need to be real conservative on this, Ed. Go to the E.R. now. He can't tell over the phone whether you are in a-fib or anything else. I'm not an arrhythmia specialist, but the only way to know for sure what is happening is an EKG. I will call ahead to the E.R. to let them know that you are coming so that you don't have to wait there forever to be seen. And make sure that Sharry drives."

As I thanked Robin, I thought, "Merlino to the rescue again!" Sharry was frightened, but relieved that Dr. Merlino had been available to provide a second opinion. Jean and Tony did not seem too alarmed - they had both had their own share of heart problems. Emily fixed dinner for them after we rushed out of the house to the emergency room.

Merlino's call had greased the skids in the E.R. Upon our arrival, one of the emergency room doctors examined me immediately and took an EKG. He looked at it closely and mumbled, "I'm not sure. Could be a-fib. I'm going to fax this thing to the arrhythmia guy on call so that he can check it out. Since you have that AICD and all that other stuff in you, I would prefer that he decide what to do."

Sharry and I waited in the examining room where the EKG had been conducted. I continued to feel terrible. We held hands and worried together.

In about an hour the arrhythmia doctor who had spoken to me on the phone arrived. He was relatively young, and his mood suggested that he was not a happy camper. We had obviously ruined his Saturday evening. I think that he was also angry that Merlino had overruled his advice to wait until Monday.

"Well," he confessed in a totally non-apologetic, and even condescending tone, "It turns out you're not in a-fib. It's v-tach, but at a low rate."

"How low?" asked Sharry immediately.

The doctor gave me the "And who is she?" look.

"I forgot to introduce you to my wife, Doctor. That's Sharon. She's a registered nurse."

Without turning to look at Sharry, the doctor stuck his hand over his shoulder and moved it up and down as if he were shaking her hand. Sharry and I looked at each other in dismay. This guy was not earning our confidence. Within the past three hours, he had given me a mis-diagnosis over the telephone, acted as if he was doing us a favor by coming to the hospital, and now offended us with his mannerisms.

"Your heart is in ventricular tachycardia at about 120 beats a minute. Your AICD is set too high to do anything about this. It doesn't sense that anything is wrong. Apparently your condition has changed. You are now going into v-tach at a much lower rate than before. I think that I can fix it right here."

To his credit, the doctor had brought the correct laptop device to interrogate and control my AICD (there are several different types and each has its own interrogation device). Within five minutes he successfully used the laptop to pace me out of the v-tach. Almost immediately, I felt fine.

"I'm going to lower the threshold settings on the AICD so that it will pace you or shock you at a lower level to keep this from happening again. I will set it to pace you at 110 and then to shock you if it gets to 120. I don't think that you need to be admitted to the hospital tonight."

"That sounds fine to me. I feel much better now. I will take it easy for the next several days. Thanks for coming in to help us."

Sharry and I left the E.R. around midnight. We stopped on the way home at a diner to eat the dinner which we had skipped. We talked continuously about everything except my medical condition, as if somehow we might fix the problem by ignoring it.

Jean and Tony left the following morning for their return trip to Arizona. I went to church, but did little else for the remainder of the day. I wanted to be able to go to school the next morning, because it was "egg drop day."

Near the end of each school year, I give the students an assignment of designing and constructing an "egg delivery vehicle." This project is an old standby for physics teachers. It has been around for years. I chose to use it as a method of raising grades prior to the final exam while also allowing the students to observe the results of each other's creativity. I had purchased eight dozen eggs so that each student could receive one to place in the egg delivery vehicle. We would then go to the bus tunnel in front of the school and drop their creations, one at a time, to a chalk target 30 feet below. If the egg survived the fall without breaking, the student would receive a double weighted 100. If the egg broke, I gave its dropper an 85, as long as there had been evidence of some effort in the design of the delivery vehicle. There were also bonus points for the longest flight time and accuracy of hitting the target.

The egg drop was always a big favorite with the students. Unfortunately, events were about to occur which took me out of the 1994 egg drop.

All went well during Sunday afternoon and early evening following the E.R. episode. I felt fine. As I lie in bed just before sleeping, I suddenly felt my heart flutter. "Here it comes!" I whispered to Sharry, who was lying beside me.

"What?" she asked with evident alarm in her voice.

"I think that the AICD is going to fire. I can feel my heart racing. I hope that the damn thing paces it out before it shocks me. I'm scared."

I tried to lie perfectly still. I did not want to be shocked. I began to sweat.

After perhaps 15 minutes, Sharry broke the silence. "I'm going to call Dr. Friehling. This is crazy."

It was now midnight. When we called Friehling's answering service, we were happy to learn that Ted was on call instead of that other guy. He returned our call almost immediately.

I explained to him what I thought was happening. Since he was unaware of the E.R. incident and the changes which had been made in the AICD settings, I gave him a brief summary.

After a short pause, Dr. Friehling responded, "I think that you are well-protected, Ed. If you go into v-tach, the AICD is there to help you. You may get shocked, but that is why we have it in there. I know that this sounds difficult, but try to get some sleep. You'll be OK. Call me right away if the device fires."

I am not sure what I expected Friehling to say. I certainly did not want to go back to the hospital. I wanted some type of miracle so that this nightmare would go away.

But it would not go away. The remainder of the night was horrendous. Both Sharry and I lie awake worrying about what might happen next. Ted's advice was not reassuring. I think that we both cried several times during the night. We did not speak at all, except for Sharry's occasional, "Are you OK?"

As I lie next to Sharry, my thoughts drifted back to the summer of 1967, when I had first met her. I was a young officer then stationed at the Naval Nuclear Power Training Facility just outside Saratoga Springs, New York. The curriculum, which involved shift work and long work days, was designed to teach us how to safely operate a nuclear reactor similar to those found aboard submarines. While on a lunch break, I spotted a note on the bulletin board seeking any officer with a sword to be an usher at a military wedding in Saratoga in two weeks. Having had no social life since arriving in upper state New York, but having a shiny new sword, I volunteered.

Sharry was one of the bridesmaids. I introduced myself to her at the wedding, and we began to talk. As the reception progressed, we enjoyed each other's company, but probably drank too much. I learned that she had grown up in New York, New Jersey, and Maine, graduated from the University of Connecticut, and was currently working as a registered nurse in New Haven, Connecticut. As the reception ended around 10 PM, we both assumed that we would never see each other again and shook hands good-bye. By midnight I was in the Saratoga Springs jail for going through a red light with my headlights out. My Navy uniform saved me because the police allowed me to sober up overnight before releasing me with no charges the following morning. My only thoughts of Sharry were fuzzy. I liked her, but she was obviously bad luck.

Several months later I was riding my motorcycle in the Berkshire Mountains in western Massachusetts and decided to continue south to New Haven to try to locate Sharry. I assumed that she was still working the evening shift at the VA hospital in West Haven. I sent a note to her floor asking if she would like to have a drink together after work. Her return note said, "Only if you're buying."

After having a few beers at a local Yale hangout, I realized that it was past 1 AM. I asked her if I could stay at her apartment. She very reluctantly said, "OK, but you are sleeping on the couch, and you better be gone before my roommate gets home in the morning."

I did exactly as she requested. Unfortunately my motorcycle was stolen during the night. I did not go back to tell Sharry. Instead, I hitch-hiked directly back to upper state New York. This Sharry person was definitely bad luck.

Six months later, while I was assigned to Submarine School in Groton, Connecticut, I called Sharry and asked, (1) would she like to go to New York City some evening, and (2) did she have a friend with whom we could fix up one of my roommates so that we could double date? She called back saying yes on both questions. On the following Saturday my roommate, "CM" Wood, and I drove the 60 miles to New Haven to pick up Sharry and her friend, Joan, and then another 60 miles into New York to visit some bars in the Bowery section of the city. Heavy snow started to fall on the way home, but we made it to New Haven. I did not even consider asking her if we could stay overnight for several reasons, not the least of which was the concern that my car would be stolen. Somehow CM and I made it back to Groton by about 4 AM. This misadventure made it three for three in terms of Bad Luck Sharry. I decided to concentrate on other women.

A few months later I received a post card from Sharry. She was in Denver and reported that she was driving across the country to take a nursing position at Stanford University Hospital in Palo Alto, California. I had no idea why she sent the card. I assumed that she must have had car problems and had nothing better to do while awaiting the repairs. It certainly could not have been spawned by her fond memories of our dates. Since I did not yet know where I was to receive my first shipboard assignment following Submarine School, the news about her move to California had no serious interest for me.

About one month later I received orders to the pre-commissioning unit of USS GURNARD (SSN 662), a nuclear powered fast attack submarine which was under construction at Mare Island Shipyard in Vallejo, California. One other recent Submarine School graduate, Mark Davis, had also received orders to GURNARD. Although we were both 1965 graduates of the Academy and had attended the same class at Submarine School, we did not know each other. Our interests were divergent, to say the least. At the Naval Academy we had run in different circles of friends. When we arrived at Mare Island, Mark and I discovered that we were the only officers who had yet reported to the unit. Although we had no official status, we decided to take daily turns as Commanding Officer of GURNARD. This lasted about two weeks until the real Commanding Officer and Executive Officer arrived. Soon most of the other nine officers reported, and Mark and I assumed our true roles as low guys on the totem pole of seniority.

Although Mark and I still had few common interests, we decided to purchase a house together in Napa, California, about 15 miles north of the shipyard. Napa was in the middle of northern California's wine country. Inflation had not yet affected property values there, and we were able to obtain a small, but very adequate, two bedroom tract house for $17,500.

Shortly before I had left Connecticut, the New Haven police had unfortunately located my stolen motorcycle, just as I was poised to collect a handsome sum from the insurance company. The Navy would not pay to ship the motorcycle to California, so I disassembled it and shipped it in a large wooden crate as "professional books." Mark was an excellent mechanic (at least compared to me). He helped me to reassemble the motorcycle, and soon I was off riding in the hills surrounding Napa.

One day I decided to ride the bike south to Palo Alto to look up Bad Luck Sharry. I am not certain why I chose to do this. I found her address in the phone book and proceeded the 90 miles across the Golden Gate bridge and through San Francisco. It was 1967 and the heyday of flower children, Janis Joplin, drugs, and anti-Vietnam war feelings, particularly in certain sections of San Francisco. I was caught up in the clothing fads of the time. On the day I visited Sharry, I was wearing orange corduroy bell-bottoms and a Mexican poncho. When I arrived at her apartment, one of her roommates answered the door. I asked to see Sharry. The roommate looked me over, closed the door in my face, and yelled, "Sharry, there is some weird-looking guy here to see you."

Sharry and I started to date, usually meeting in bars in San Francisco, which was approximately half-way between our respective residences. I continued to be a heavy drinker. It was not unusual for me to drive back to Napa in my LeMans convertible with the top down and a magnum of cheap champagne as my companion.

During the period that we were dating, Sharry was doing shift work as a staff nurse at Stanford. It was an exciting period to be there because Dr. Norman Shumway and his cardiac team were performing some of the pioneer work in the U.S. in heart transplant operations. Little did Sharry or I realize at the time that this experience gained by the medical community from Shumway's work would have such a direct impact on us 25 years later. In fact, one of the young cardiologists later involved in saving my life received his training at Stanford under Shumway.

As the construction of GURNARD progressed, Mark and I found ourselves in shift work, typically involving 12-16 hour days, usually seven days a week. This routine certainly cut into my social life, but I was young, foolish and determined not to cut back completely. Sharry and I continued to see each other, although on a less frequent basis. We both dated others. There was no indication of a lasting relationship. GURNARD completed construction and was commissioned in mid-1968. The submarine went directly to sea to conduct tests off Hawaii and later near Bremerton, Washington. Sharry and I wrote each other occasionally, but it was a fragmented relationship with little opportunity for dating.

GURNARD was then assigned to San Diego as its homeport. Mark and I sold the house in Napa for a considerable profit. He bought an airplane, and I bought a 30 foot cabin cruiser. By now I also had a second car - a white on white 1957 Chevy convertible. I never considered it excessive for a 25 year old Navy Lieutenant to own two convertibles, a motorcycle, and a cabin cruiser. Sharry flew to San Diego occasionally to see me for a weekend, but we both continued to have other social interests.

In December of 1968, my father became seriously ill with pneumonia. His years of smoking-induced emphysema heightened the problem. I took emergency leave from GURNARD and flew back to Kentucky to be with him and Mom. When Sharry heard the news, she immediately flew from San Francisco to join me. As a nurse, she helped me understand the seriousness of Pop's condition. She was also able to assist my mother during the long hours in the hospital.

One evening after Pop had shown improvement, I took Sharry to Cincinnati's Eden Park which overlooked the Ohio River. It was a beautiful, cool evening and, as we looked at the lights across the river in Kentucky, I asked Sharry if she would marry me. She was sufficiently surprised that she almost pushed me over the edge of the cliff toward the river below. She then said, "Yes."

We decided to fly to New York City to share our news with Sharry's family, who lived in suburban New Jersey. I wanted to formally ask her father for his blessing for our marriage.

I had met Mr. Madigan once before at a lunch with Sharry in San Francisco. He was the Executive Director of News and Special

Events for ABC and was traveling to Japan on business. Our conversation was pleasant until I asked him what it was like to be working for the "number three" network. Sensing by his reaction that I may have just committed a mild faux pas, I attempted to recover by telling Mr. Madigan of my plans to leave the Navy to become a professional gambler. Although I carefully explained why such a move was essentially foolproof because of my "secret system," he was obviously skeptical. After the lunch Sharry told her father how wonderful it had been to have a meal together with the two men in her life. She later told me that he had dryly replied, "*Surely* there is someone else besides him."

While at Sharry's home, I talked to Mr. Madigan about our plans to marry. He was not overly enthusiastic, but he did not openly express regret or indicate his opposition. In retrospect, I think that he regarded me as a rather foolish young man, but acceptable, if Sharry loved me.

We set a wedding date for June 26, 1969 to be held in Sharry's home church in Short Hills, New Jersey. Arrangements began immediately since there were only four months to prepare. I was involved in none of this. I immediately returned to further sea duty on GURNARD in San Diego. Sharry flew back to Palo Alto.

Three months later Pop became seriously ill again while I was at sea. He struggled valiantly, but his lung function had deteriorated to essentially zero due to his lifetime of smoking. Before I could return from sea, my father passed away.

I flew home for the funeral. It was a very emotional experience for me, because I felt guilty about not being there when he died. I had long talks with Mom. I told her that I was confused about where my life was going. I explained to her that I was very nervous about getting married in three weeks. I talked to a local priest, who was absolutely no help. He told me to pray to my patron saint for guidance.

I decided to telephone Sharry in California to tell her that I wanted to call off the wedding. My ego was so distorted that I imagined her killing herself upon hearing the news. We decided to meet in Los Angeles to discuss the matter further that weekend at the wedding of Sam Dutrow, one of my Academy roommates. I felt like a total jerk. I knew that all of the preparations had been made for our wedding and that I was causing considerable grief and embarrassment for not only Sharry, but also her family. Wedding announcements had been sent out, dresses had been purchased, the wedding was imminent. Sharry was very angry with me, to say the least. I was a true rat. We left Los Angeles with her heading north to Palo Alto, while I returned to GURNARD in San Diego.

It was doubtful in my mind that I would ever see Sharry again. Upon reaching GURNARD, I decided to sign on for a large cash bonus to remain in nuclear submarines for four more years. The ship sailed shortly for an extended sea cruise to the western Pacific. For the next 15 months, I became involved in the intense pressure and activity aboard the submarine. Although I was still a junior officer, I was given considerable responsibility and loved every minute of it. We visited ports throughout the Far East and experienced several exciting submerged adventures involving Soviet submarines.

In late September of 1970, GURNARD returned to Pearl Harbor, Hawaii for repairs and torpedo testing. I was assigned to study all day, every day, for the Nuclear Engineer's examination. It was mandatory to pass this extremely difficult two day, written and oral exam, if an officer wished to continue in nuclear submarines. The examination was held at periodic intervals in Washington, DC by the czar of the Navy's nuclear program (and many claimed, the entire Navy), Admiral Rickover.

I threw myself into an intense study program, but I continued most of my self-destructive drinking and social habits. One evening I found myself examining exactly what I had become. My conclusions both embarrassed and frightened me. I was indeed well on the road to becoming a genuine "burnt out case" at age 27. As I thought about this, I went over several options. The most appealing was to try to regain control of my personal life. Perhaps I should see if I could marry and begin a family.

Unfortunately there was no one that I could think of who might take me. I had enjoyed a great relationship only with Sharry, and I had blown that opportunity nearly 18 months ago. I decided that the only option which I had was to contact her, beg forgiveness, and ask if we could resume a serious relationship. The telephone call to her from Hawaii to California was the most difficult of my life. Not only did I ask her to forgive me, but I also told her that I wanted to marry her if she would still have me.

Sharry's initial response was understandably cool and skeptical. She did not say no, but she certainly did not seem to be terribly excited about my offer. We agreed to talk later on the subject. I was not very optimistic about my chances.

Several days later I telephoned again. She said that she had considered my request for marriage, and that it might work out. I asked her if that was a "yes." After several statements warning me about dire consequences if I were to call off this wedding, Sharry agreed to marry me. I did not realize at the time that her decision to give me a second chance would have such incredibly positive repercussions throughout the remainder of my life.

Because of my Navy schedule, we had to arrange for a very short notice wedding. I had orders to fly to California the following week to visit Navy Reserve Officer Training Corps (NROTC) units at four universities, starting with UCLA in Los Angeles. Sharry recommended that we meet there to finalize plans for the wedding to be held the following weekend in Palo Alto. Our brief time together in Los Angeles was not uncomfortable, considering the circumstances. We enjoyed each other's company, and both of us were pleased with our decision to marry. We were not concerned about the short time frame involved. All of the key players (her parents, my mother, and our California friends) would be there. Sharry had arranged for the use of Saint Ann's chapel at Stanford University, she still had her wedding dress, and I would be wearing my Navy uniform.

Our wedding took place on Halloween, 1970. We always kidded about the date, but at least I was never guilty about forgetting our anniversary! Spurway was my best man. In keeping with his bohemian style now that he was a civilian and living in a tent near Monterey, he did not wear a suit. He did, however, offer some very moving words during the service when he read about five minutes of remarks. It was a great wedding - no dictatorial photographer, no consultant to over-organize, - just a cozy, fun celebration for everyone involved.

Sharry's roommates helped to host a highly informal, but very enjoyable, reception at their home that evening. We then flew to

Hawaii for our honeymoon. It was not a typical honeymoon, because I had to return immediately to my daily study in preparation for the Engineer examination. We were living in a furnished apartment in downtown Honolulu. It was not exactly fancy living. Some guy was murdered in the basement garage our first week there. We had a 1960 Oldsmobile convertible which burned nearly as much oil as gas. I had bought it for $150 from a sailor going to sea and sold it two months later to a different sailor for $160 and a ride to the airport on our departure from Hawaii.

One week into our Hawaiian experience I made one of the most ill-advised decisions of my life. To this day Sharry has not forgiven me, and I do not blame her. I asked my mother to come to Hawaii to stay with us so that she could see the islands. I had not even discussed this with Sharry. For her part, Sharry was amazingly calm, at least for the first week. After a few days together while I was at work, the tension between the two increased dramatically. Of course, I was oblivious to this development. Mom stayed two weeks, a full dose for anyone, much less a new bride. For the remainder of our years together Sharry has always told everyone how she had to spend her honeymoon with the mother-in-law.

All of these memories flooded my mind as I was lying next to this wonderful person who had somehow found something in me to love for over 20 years. It was primarily her steadfast support and strength of character which had enabled us to make it this far together. Now, however, we both knew that we were facing the unknown. Was this the final crash? If I did go into sustained tachycardia, would the AICD fire properly? What would happen if it did fire, but my heart continued in v-tach? How many firings would take place before it quit? Would I then die?

Although each of these questions had been valid for the past several years, I was now forced to confront them in the reality of a hot sweat, lying in my own bed, next to my equally terrified wife. Sharry has never discussed the details of her emotions that night. Her only comment has been, "It was the low point of my life."

I got out of bed just before 6 AM. I had slept little, if any. After taking a lengthy shower, I was dressing in front of my chest of drawers. Sharry was in the shower. Without warning, I felt the unmistakable bolt of the AICD firing in my chest. I instantly yelled out, **"Oomph!"** as I doubled over in shock. My scream must have been very loud, because Sharry came running naked from the shower and Emily immediately appeared from her bedroom with a look of horror on her face.

"It fired. I'm OK now, I think," I said softly as I straightened up. "I'm going to sit on the bed for a few minutes."

Sharry paused and then said, "We **have** to call Friehling."

"I'll call him from work after his office opens. He said that I should expect this. The device is working."

It was obvious that Sharry did not agree with my plan, but she did not argue. In a few minutes, I finished dressing and went downstairs.

After placing a bagel in the microwave, I went to the dining room to pick up my wallet and keys. I was planning to load the eight dozen eggs into the truck to take to school. Just as I reached for my wallet, the AICD fired again. It was as if I were in the midst of an instant replay of the scenario upstairs just ten minutes earlier. My scream of pain brought both Sharry and Emily running downstairs. They both now knew what had taken place and were coming to help me.

"It happened again. I wasn't doing anything special. It just fired. I think that I am back to a normal rhythm again." For some reason, I was defensive, as though I was begging my wife and child to understand that this was not my fault.

"You're **not** going to work. This is serious," said Sharry sternly. She was definitely lecturing me.

My reaction was confrontational. "Oh, no, I'm going in. The egg drop is today, and I'm going to be there. I'll call Friehling later."

I glanced at Emily. She was standing rigidly as if she were a white granite statue. It was bad enough that her father was in serious medical trouble, but now he and her mother were arguing about it.

Before we could continue our debate, the AICD fired again. This time I slumped into one of the kitchen chairs and started to cry. I knew that I was headed to the hospital. I had no way of knowing whether the setpoints on the AICD had been set too low in the E.R. or my heart condition had further degraded.

Sharry telephoned Friehling's answering service to tell him that the device had fired three times in the past twenty minutes and that she was taking me to Fairfax Hospital immediately.

Before we left the house, Ted called to tell us to go directly to admitting instead of the emergency room. He had called them to expect me and to place me in a room on the second floor where I could be continuously monitored.

I felt safer once I was in a hospital bed, but I was still frightened. I was now acutely aware that I might be in the final stages of my life. I found myself praying frequently throughout the day. At 11 PM that evening, my confidence was totally shattered when I received another series of three shocks approximately five minutes apart. The hospital heart monitoring system indicated that I had indeed been in v-tach each time and that the AICD was functioning correctly. Each time it had attempted to pace me out of the dangerous rhythm, but the heart did not respond and a shock was required. I lay awake most of the night in spite of receiving medication (Valium, I believe) to calm me.

Al Del Negro came in to see me before breakfast. "You had a lousy night," he said. "I looked at your trace. We're going to do an EP study on you later this morning. We are going to try a drug called Mexitil on you to see if it will help. The problem is that you are now going into v-tach at a very low rate - probably around 110. We'll see what we can do for you."

The Mexitil did not work. The EP study showed that it exacerbated the problem. My arrhythmia doctors now decided to try an IV approach involving 30 cc/hr of Pronestyl. I would remain on that drug for two days and then another EP study would be conducted to assess its effect.

The Pronestyl did not work either. Ted and Al were able to induce tachycardia at an even lower rate during the EP study on Thursday. The only good news was that my heart was remaining stable at all other times. All medication avenues were exhausted. The only option was to go home, take it easy for several days, and see how my heart responded.

When Nelle heard that I was in the hospital, she flew home immediately from Indiana where she was working two summer jobs to help pay for her college expenses. We decided that Sharry should work on Friday and that Nelle could drive me home. Tom Cindric, one of my teaching buddies at Woodbridge, had given the final physics examinations to my students for me. Because the exams were all essays and problem solving, I had to grade them over the weekend. Graduation was the following Friday, and grades for the seniors had to be in to data processing the next school day after each final exam. I "took it easy" by grading the examinations and compiling quarter, semester and final grades for over 120 students during the next several days at home.

I did not go into school on Monday or Tuesday. Nelle shuttled the exams back and forth for me. The last section of exams were held on Tuesday. After grading them at home that evening, I decided to ride with Nelle to Woodbridge as she returned the last set of grades to the office.

"I feel funny. I think that I will stay here in the van while you take the grades into the school, Nelle," I said as we entered the Woodbridge High parking lot. Nelle stared at me, obviously trying to decide if it would be safe to leave me. "Go ahead. I'll be OK. Then we can go straight home."

Nelle ran to the school office with the grade sheets. She was back at the van in less than two minutes. As we backed out of the parking space, the AICD fired.

I screamed, "Oomph!" and doubled over momentarily.

"Dad, are you OK?"

"Drive home Nelle. Be careful. If this thing goes off again, we'll go straight to the hospital. If I pass out, pull over and use the car phone to call 911."

Nelle was incredibly calm. She simply nodded and stared at the cars ahead. I was very proud of her.

In less than a mile I suffered another shock.

"We're going to the hospital, Dad. I will call Mom. Are you well enough to be able to call Dr. Friehling's office?"

"I think so."

The connection with Friehling's office was intermittent as we passed through a cellular dead zone while crossing the Occoquan River. I had reached Al Del Negro. I was able to pass enough information to him so that he understood that I was being shocked. He concurred that I should head to Fairfax Hospital.

It was Wednesday, June 15, 1994. I asked Nelle to drive past our home on the way to the hospital. I did not tell her why, but I was convinced that I might not see it again. Nelle did not slow as we passed by. Emily was in school, Sharry was on her way from work to meet us at the hospital, Sydney, our Australian cattle dog, was the only family member at home. I remember how nice the yard looked. Then I openly cried.

Upon arriving at the hospital we learned that there were no open beds on my usual spot, the second floor. I was admitted to a room on the third floor. It had less sophisticated heart monitoring facilities, but there was a system in place and I would be closely observed. During the afternoon I had one episode of light-headedness, but no shocks. In the early evening, while Sharry was still with me, I was paced out of an arrhythmia by the AICD. It did not have to shock me. As I felt the pacing taking place, I gripped my sheets tightly in anticipation of the coming shock. A nurse ran into the room and asked excitedly, "Mr. Linz, are you OK?"

"I think so. I believe that I have just been paced out of an arrhythmia. Can you check the trace to see what it says?"

There was no shock this time. The nurse returned quickly to the room after going to the monitoring unit at the nurse's station. "You were right. I will call Dr. Del Negro."

Sharry and I spent the next two hours in a tense atmosphere. When would it happen again? At 10 PM I insisted that she go home. I was now feeling better than I had felt all day and she desperately needed sleep. I told her that I would telephone home if anything else happened.

As soon as Sharry left, I gathered a stack of student essays and went to a small empty room at the end of the hallway. There I read the essays for the next hour and a half. Each year, sometime in the final two weeks of class, I give the students three questions to consider:

(1) What would you like to be doing ten years from now? (job, family situation, locale, etc.)

(2) What will you have to do to make your answer to question #1 happen?

(3) What do you think that you will remember most about this class ten years from now?

I always enjoy reading their responses. Almost all are genuine and sincere. Most want a great job, at least half would like to be married and have a family, and nearly all believe that they will remember my corny jokes and how much I hate hamsters. As always, I became rather emotional as I read their hopes for the future. It was particularly wrenching, because I could not help thinking that I might not see any of them again. Their graduation would be in less than 48 hours, and I would definitely not be there.

Shortly after returning to my room at 11:30 PM, I heard a loud commotion in the hallway. The noise was rapidly getting louder and apparently approaching my room. Suddenly, just as at least five people entered my room with a cart in front of them, the AICD fired. I screamed in pain as several nurses grabbed me to keep me from falling over.

"Your monitor alarmed, Mr. Linz! We came to help you. Are you OK?"

"I think so. I need to sit down."

As I sat on the edge of the bed, I noticed that my roommate, an older man recovering from open heart surgery, had remained asleep through my ordeal. I also decided that I now had a good estimate of how long it took the capacitor inside the AICD to charge up and fire after its computer recognized an arrhythmia situation: about the length of time for five people to race fifteen yards to my room from the nurse's station after my monitoring alarm goes off. All of the nurses except one left the room. As we talked, I said quietly, "Here it comes again."

I was correct. **BOOM!** I was hit with another shock. The nurse appeared to be in shock herself. There were few AICD patients on the third floor and she had never seen a patient in the midst of being shocked by the device. She grabbed my hand and said nothing. She held my hand for at least ten minutes. Two other nurses had come to the room immediately after the second shock, but left when they saw that I was being cared for. I was now terrified. Would I live through the night?

I did, but it was the worst night of my life. I thought about calling Sharry as I had promised her, but I rationalized that she could do nothing to help, and that she desperately needed the sleep. After the nurse left the room, I tried to remain absolutely motionless. I was afraid to move, even slightly. I certainly did not want to go to sleep. If I were going to die, I wanted to face it directly. Most of the night I prayed for God's help. I believed that I was ready to go if He wanted me.

There were no shocks or recorded arrhythmias through the remainder of the night or the next day. I telephoned Sharry at her office early in the morning to tell her about the shocks. She was extremely upset that I had not called her, but I was not sorry about my decision. Each of my doctors seemed concerned about my worsening condition, but there was no discussion of new treatment or medication. I felt terminal.

At 11 PM that evening a nurse came to my room and said that I needed to go to x-ray for a chest x-ray which had been ordered by Dr. Matthews earlier in the day.

"Now?" I asked incredulously. 'Why 11 o'clock at night?"

"This is the first available time today. They've been busy with emergencies."

"This is crazy," I protested. "Is anyone going with me? I will have to be off the monitor while I am down there."

"We don't have anyone. You'll be OK. It will take only a few minutes. I have called for a transporter to take you down there in a wheel chair."

I should have protested more rigorously, but I was worried that I might become upset in the process and trigger the AICD to fire. I did not want that.

The transporter, a young East Asian who spoke little English, arrived shortly. The nurse disconnected me from the monitoring system. Within minutes, I was headed to the basement of the hospital for a midnight x-ray.

Radiology was empty when the transporter and I arrived. He left me sitting in the wheel chair in the hallway as he searched for a warm body. We could hear laughing and voices, but it took at least five minutes to locate a technician.

"Chest x-ray, huh? How come now?" the technician asked me when he came to take me into the x-ray room. The transporter had left long ago. I had been alone for at least ten minutes.

"Just take it. The nurse on the floor said that you have been busy. I don't feel too good. I think that I need to get back to the floor."

The technician was excruciatingly deliberate as he walked through the x-ray procedure. "Can you stand up by yourself?" he asked.

"I think so. But I don't feel very good."

The x-ray was completed and I was wheeled into the empty hallway to wait for a transporter to take me back to my room on the third floor. As the technician left me, I said, "How long will I be here? I really need to get back to the third floor where I can be monitored."

"I called them. Sometimes it takes a while this time of night for someone to come."

The technician disappeared into a room down the hall. I immediately heard laughing and loud conversation. I never felt more alone.

At least twenty minutes passed. Suddenly I felt my heart begin to race. As I braced for the inevitable shock, I felt the strong beat of the pacing mechanism in the AICD. Fortunately, it was successful in reversing the arrhythmia and I was not shocked. As I regained my composure, I began to sweat heavily. I yelled, "Would someone **please** help me?" I began to sob as I realized that I might die unnoticed in an empty hospital basement hallway.

After three more screams for help, the technician looked out of the room in which he was partying and asked, "You still here? What's wrong?"

"I think that I may be dying. Where is the transporter?"

"I told you. They are busy this time of night. I will call them again."

"No! Please don't do that. Will you please take me yourself to the third floor. I'm in trouble! I have a heart problem. I need to get back there now!"

The technician was not impressed. He looked back into the room where his friend was apparently located, looked at me, and then shrugged and said, "OK, but it's not my job. I'll take you up there."

He did, but with a major attitude. When we arrived on the third floor, the nurse looked as if I had hit her in the stomach when I told her what had happened. "Oh my God!" she said. "I knew that we should have sent someone with you."

Dr. Friehling had an even stronger reaction the next morning. From what I could determine, he went ballistic. Apparently, when he had gone to the nurse's desk to find out what had happened during the x-ray incident, he had found that the technician who was supposed to be watching the monitoring system was not at his station. This negligence, coupled with the error in judgment by the evening nurses in allowing me to go unattended by a nurse to x-ray, had caused Friehling to explode, "I want my patient off this floor immediately. Put him on the second floor where someone will take care of him." I did not hear his exact words myself, but when I was transferred to the second floor less than twenty minutes later, all the nurses were abuzz about the incident. Dr. Friehling had apparently spared no expletives in conveying his message. As far as I know, he never apologized for his outburst. He felt that he was protecting his patient's interest. He had lost confidence in the staff on the third floor and wanted me where he was comfortable that an arrhythmia patient would be properly monitored and cared for.

All went reasonably well on the second floor. I thought of my students when they graduated from Woodbridge the following evening. I wanted to be there to share their excitement. I had not missed a graduation ceremony since I began teaching in 1985. On Sunday evening I had another pacing incident in my room, but no shocks. I wondered what was going to happen. I could not remain here indefinitely. What could we do?

Friehling answered this question as he and Al Del Negro entered my room on Monday morning, June 20. "You need a new heart," he said enthusiastically.

"A new heart? What do you mean?" I asked.

"A transplant. Your heart isn't going to make it much longer. I have talked to Bob Matthews and Kevin Rogan and we think that we can get you on the list for a transplant. You and Sharry need to talk this over with the transplant team. They will be in to see you today."

Before I could respond, Al broke in, "We think that we can keep you stable with the Procainamide which you have been taking since last Wednesday and a drug, Dopamine, which we will give to you intravenously. We cannot do much else. The sarcoid is winning. You need a new heart."

We talked for several minutes. I thanked both of them for all of their efforts to help me during the past three years. "I'm alive today because of you guys. I will talk to Sharry. The transplant sounds like the only option left."

Sharry arrived at lunchtime. Our discussion of the transplant decision was surprisingly brief. We both realized that it was our only remaining hope. When Dr. Rogan, a cardiologist on the transplant team, arrived later in the afternoon to discuss a possible transplant, we were ready with our answer.

"Let's do it, Doctor. Do you think that we can get one?"

Dr. Rogan was cautious. "Our transplant team has to evaluate you, both medically and psychologically, before we can place you on the list waiting for a donor heart. There are far more people waiting for hearts than donor organs. We will have to follow specific procedures, but I believe that you will be judged to be in Category 1. That means top priority."

A series of doctors and nurses came to see me during the next 24 hours. Each was an expert in a different specialty. I was thoroughly examined several times, but always from a different perspective. A female psychiatrist, for example, seemed to be very intent on determining whether or not I would be compliant with a challenging medication regimen. No one would promise that I would be on the list. By evening of the next day, Sharry and I were becoming anxious. We knew that my case was now being evaluated by a committee. Would they consider me to me a good candidate for a transplant? Or was something unforeseen going to dash this last hope?

The answer came from Dr. Matthews the following morning. "Kevin Rogan just called me," he said. "The committee has decided in your favor. You're now on the heart transplant list. It could be today, next week, next month, or maybe a year, but you are going to get a new heart. You will have to stay here until then. You're too sick to go home to wait. We have to monitor you continuously and keep you on the Dopamine drip. I think that you have made the correct decision."

When Dr. Merlino saw Sharry and me later that afternoon, the three of us openly wept together. She was expecting twins in less than three weeks and had not been working. I was overwhelmed that she had come to the hospital to see us. Her message was, as always, straightforward, "You've crashed, Ed, but I think that we can pick up the pieces."

I had no idea how long that process would take.

Chapter 11

ROOMMATES

I was now in Room 277 in Fairfax Hospital. In a few days I knew all of the nurses on the second floor. They were a friendly, competent lot. Each had a distinctive approach to nursing. Of course, I tended to develop favorites, but I felt safe with any of them.

Safety had become the overriding consideration for me. I was definitely no longer "safe" at home. Although the AICD had kept me alive several times in the past week, the sarcoidosis was now a constant threat to my existence. It was causing frequent arrhythmias, any of which might be the one to kill me. Room 277 became my remaining "safe haven" on Life Row. Here my heart was being monitored continuously by both a technician and automatic sensing equipment. If I were to slide into life-threatening tachycardia, a team of nurses were but a few yards away at any time to render assistance. Obviously, all of the medical expertise in the world would not be helpful if my heart were to quit altogether, but I refused to consider this possibility - at least, not at the moment. I was determined to do whatever would be necessary to stay alive long enough to receive a new heart.

I was initially placed in the bed away from the window, but closer to the door. Although I wanted the bed next to the window, I did not complain, because I knew from experience that I would be able to move to the preferred location as soon as my current roommate was discharged. On a cardiac floor, especially in these days of "managed care," the wait would not be long. In fact, the next day my wish came true. As soon as I was moved, I dug in. I placed at least ten photographs, a piggy bank, five books, and miscellaneous other personal effects on the window sill. I wanted to ensure that anyone entering the room would immediately understand that he was now on my turf.

As each new roommate was wheeled into 277, I greeted him, "Welcome to Fairfax Hospital. I am Ed Linz, your coronary concierge. Please feel free to use my services at any time."

I soon developed rather strong feelings about these individuals whom fate brought into such close proximity to me. I decided that hospital roommates can be divided into two distinct groupings: OK, and not OK. There seems to be little middle ground. In my opinion, there is only one criteria to determine placement in the group: are they quiet or not?

During my several extended stays in the hospital, I had occasion to observe a significant number of roommates. According to my definition of OK, less than half could be considered in that category. Most were nice people, but that attribute is not a sufficient, or even necessary, condition to being a good roommate.

For example, there was Don. He was a very nice man of about 65 years, but he was a talkaholic. It did not matter to Don what I was doing. Whether I was trying to read the newspaper, talk to someone on the telephone, discuss medication with the nurse, or sleep, Don talked. I tried to discourage him by totally ignoring his banter, but the relief was brief, and he was soon on to another topic. Whenever I was able to move around, I found myself going for a lot of walks in the corridor. Fortunately Don was in my room for only two days before being discharged in the care of his wife, whom I pity to this day.

There were other examples of "not OK." A large number of my roommates were over 50, and most seemed to have a cruel snore at night. A small percentage were soft-toned rhythmic snorers. This type of malady was troublesome for me at first, but I quickly adapted to the environment and could proceed on to sleep with little difficulty.

The next step up my ladder of snoring angst was the intermittent wheezer. On the intake breath the typical guttural sound is made, but the output phase would be a whistle of variable pitch. I found this to be a difficult situation because my brain never could gain synchronization with this unpredictably changing sound. The torment could generally be overcome only by my wearing a Walkman playing a book on tape narrated by a melodiously voiced reader. Two of my favorite tapes were recordings of books by Peter Mayle,

A Year in Provence, and its sequel, *Toujours Provence*. The Walkman was generally a successful antidote, so much so, in most circumstances, that it took me two weeks to make it through one side of a tape. I would fall asleep fairly rapidly only to wake during the night to find my headphones still on, but the tape at the end of the side . If the wheezer was still at it, I would have to reverse the tape to find the last location in the story which I remembered. But the Walkman approach was effective in providing some insulation.

A particularly bothersome category of snorer was the "silent-but-deadly" type. These individuals would be very quiet for x number of minutes, but then would suddenly, without warning, blast the room with a loud grunt very similar to a hog with an attitude. I would be lulled into a sense of security and peacefulness by the silent phase, approaching the bliss of sleep, only to nearly jump out of the bed upon hearing this terrible sound. Generally the Walkman reinforced by a pillow on each ear could handle this situation.

The deepest corner of snorers' hell was reserved for only a select few who were loud, wheezing **and** intermittent. These individuals were unique and beyond effective countermeasures. In this category there was a clear champion - a man whose snore could be heard round the world, or so it seemed. "The Champ" (as I labeled him after our first night together) would produce a sound several decibels above the threshold of pain on his intake stroke. He would sometimes follow this with a whistling sound akin to fingernails scraping across a classroom blackboard. I tried all known techniques to combat the Champ, but by three in the morning, he would still be firmly in control of the situation, and I would be tossing and turning in bed trying to understand what I may have done wrong to merit this torture.

After two nights of no sleep with the Champ, one of my doctors came in for his daily visit and exclaimed, "You look terrible!"

He then said quietly, "A snorer?"

"Yes," I nodded, and pointed my thumb in the Champ's direction. He was watching television in his bed and was unaware of my conversation with the doctor.

The doctor spoke abruptly, "I'll take care of it. Who is your nurse?"

I have no idea what happened next, but within 30 minutes, the Champ was headed out of my room and down the hall to a new room to drive someone else crazy. At first I felt just a little guilty about the situation, but it quickly faded as several rationalizations took over. I think that the primary one was: "It's a dog-eat-dog world out there."

I did occasionally think of the Champ, because he remained in the hospital for several more days. Every time I passed a member of his family in the hall, they would glare at me as if I had sentenced their father/husband to a lower form of life. I still think that they were simply envious of me. I had been able to escape the Champ, but they were stuck permanently with this guy and his foghorn.

There were other categories of noise-producing roommates. A large number were television addicts. Many of my roommates were older and had poor hearing. Fairfax Hospital offers an individual bedside television for each patient, so I was always very aware of my roommate's viewing tastes, or lack of.

I quickly learned to despise daytime television. Most of my roommates were TV junkies. They would turn on their set immediately upon waking and then listen/watch for the remainder of the day. From 9 AM on, the shows were inane and hideous, if not totally disgusting. Listening to hour after hour of "talk shows" in which each host tried to outdo the next for sheer sensationalism left me worrying about the American condition. I certainly could detect no socially redeeming value to this trash. I tried to concentrate on my own activities, such as reading the newspaper, writing letters, or sending e-mail messages, but it was difficult to think over the electronic din.

Afternoon television was slightly better. I grew to be able to tolerate soap operas, not because of their content, but because the dialogue, although inane, was generally conversational and more pleasing to the ear than the morning stuff. Fortunately, my bed was in a location so that I could not watch my roommate's television, and I found that I could actually read and write during these shows.

The addictive nature of the soaps was particularly interesting. One of my roommates, a 65 year old taxi driver named Bennie, bragged that he had **never** missed *The Young and the Restless* for the past twelve years! In an excited voice he told me, "One way or another, Ed, I get home every day from 12:30 to 1:30 so I don't miss it. Just in case, though, I got my VCR set to record it if I get stuck in traffic somewhere." After several days together, I realized that Bennie was a true soap junkie; once he had his daily Y&R fix, he was one happy cabby.

"Evening" news began at 4 PM on one of the local stations. The same stories would then be recycled for the next three hours, and many of my roommates watched every minute. I often wondered how much actual news was breaking each day to keep people listening for three hours while being bombarded by commercials. Of course, there was always CNN, and, naturally, I had one roommate who watched it all day long. Fortunately, he stayed with me only one day. As he was being wheeled out of the room to be discharged, I had a strong urge to yell, "Get a life!"

Early evenings brought the game shows. Several of my roommates seemed to get genuinely thrilled yelling encouragement, admonition, or answers at the game show participants. What was amazing to me was that they did this while carrying on a steady stream of conversation with their visitors. Judging by how most of the visitors seemed to regard this behavior as not only acceptable, but appropriate, I theorized that the same process took place in their own homes on a nightly basis.

For those whose tastes favored the lurid, there was always the option during this period of watching the "news magazines." I am the first to admit that "news" is a very subjective term, but most of these shows were simply electronic variants of tabloids such as *The National Enquirer*. Apparently this genre is also difficult to watch in silence, because many of my roommates would periodically yell, to no one in particular, "Did you see that?" or "They ought to kill those bastards!" or some even more profane announcement.

The early evening shows would be followed by a series of situation comedies. The canned laughter was really annoying, but the winner of the "Best Way to Drive a Sane Person Crazy" award was the extremely high pitch "Woo-oo-oo-oo-oo!" whenever some sexually suggestive situation occurred in the script. Real subtle. No television producer ever lost his job by underestimating the intelligence or taste of the American viewing population.

I soon developed a minimally acceptable (to me) sets of rules which I would ask my roommates to follow. All I requested was that the television be off before 8 AM and after 11:30 PM. Most honored this request. However, several would fall asleep with their set on. This created a problem, even if I was mobile. Should I sneak over and try to turn off the TV without waking the sleeping offender? What would I say if he woke up to find me by his bedside? I would definitely be "in his space." On the other hand, I did want to sleep. I generally finessed this problem by calling my nurse and asking her to turn off the set. This embarrassed me at first, but I soon regarded this as a routine event.

There was, however, one roommate, who, although a reasonably polite individual, absolutely, positively had to have the television on so that he could go to sleep, or so he claimed. He was one of my numerous roommates who was recovering from angioplasty (the procedure in which an inflated "balloon" is inserted to re-open a clogged artery in the heart). One of the annoying aspects of this procedure for the patient is the requirement to lie flat on your back for several hours until the catheter which was used in the procedure can be safely removed from the insertion point in the groin. After over six hours of this agony, the catheter is removed and a dressing is applied to ensure no bleeding from the artery. A small sandbag is then placed on top of the dressing, and the patient must remain flat for several more hours. Most of these patients remain only one night and are able to return home the following afternoon. In short, they are generally acceptable roommates.

This guy, whom I will call Chuck, was not. He would fall asleep with the TV on, I would get out of bed, go to his bedside to turn off the torture, return to my bed and try to sleep. Chuck would wake up as if he sensed when I was almost asleep, turn on the TV and then shortly fall back to sleep, as indicated by his snoring. I would toss and turn for about 20 minutes using all of my normal antidotes, before getting up once again to begin the entire process over again. I tried the "get the nurse to help" strategy, but Chuck simply turned the set back on shortly after she left. I then asked for a Valium, although I disliked taking drugs additional to those I already had to receive each day. The Valium did knock me out for almost three hours, but when I awoke during the night for one of my necessary visits to the bathroom, I found Chuck still at it with his annoying routine. At 5 AM I had reached the breaking point. I rolled out of bed, shuffled over to Chuck and spoke slowly to him through clinched teeth, "Turn it off, Chuck. I haven't slept the whole night. I have to sleep, or I become **very** strange, if you know what I mean." Standing over a patient who cannot move and issuing a firm, but vague, threat had immediate results. I have no idea whether Chuck was simply being polite, or if he suddenly had visions of becoming chopped liver. The TV went off, Chuck went home later that day, and I napped during most of the afternoon. The nurses mercifully did not give me a new roommate that night.

My ultimate daytime avoidance technique (when I was mobile) was to leave the room and seek the relative serenity of the halls. The hospital waiting rooms, I learned, are definitely not a safe haven. Each has its own TV, and it is **always** on, matter what is being shown, day or night.

As a teacher I had long ago developed an intense dislike for television. I even came to the eventual conclusion that there is no such thing as "good television" (such as, some informative PBS series on Australian sheep and the quaint villagers who tend them). My complaint is that television, no matter the content, is an intellectually passive medium. Images are shown with accompanying dialogue, and the viewer's mind has little to do. With books, newspaper, or radio there is a requirement for your mind to form a mental picture to go along with the associated words. Children are particularly vulnerable to this inherent shortcoming of television, because their minds are still developing. If they do not have to think, they are missing valuable opportunities to exercise the mind. I do not know whether or not intellectual inactivity leads to brain atrophy, but if the mind behaves as other body organs, there is a strong argument that such may occur. As a teacher, I have always regarded the ability to think as a "use it or lose it" situation.

Numerous studies for the past 30 years have shown that the average American spends at least 20 hours each week watching television. The number of hours spent by children in front of the TV is even more staggering. Some studies cited surveys in which **pre-school** children spent over 30 hours a week glued to this mind numbing device! Often many parents and pre-school staff use television as a baby sitter for children while they do other activities. Even if the content is "educational," the child's mind is not being exercised during its most formative years.

I first began to develop some critical thoughts about television after I had spent several years aboard submarines. I noticed in the mid-70's that many of the junior officers on board ship seemed to have little intellectual curiosity. Their only form of entertainment during the evenings was to watch a movie in the wardroom (officer's dining area/lounge). Most did not know how to play **any** card games other than poker. Bridge, and even hearts, required too much thinking. Few, if any, of these college graduates could play chess, or even a reasonably competitive game of checkers! When the submarine pulled into a liberty port, even one in a foreign country, some of these young officers would remain aboard ship to watch movies all night long. While the "old hands" were immediately across the brow searching for adventure in various forms, many of their younger counterparts were spaced out on the ship watching a movie which they may have already seen several times!

In trying to analyze what may have caused this difference between two groups of officers involved in the same high-pressure, at-sea environment, it came to me that most of these younger officers were born in the 1950's when television first came to the mass market. Although it is impossible to develop a valid cause-effect relationship based upon such a theory with no statistical analysis, I came to firmly believe that they were some of the first true intellectual casualties of the age of television.

As a teacher I subsequently saw further evidence among my students. Most had few critical thinking skills and were unable to read a section of a textbook and then, the next day, describe verbally or in writing the essence of the article. Asking them to critically evaluate a reading on a subject was an exercise in futility; most saw "critical analysis" as simply a re-telling of what was written. This deficiency had become so wide-spread by the 90's that the education industry started to tout courses in critical thinking, problem solving, and other jargon-laced topics, as if one had to have a special course in order to think.

What really concerned me was that I was now seeing the second generation of these non-thinking television addicts. How can parents who have no thinking skills promote activities for their children when they themselves have no experience in this area, other than to figure out where the remote channel changer is located? Most video games are little, if any, improvement. Some of these activities do promote hand/eye coordination, which may make driving easier, but which does little to stimulate the intellectual portion of the brain. As I watched most of my roommates willingly surrender all of their free time to this addictive medium, I began to wonder if we are in the process of unwittingly undergoing a type of Darwinian change in the species in which the thought process is being lessened, perhaps permanently.

There were other variants of hospital noise-producers. One annoying group included those individuals who are connected to an intravenous (IV) monitoring device which makes a BEEP-BEEP-BEEP sound at regular intervals until action is taken to restore the alarm condition. This is typically a low flow alarm indicating that something has occurred to lessen the desired quantity of IV solution flowing into the vein. Usually this is a temporary situation which will clear itself with no action, but the alarm continues until it is reset. The devices in my room required someone to push two buttons in sequence, first a yellow one labeled HOLD, and then a green one labeled RUN. Obviously someone has to hear the alarm to reset it. Therein lies the problem. The alarm is loud enough for most people to hear it and wake at night, but the heavy sleepers hear nothing. One of my older roommates heard well enough at lower frequencies (such as typical male voices), but could not hear higher frequencies sounds (such as many female voices). Guess what frequency the BEEP-BEEP-BEEP is closest to? This fellow could not hear his IV alarm when he was awake, much less when he was snoozing. So the alarm goes off at night, I wake up, he does not wake up, I call the nurse, and ten minutes later, the problem is corrected - until it goes off two hours later.

Some of my other roommates on the IV monitoring device heard the alarm, but had no idea how to reset and silence it. In this case the BEEP-BEEP-BEEP would continue until the nurse appeared. If she was occupied with another patient, re-setting an IV alarm was not a high priority for her. If this situation occurred several times during the night, the next day I would tell my friends that I was suffering from "Road Runner Syndrome."

In addition to the OK/not OK labeling, there are some roommates who are so unique that they fall into special categories, such as exceptionally weird, dangerous, really pleasant, incredibly sad, genuinely pathetic, and superbly entertaining.

By "weird" I mean someone who goes far beyond the normal broad definition of reasonably sane. Let me give you an example.

It is one in the morning and I am soundly asleep with no roommate. Suddenly I am awakened by the sound of the curtain between beds being rapidly pulled shut. It is a nurse, and the sounds of a night-time admission begin. While the medics maneuver the gurney alongside the bed, the nurse raises the other bed to an elevated position for a transfer of the patient. When the beds are lined up properly, a plastic board is inserted under the patient and the nurse says , "1, 2, 3, PULL !!"

The patient is slid from the gurney to his bed, the plastic board is pulled out from under him, and his hospital stay begins. The nurse rushes about doing various things, such as ensuring that the patient knows where he is, and that personal belongings are safely stowed in a closet with his name on the bag. Then the nurse attempts to obtain a medical history from the patient. Everything went reasonably well and quickly up to this point with this guy whose name was Anthony. The nurse was one of my favorites, Teresa, who was originally from India.

Teresa speaks with a slight accent and has incredible patience when dealing with patients. Anthony was to set a new standard of intransigence. Teresa began by asking him what his symptoms had been upon coming to the hospital. He mumbled an incoherent reply. In fact, all of Anthony's responses were mumbles, except when he rather proudly said that he had tried to kill himself with a drug overdose because his girlfriend left him. This was interesting, but not particularly helpful to Teresa. My ears did perk up, however. If this guy was suicidal, could he also be homicidal?

I had trouble getting back to sleep. After Teresa left the room I spoke loudly across the pulled curtain to Anthony, "Welcome to Fairfax Hospital. I'm Ed Linz." Considering the circumstances, I decided to leave out the coronary concierge part.

Surprisingly Anthony replied in a very clear voice, "Thanks, Man! I'm Anthony." For some reason this exchange served to re-assure me that Anthony would probably not kill me during the night.

Later that morning I awoke at seven. Anthony was talking rather loudly on the phone to some woman. It was a long conver-sation. I assumed that it was a woman because Anthony kept using the term, "Baby." This call lasted about 30 minutes and consisted mostly of Anthony saying how much he wanted "to get out of here."

The next call went to a person named Judy. Judging by the con-versation, Judy was not the same woman with whom Anthony had been previously speaking. Many of the same themes were struck, except that Anthony asked her to pick him up when he got out.

About 10 minutes after this call ended, the phone rang and I an-swered it. (In a typical Fairfax Hospital double room there is a single phone line shared by two receivers located near each bed). A female voice said, "Is Anthony there?"

This caller was Rochelle. She talked for about 45 minutes with Anthony, but I could not hear most of the conversation because he had switched to more of a whisper mode. I left the room, took a few laps in the hall and returned . Anthony was still talking on the telephone. I could not determine if he was speaking with Rochelle, or if he was having a second conversation with Judy or "Baby," or yet another new female. Being incredibly tired from the no-sleep scenario of the previous night, I lay down to catch a nap.

I fell asleep almost immediately. In less than 15 minutes I was awakened by the regular cleaning lady, a lovely Korean woman named Myong. She excitedly asked, "Where your roommate?"

As I rubbed my eyes to try to wake up, I looked at Anthony's empty bed and said, "Did you look in the bathroom?"

"He not there either. Look! Over here on the floor!" Myong left the room quickly in search of our daytime nurse, Rachael.

I rather tentatively edged over to see the far side of Anthony's bed. There on the floor was his IV, needle and all, which he had obviously ripped out of his arm before making his get-away! As far as I know, no one in the hospital saw Anthony leave. He certainly did not stop at the cashier's office on the way out. He did, however, obtain free lodging and breakfast out of his ordeal, causing me to wonder how often Anthony used the Fairfax Hospital Bed and Breakfast.

Anthony, I concluded, may have been involved in a drug overdose, but I doubt that it was in response to his girlfriend leaving him. He struck me as a rather typical crack addict who had taken a sufficient quantity of drugs to develop a heart arrhythmia. The E.R. personnel had apparently decided to send him to our floor so that his heart rate could be monitored by the telemetry connected to the leads on his chest. Surprisingly, as he left, he had not "borrowed" the expensive telemetry unit in the front pocket of his gown, which he left lying on the bed. I was guessing, but it certainly appeared to me that Anthony had a sizable stable of girlfriends, or was gainfully employed as a pimp. I wished that he had stayed longer so that we could have talked about the economics of his profession, whatever it was.

I never had a truly dangerous roommate, that is, one whom I felt might cause me or the staff actual bodily harm. I did, however, have one guy who was totally irrational. From the moment of his admission, he continued to yell and curse at every opportunity. His favorite targets were nurses and doctors. The staff resident assigned to him actually walked out in disgust after absorbing more than a safe annual dose of bile from this guy's mouth. His condition was serious enough for me to have some concern about what might happen to me when I went to sleep. Fortunately he was transferred the following morning to somewhere else in the hospital, - hopefully the psychiatric section. I never learned this person's name, nor did I care to. As he left the room on a gurney accompanied by two rather large hospital security guards he delivered a loud stream of obscenities to the nurses.

There were also many really pleasant roommates. One of my favorites was a true gentleman named Dick. He had worked for the CIA for 30 years and now was an Adjunct Professor teaching communications at George Mason University in Fairfax. "Adjunct Professor" is a euphemism for "Rent-a Prof." George Mason was notorious for staffing many of their teaching positions with adjuncts, because they receive no benefits and are not a concern with respect to tenure decisions. Since the metropolitan Washington,

D.C. is awash with Ph.D.'s, many of the local universities love to hire adjuncts.

Dick was a very interesting conversationalist. He did not spend the days telling CIA stories. In fact, he was relatively mum on his days with "the agency." He did indicate that he had been stationed all over the world. I suspect that his specialty had been disinformation, but I never asked. What Dick did talk about openly was his love of salmon fishing and literature. He was exceptionally well-read in a broad array of subjects. Our conversations still form fond memories of my days in the hospital. Dick frequently telephoned me after he had been discharged. He also came in to visit me during my long days on the transplant list in spite of the fact that his own recovery from a heart attack was not going smoothly at home.

Dick, as with many of my roommates, was not married at the time. He did have a very pleasant, long-time girlfriend, Linda. She was a few years younger than Dick, who was in his early 60's. They had separate apartments, but were obviously more in love than many of the married couples I had seen in the hospital. This situation sometimes presented a delicate situation for Dick and Linda. Whenever someone would come into the room and assume that she was his wife, Linda would be addressed as "Mrs." Generally both Dick and Linda chose to let this ride, but sometimes, such as when consent forms had to be signed, it was a problem. Linda was not a next-of-kin, and the hospital did not recognize the term "significant other" for legal purposes. A niece had to fill the next-of-kin gap for Dick. Whether or not this engaging couple ever married I do not know, but I thought that they were wonderful together.

Some of my roommates were in extremely sad situations. One of most depressing cases involved a 65 year old named Gene. Due to arrhythmia problems, he had received an AICD like mine to shock his heart back into a normal rhythm whenever a dangerous situation occurred. The first time Gene was admitted as my roommate, he was being returned from the EP lab. Drs. Friehling and Del Negro had done an EP study on him to attempt to find a medicine which would better control his arrhythmia problem.

Gene was frightened, and with good cause. He had been at home and had received 14 shocks from his AICD in one day. Since the most I had ever received was 6, I could imagine Gene's terror. The force of one shock is more than considerable. In my case, I always doubled over and let out a yell as if I had been kicked in the chest by a mule. The worst part of an AICD shock for me was never the physical pain, but the immediate fear that my heart would not respond to the shock and I would die immediately. The six shocks which I had received in one day had occurred only after my heart had deteriorated into a very dangerous condition. I cannot imagine the terror of 14 shocks! Gene's solution was to lie in bed in the fetal position all day trying to ensure that his device would not fire again. I probably would have done the same thing.

After a few days on a different medicine, another EP study was conducted on Gene with apparently good results. It was determined that he could safely go home because the new medicine had prevented the EP specialists from being able to induce an arrhythmia in the lab.

Gene was discharged that evening. He was unmarried, and all of his brothers and sisters were elderly and could not drive. Three of his sisters had never even learned to drive! A neighbor took Gene to his home.

Two days later, Gene was back on the floor, but in a different room. I was reluctant to go to see him, because I knew that I would have trouble handling the news. I finally mustered up the nerve and went to his room. It was worse than I had imagined. Gene was again curled up in the fetal position on his right side fearing any movement which might set off his device.

It seems that Gene had done well during his one night at home (he lived with an older brother who was at least as sick as Gene), but had started to suffer multiple shocks from his AICD in mid-morning. Near death, he had been brought to the hospital by the 911 team. He was stabilized in the E.R. and placed in the Cardiac Care Unit. The following morning Gene was returned to the EP lab for yet another study. This time the EP team again found a different combination of drugs which apparently were effective in preventing the arrhythmia.

Gene remained on the floor for two more days. He was encouraged to get out of bed and to try to simulate some of his daily activities while he could be monitored closely by the telemetry on the floor. His attitude by now had shifted to where he would rather have the AICD turned off (by a special magnet) and take his chances at home with no electronic protection as opposed to facing the terrifying shocks. "It's a quality of life issue, Ed. I'd rather die at home peacefully. I can't take those damn shocks anymore," he told me. However, two hours after our conversation, he changed his mind and decided to have one more go at it with the device on. The next morning he was discharged and, as before, his neighbor drove him home.

I never saw Gene again. I have been too cowardly to ask Friehling or Del Negro whatever happened to him. Although I hope for the best, I suspect the worst.

Occasionally I would encounter a truly pathetic situation. I was walking in the hall one afternoon when I saw a new roommate being maneuvered into my room. This was an obviously very elderly man who had more tubes sticking out of him than most patients in critical care units. My nurse cautioned me that my new roommate was "a bit confused."

I never learned his name. He was receiving oxygen and multiple medications, if the number of IV lines was an indication. I was told that he was well over 80, that he was Romanian, that he spoke no English, and that he had been in and out of consciousness for several hours. Our night together seemed exceptionally long, because each of his desperate gasps for breath seemed as if it might be his last. "This man is a fighter," I worried to myself as I prayed for him.

Early next morning I asked my nurse why this man was on a cardiac care floor instead of one of the intensive care units. She said that she did not know. He was, she said, in a "no code status," meaning that no extraordinary effort would be made to save him in the event of an emergency. I said that it appeared to me that any heart problems were the least of his worries. She agreed, and said that she heard that he would be moved "sometime today." When nothing happened by noon and the man seemed to be in an even worse condition, I panicked and asked that he be moved immediately to Intensive Care. I went back to my room feeling terrible that I had been so self-centered. This man was not a snorer, he was simply very sick. "Perhaps", I thought, "I have been in here so long myself that I am losing my sense of humanity."

Two hours later I was reading in my bed when I heard the nurse shut off the Romanian's oxygen. He had died while I was reading. Now I felt really guilty. I did not fully understand how the "no code" policy worked. Did the staff pull his plug? Were my complaints instrumental in such a decision? This paranoid nonsense kept going through my mind. For the first time since being in the hospital, I felt that I might be losing control of my own mental state.

Two of my nurses, Mary and Jana, suddenly appeared in the room. "Let's go for a walk, Ed," they said. "We'll talk." Both nurses stayed with me for nearly an hour, helping me to cope with the fact that my roommate had passed away within three feet of me. When I returned to the room, the curtains were totally closed around his bed. I could not help but peek inside. A sheet was pulled over his entire body. I quickly pulled the curtain shut and grimaced. He had died cruelly and alone. Several more hours passed before his body was removed, apparently due to requirements for the man to be pronounced legally dead and the lack of any available next of kin.

I felt particularly bad about the Romanian's death. What especially stuck in my mind was an event which occurred shortly after he had arrived in my room. We were alone, and, as I stood in front of his bed, I waved my hand back and forth to signal hello. I never will forget how this supposedly comatose man raised his right hand and feebly waved acknowledgment. "He isn't unconscious!" I gasped. The thought that he had endured such terrifying final hours, alone and aware, seemed to multiply the tragedy of the situation. The other thought which haunts me is how, in spite of all the tubes down his throat, he kept repeating throughout the night, "Oh, Mama!" When his body was finally removed, I found myself waving again. This time all I could think of to say was, "I never knew you....but, good-bye, my friend."

Perhaps my most unusual roommate was an apparent schizophrenic who had multiple personalities. I privately referred to him as Dr. Jekyll and Mr. Hyde. In his bad phase, I considered him to be Jack the Ripper. When he was good, he was Mother Teresa.

As Jack the Ripper, he was a saturation bomber. This guy had so many different weapons with which to bombard the senses. The first characteristic was his incredibly loud, and irregular snoring. He was not in the same league as the Champ, but he was definitely on my top ten list in terms of sheer obnoxiousness. If this was the Ripper's only weapon, I could have handled his attack. The problem was his simultaneous assault on my sense of smell.

During my days in the Navy I had occasion to encounter some really bad odors. The inherent smell of the atmosphere inside a submarine which has been submerged for over a month without a supply of fresh air from outside is totally disgusting. This punishing scent was a combination of diesel fumes, cooking odors, body sweat, flatulence, and fumes from blowing our "sanitary tanks" overboard (i.e., flushing a day's worth of toilet collections off the ship and into the sea). This nauseating odor permeates everything on board, including clothes, bedding, hair, etc. Those Navy PR photos showing husbands and wives running toward each other to embrace when the submarine returns to port never show what happens next. After a few kisses and hugs, the wife says, "Honey, we have to go home and get you changed." Most of the time the windows were open in our car on the way home, - even in winter.

There were other really evil odors which one could encounter in the Navy, often when overseas. The smell coming from the "river" between the Subic Bay Naval Station and Olongapo, the Philippine city immediately adjacent, was particularly deadly. The river was actually an open sewer, except that Filipino children would swim in it to dive for coins thrown near them by sailors crossing the bridge. We learned to try to hold our breath for the length of the bridge.

Overseas had no monopoly on bad smells. I know this because we had lived in Moss Point, Mississippi during the mid 1970's. Our home was located at what Sharry referred to as "the confluence of five of the most obnoxious odors known." Most were identifiable and were standard fare: an oil refinery, a paper mill, a cat food factory, and an operation which processed pogy (a species of fish which were plentiful in the Gulf Coast area). There was one odor for which we were unable to identify the source. It had, as Sharry liked to describe it, the smell of burnt Brussels sprouts. When the wind brought this one over the house, usually at night, we would waken with our eyes watering - even with all the windows shut and the air conditioning on! The real problem with Moss Point was not any one individual odor, but the fact that no matter which way the wind blew, the smell was annoying.

The odor from the Ripper made these inconvenient moments seem like a walk in the park. The night after he came to my room the smell from his side of the room was indescribable. The "scent" was unique. It turned out to be due to bleeding in his throat from an operation on his esophagus. The blood traveled through his system acting as a mega-laxative causing continuous diarrhea. Hence the killer odor.

As I tried to go to sleep around midnight, I asked my nurse, Kathleen, if she knew of anything which might help. "We have something down at the nurse's station which we sometimes use. It's a liquid and it smells like peppermint."

Before I could ask her more about this possible antidote, she had to leave the room for an emergency situation with another patient. Around two in the morning I was still awake, suffering from the snore and the smell. I rang the call bell and yelled over the intercom, "Kathleen, the peppermint!! **Please** bring the peppermint!"

Another nurse arrived with the magic potion and liberally dosed five balls of cotton with several drops each of the supposed cure-all. I immediately felt as if I had been dropped into the peppermint chewing gum vat at Wrigley's. This new odor was intense, but it was a definite improvement. The bad news is that the Ripper was stronger. After about only 30 minutes of acceptable conditions, his stuff overwhelmed the peppermint stuff in a pitched battle of odor molecules.

I slept very little, if any, that night. In the morning I awoke gagging and desperate. I immediately hopped out of bed, grabbed my IV pole, and headed straight for the door. I spent the next two hours pushing my IV pole back and forth through the hallway, going with a very quick step whenever I passed the door to our room.

The good news is that by late morning the Ripper had stopped bleeding and his diarrhea eased. The nurses washed him (I bet that they had drawn straws for this one) and soon Mother Teresa appeared in the same bed where the Ripper had been lying. The man turned out to be exceptionally pleasant and enjoyable. He listened to classical music on headphones and was never a bother during the day. Unfortunately, when night fell and he slept, the Ripper returned, but in a less dangerous mode, torturing me only with his snoring. I came to like the guy, but was happy to see him go after four days.

Fortunately, I also had several highly entertaining roommates. Two were particularly memorable. The first was a gentleman from Brazil, whose first name I did not obtain. He seemed to be more comfortable calling me "Mister Linz," so I reciprocated and used "Mister _____" with him. We liked one another, but we just never proceeded to first names.

The Brazilian was my roommate for six days during the 1994 World Cup soccer tournament. Since I like soccer very much (having played, refereed, and coached), I was really pleased to watch a true zealot. This man knew soccer. Surprisingly, he was remarkably objective in his analysis of each team in the Cup. He wanted Brazil to win, of course, but his passion was controlled. He could admit when his team was playing poorly and discuss its strengths and weaknesses. The two of us had some interesting conversations with an EKG technician who came to our room daily. He had played soccer professionally in his native Ghana and was very articulate and animated. After my Brazilian friend was discharged, I smiled through the remainder of the tournament whenever I recalled how a Ghanaian, a Brazilian and a North American were brought so closely together in a hospital room by a mutual love of sport.

Another entertaining roommate was a "good ole boy," named Sandy. He was only 32, but he had suffered a heart attack during a softball game. It turned out that Sandy was an excellent softball player. He was a catcher and a first baseman and played in four different slow pitch leagues weekly. Having played considerable softball myself, both slow and fast pitch, in some very competitive leagues throughout my years in the Navy, I had a lot to talk about with Sandy.

Sandy and I also discussed hunting. Although I am no longer a hunter (I gave it up as a teenager when I decided that I enjoyed watching squirrels more than shooting them), I do enjoy listening to others describe their experiences. Sandy was primarily a deer hunter. In fact, much of his life apparently revolved around hunting (when he was not playing softball). He loved to get his limit each season. He would even travel to different states with different hunting seasons to get his limit there also. "I don't mount 'em, I eat 'em, - all of 'em," he explained. "Venison burgers and stew are my favorite foods!" I enjoyed the animation in his voice and facial expressions, but, in view of Sandy's heart problems, I found myself wondering about the fat content of venison. Was this Bambi's revenge?

While walking the halls daily with my IV pole as a companion, I met several female cardiac patients who would have apparently made "OK" roommates. One was Sidney, a lady around 50, whose lifestyle was interesting. She no longer worked and was married to a retired Naval Officer, who had recently retired from a second career. They traveled together all over the world to keep themselves busy. Just in 1994 alone, they had been scuba diving in St. Lucia, climbing mountains in Switzerland, taking in plays in London, and relaxing in Corsica. I did not have the opportunity to ask Sidney how they afforded all of this, but I was envious. Sharry and I have been to many places around the world, but not all in the same year! I did develop a theory as to the financing: the husband was not exactly retired. He was an international drug dealer/arms merchant who shuttled between the Caribbean and Switzerland and God-knows-where-else laundering money and striking deals. Perhaps I have read too many post-Cold War spy novels.

My favorite roommate, by far, was Siobhan. She was not actually a roommate, but of all the patients I met during my stay in Fairfax Hospital, she made the greatest impression, and became my "soul roommate."

Siobhan (pronounced "Shuh-von) was a beautiful 21 year old who had suffered through four years of serious heart problems. By the time of her arrival in Room 271, she had undergone an open heart surgery, numerous electrophysiology studies, the insertion of a pacemaker, and countless different doses of powerful medicines in an attempt to alleviate her heart condition.

She had initially learned of her problem at age 18 early in her first year of study at McGill University in Montreal. While working out with teammates on the crew team (she was a coxswain), she had gone into a life-threatening arrhythmia. She was saved from death in the emergency room of the nearby hospital by the use of shocking paddles, which converted her heart to a normal rhythm. This near-miss occurred in September of 1990, nearly a year prior to my first heart-related hospitalization. Strangely, the Canadian doctors initially assured her that this had been a one-time incident and that there was little cause for concern.

Over the next several months Siobhan suffered numerous other instances of ventricular tachycardia. She was hospitalized frequently. Numerous drugs had been tried to eliminate, or at least control, the arrhythmia. None had been successful.

By February of 1991, Siobhan's illness had been diagnosed as right ventricular dysplasia, a relatively rare disease of unknown cause. Dysplasia itself is a general term for the abnormal development of tissue. In Siobhan's case, her doctors felt that the tissue in the lower portion of the right ventricle of her heart had developed improperly, causing electrical signal conduction from the AV node to the ventricle to be diverted or blocked. This situation, as in my sarcoidosis, creates auxiliary signals leading to a dangerous heart rate at random and unpredictable intervals.

On Valentine's Day, 1991, Siobhan underwent open heart surgery in a hospital in London, Ontario. Her doctors had previously attempted an ablation of an infected section of her right ventricle in an EP lab, but it had been unsuccessful. Within two weeks Siobhan had recovered from the major effects of the open heart surgery, but it soon became evident that this operation had been unsuccessful. Her heart was not well. During the surgery, the doctors had seen considerable fatty tissue instead of muscle in many locations in her heart.

Siobhan returned to her home in Bethesda, Maryland to recover. She spent most of the next year seeing different doctors in several local hospitals. By the fall of 1992, Siobhan was well enough to return to higher education, this time at the University of Vermont. She was now taking an experimental drug, Sotalol, which was being relatively successful in controlling her arrhythmia. During that school year she experienced only 2-3 episodes of tachycardia, and each was converted by the drug, Procainamide, when given through an IV in a local emergency room. In spite of these continuing medical problems, Siobhan referred to this phase as "normal campus life."

While at home in Maryland for the Christmas holidays in 1992, Siobhan suffered another serious episode of v-tach, but was successfully converted to a stable heart rhythm in an emergency room. By this time she realized that she was living with a dangerous disease, but wanted to enjoy as much normalcy in her life as possible. She soon moved from her parent's home in Maryland to an apartment in Alexandria, Virginia to attempt to assume the lifestyle of any young woman her age. She obtained employment in a photography related job and worked from January to November of 1993 with no significant medical episodes.

Suddenly, around Thanksgiving, events turned bad. Siobhan began to suffer serious v-tach at least every two weeks requiring visits to a local E.R. for conversion using intravenous Procainamide. By this time, several cardiologists in the electrophysiology specialty had become aware of Siobhan's case. She was referred by her original cardiologist in London, Ontario, for treatment at the National Institute of Health (NIH) in Washington, D.C. For some still unknown reason, the doctors at NIH recommended installing a pacemaker, and after considerable uncertainty due to communication problems with the NIH staff, her parents agreed to the procedure. Subsequent events showed that the pacemaker was of little assistance.

During this period in the Washington, D.C. area, Siobhan had been taking Quinidine to control her rhythm disturbances. In July 1994, she developed a severe allergic reaction to the drug and had to be rushed to a local hospital in Maryland. She was stabilized, but it was decided that her best hope was to fly to Boston to be seen by Dr. Mark Josephson, a renowned expert in the field of electrophysiology, who was currently at Beth Israel Hospital there. Dr. Josephson performed 19 separate ablations on various locations of fatty tissue in Siobhan's heart during a very lengthy session in the EP lab. Once again, her heart seemed to be stable.

Siobhan returned home to be with her parents. Only a few weeks later, she again went into a dangerous v-tach. She was rushed to the emergency room at Sibley Hospital in Maryland and was successfully converted using the shocking paddles. Sibley had no EP lab facilities, so plans were made to fly her to Boston to be treated by Dr. Josephson. By this time Siobhan had relapsed into sustained v-tach at 240 bpm. She was converted again with the paddles. Although a private jet was already in the air from New York to pick up Siobhan for an emergency transfer to Boston, her parents canceled the aircraft on the advice of the Sibley cardiologists who unanimously agreed that the uncertainty of the commute to the airports and the flight itself was too dangerous. Instead, she was transferred by ambulance to Fairfax Hospital across the Potomac River in nearby Virginia in order to receive immediate assistance from the arrhythmia specialists, Friehling and Del Negro, who also had national reputations.

I first met Siobhan and her family two days later. Kathleen, my good friend and nurse on the second floor, asked me to talk to Siobhan because our conditions and case histories were so similar. I was immediately struck by Siobhan's beauty and outgoing personality. She had long blonde hair and was obviously an expert at charming people. It was also immediately apparent that she was knowledgeable and articulate about her medical condition.

Over the next several days we became friends. I had the opportunity to observe her closely as she scheduled visits by her many boyfriends so as to avoid an overlap. In view of the sheer numbers, this was not an easy task. Hers was a wide assortment of suitors, ranging in personality and appearance. At least two were, as she described them, "former fiancés."

We pushed our IV poles in front of us as we walked the halls together, sharing thoughts about our common medical experiences and our mutual bad luck. I also became her official love-life advisor (a position for which I was uniquely unqualified). However, the lack of meaningful experience had never before stopped me from commenting on a topic.

I gave her the same advice which I had given to my classes at Woodbridge each year, "Only two things are important in life for someone your age: color coordination and marrying rich, at least the first two or three times. If you have to choose, color coordination is the more important."

"It would be difficult to accomplish either of those objectives in this stupid hospital gown," she lamented. I had to agree.

It soon became apparent, however, that Siobhan's ability to attract young men was not hindered by a hospital gown. One of the monitor technicians, an exceptionally nice young man, became instantly infatuated with her. He had to take a number, because even the construction men who were remodeling the area would typically stop their work to gawk at Siobhan as she passed by in the hall. I frequently kidded about her ability to overwhelm these defenseless guys. "You have intoxicated them, Siobhan," I teased. "They've become Siobhanaholics, and there is no known cure." In response, she would just smile and change the subject.

Siobhan had another side to her. She was absolutely one of the bravest people I have met. She rarely complained about her condition. Instead, she tried to concentrate on the positive. During her free time she was drafting an outline for a fictional novel (about a murder in a hospital!), sketching objects, corresponding with several long-distance admirers, and throughout it all, smiling endlessly.

As I watched Siobhan's medical treatment, I began to feel a strong sense of deja vu. The same arrhythmia team, Drs. Friehling and Del Negro, placed her on a loading dose of Amiodarone similar to that which I had undergone almost exactly three years earlier. During the week-long period she was receiving the initial large doses of the medication, I recommended that she and her parents contact one of the hospital's transplant coordinators to receive information about a possible heart transplant if such became necessary in the future. Sharry and I had benefited greatly from our talk with members of the heart transplant team when I had been hospitalized earlier for the Amiodarone therapy. A meeting was held, but, as in my case, no immediate decision was made.

The EP procedure by Friehling and Del Negro on Siobhan following her Amiodarone loading consisted of ablating the location which was producing the dangerous rate of 240 bpm and then doing tests to insure that the Amiodarone was preventing other sites from producing severe v-tach. Basically, under the circumstances, the procedure was a success. As the result of this study, both doctors strongly recommended the removal of the ill-placed NIH pacemaker lead, which would also be a problem if a defibrillator might be required in the future. The following day, the lead, which had been screwed into the inside of the heart, was removed. Because there was some possibility of creating a fatal bleeding scenario, the complex procedure was performed by Friehling and Del Negro in an operating room with a heart surgeon standing by in the event that he might have to open her chest for emergency heart surgery to stop the bleeding.

Fortunately the misplaced lead was successfully removed, a new one was installed, and Siobhan was returned to her room the next day following a difficult night in the Cardiac Care Unit. After a day's rest and recuperation, she was given a standard treadmill stress test, which she passed satisfactorily. She was discharged later that day.

As she left for home, I prayed that Siobhan would never again have to see the inside of a hospital. I was also experienced enough to know from my own condition that such was not likely to be the case. Medicines are often only a stopgap measure to attempt to delay the inevitable. In the event of a progressive heart disease, there would probably be a point when chemicals were no longer effective and she would need a new heart.

I identified closely with Siobhan. She was enduring an equally dangerous heart disease. Her disease had manifested itself before mine, and she had undergone far more procedures than I. She had experienced the same fear and terror which I had felt each time my heart began to race out of control. The tragic point from my perspective was that this young fighter was almost exactly 30 years younger than I.

Siobhan proved to be a great source of strength for me. Whenever I began to feel sorry for myself, I would think of her smile and her courage. I had enjoyed a long run of good fortune before my medical disaster occurred. I had a wonderful family, had enjoyed considerable professional success in two different fields, and had seen the world. This girl still had her entire adult life in front of her. Siobhan had helped me to realize how incredibly lucky I have been. She became one of my most effective sources of inspiration. I now think of her and pray for her daily. She deserves a break.

One day a nurse on the floor told me that she thought that hospitals should be built only with private rooms. In spite of my unfavorable experiences with some roommates, I disagreed with her. It would be very lonely, and sometimes frightening, to be sick in a room by yourself. While I did enjoy the quiet of the occasional day without someone in the bed next to me, I was generally eager to have another patient assigned to my room so that I could have someone to talk to. There is also a sense of security provided by having a roommate. I felt, in most cases, that if I had a problem during the night, I could get help by yelling to the roommate, - unless he was a very sick Romanian, or a snorer who was out cold, or an older man with no hearing, or.............

So how would I evaluate myself as a roommate for someone else?

Perfect, of course!

Chapter 12

THE WAIT

As I looked out the window from my hospital bed in Room 277, I mentally surveyed the situation. Other than the IV lines running into my left arm, I had no outward appearance of a person dying, or even seriously ill. My coloration was good, I looked "healthy," my mind was alert, I had a good appetite, and I was mobile. Perhaps because of these positive external appearances, I myself had not given much thought to what might lie ahead in the future. Even though all of my doctors had told me that my only remaining chance for survival was a new heart, I had not considered in detail the mechanics of a heart transplant, much less the logistics, the risk, or the moral and ethical issues. Now that I was apparently in an indefinite holding pattern, I had time to reflect on many such concerns. I had entered "THE WAIT." It could be days, weeks, months, or even over a year before I might receive a new heart. Of course, I could also die while waiting. The only certainty was that I was not in control.

Because I now met the appropriate criteria, including continuous hospitalization to keep me alive, my doctors were able to list me as a "Category 1" candidate. At the time (June 22, 1994) there were two categories, 1 and 2, on the national list for those awaiting heart transplants. Category 2 candidates had serious, but not immediately life-threatening, heart diseases. I interpreted my status to mean that I was at, or very close to, the top of the heart transplant list in the Washington, D.C. area, at least for my blood type, O+. There were different lists for each blood type; a heart from a person with A- blood, for example, would not help me.

"Surely the next O+ heart will be mine!" I thought.

Then I learned that this was not exactly the case. There was one other O+ ahead of me on the list for the Washington area. He was a young Korean, who was also hospitalized at Fairfax. One of the transplant coordinators, Paige Roberts, assured me that he was not really ahead of me on the list, because we were not "competing" for the same heart. In addition to blood type, Paige explained, the donor's heart has to be able to physically fit in the recipient's body. Due to the Korean's small size and weight (120 pounds), he required a small heart. My body (185 pounds) necessitated a larger organ. There is generally a ± 30 percent factor on the weight issue (although this number is being frequently debated and changed in the heart transplant community). I could probably successfully receive a heart from a donor ranging in weight from approximately 130 to 240 pounds.

I did not feel strongly one way or another about this until three weeks later when the fellow received a donor heart and **walked** out the front door of the hospital 10 days later. I was still waiting. For the next few days I felt cheated, but then the rationalization process took over, and I was able to put aside my disappointment. I did not think often about the fact that someone else would have to die for me to live. In my state of mind, I was worried only about myself.

Shortly before being placed on the transplant list, Dr. Friehling, working together with Dr. Matthews, decided that I should be placed on a powerful drug, Dopamine, which must be given intravenously. A new dedicated IV line was started just for the Dopamine, which was being given in a very small quantity (3cc/hr). The new IV turned out to be a major problem, because the low flow rate made it susceptible to clogging in the feeder line. Instead of the normal three day interval after which the IV site must be changed (to minimize the risk of infection), I found myself getting poked in the arm at least every 36 hours because of these flow problems.

An additional problem with Dopamine is that it is very damaging to flesh if a portion of the drug somehow escapes out of the vein. When this occurs, the patient must receive an antidote, which is administered by inserting a needle into several locations in the affected area. This is a particularly painful process. I also noticed that the vein in my arm into which the Dopamine IV line was inserted would start to turn white as the drug worked its way into my circulatory system. This did not hurt, but it always worried me.

By the end of one week on Dopamine, my left arm was a total mess. It had become entirely purple from wrist to elbow. I was beginning to experience pain throughout the arm. My doctors and nurses had been following the situation closely. Dr. Rogan, the cardiologist on the transplant team, became involved. In view of the uncertainty of how long I might have to wait for a donor heart, he recommended that I undergo a minor surgical procedure in which a "Groshong" catheter would be inserted directly into a central vein, the superior vena cava, in my chest. The procedure is named after Dr. LeRoy Groshong, a surgical oncologist, who developed the procedure in 1978 to provide an improved lifestyle for patients requiring long-term IV treatment. In my case, such a device (basically a tube made of soft, silicone rubber) would allow the Dopamine to flow directly into the large vein returning blood to the heart. Other drugs, additional blood, or even nutritional fluids, could also be added through the Groshong, thus eliminating the need for routine IVs in the arm.

Although there is always a risk associated with any surgery, Sharry and I quickly agreed to the procedure. We both knew that my arms would become progressively worse due to the IV damage unless something was done. Our response was, "The quicker, the better."

A general surgeon performed the procedure on June 28, the 7th day of THE WAIT. The entire process took less than an hour. After the tip of the catheter was put into place in the vein, the other end was tunneled under my skin to an exit site further down my chest to allow for easy access and care. When a liquid medication, or any IV fluid, is introduced into the lumen (tubing) of the Groshong, an internal valve opens allowing the fluid to flow directly into the bloodstream. When suction is applied from the outside, the same valve now opens in the opposite direction to allow blood to be drawn into a syringe. At all other times the valve remains closed. The Groshong is designed to be used for a long haul, from several weeks to a few years. I was hoping for the former.

I was sore for the next several days in the area of the chest where the line had been implanted, but the pain was minor compared to what had been taking place in my arms with the Dopamine IV. I now no longer had a need for IVs in my arms, because of the Groshong's two lines. I could receive two different drugs simultaneously, if required. One line could also be used for drawing blood.

The Dopamine would be shut off temporarily, the line flushed with a saline solution, and then the blood was drawn directly from the central vein. This meant no more needle sticks!

Throughout the remainder of THE WAIT I was always very happy to have my new friend, the Groshong, as part of me. Jean, my daytime lead nurse, hung a handwritten sign above my bed saying, "RN DRAW." This meant that the only people who could draw blood samples from me were RNs trained to use the Groshong. It always gave me great delight each morning when the lab tech would come into the room with a cart full of needles and other blood sucking paraphernalia, because I would smile, point to Jean's sign, and say, "Sorry, RN Draw." Under my breath I would add "See ya" or some other more crude admonition. In order to keep sane, I tried to grasp whatever small pleasures that became available. Small was definitely the operative word here, but I continued to look forward to such encounters.

The Groshong did become clogged once due to clotting caused by the extremely low flow rate of the Dopamine. Dr. Rogan fixed this by ordering that Urokinase, an enzyme to break down the clotting, be inserted into both lines of the tubing. It took about two hours for the Urokinase to be successful. I liked to think of it as sort of a medical version of Liquid Plumber. In order to help prevent a recurrence, Rogan ordered that another IV solution, "half normal" saline, be added through the second line of the Groshong to keep the Dopamine flowing in the future. This worked out very well, and I had no other clotting problems.

What was not working out well was my digestive system. I became constipated (for the first time in my life) because my right-side heart failure had decreased blood circulation to my bowels. My favorite first year resident (the term "intern" is no longer used at Fairfax Hospital), Jon Sheinberg, took it upon himself to fix my problem. He began with milk of magnesia, which did absolutely nothing. We rapidly progressed to milk of magnesia with cascara. I referred to it as "Super Milk of Magnesia", but it did not work. I had also been taking a stool softener pill daily for over a week, but it had produced no help. The next step ordered by Jon was another medication, Dulcolax, which was also ineffective. Suppositories, the missile shaped slippery variety, were then inserted you know where.

They also failed to help. By this time I was feeling fairly miserable and had developed considerable empathy toward those who are perpetually inflicted with bowel problems.

I had now begun to throw up at least once a day. I received several Fleet enemas, but in spite of producing some rather dramatic noises, they were also not helpful. By the fifth day, Jon told me that we would now try "the final solution." He prescribed Magnesium Citrate, which looks like a 7 Up in a green bottle. I assure you that this stuff does not taste like 7 Up! After pouring it over two cups of ice, I drank the entire bottle, sip by disagreeable sip. It was your basic laxative on-the-rocks cocktail. Six hours later my constipation was history, at least for a few days. For the next two weeks I had to take this potion several times, but then, with no apparent change in my routine or other medications, the constipation problem disappeared.

There were other new experiences for me during THE WAIT. I had to learn how to endure "life on a rope." Because I was permanently on the dual IV regimen of Dopamine and the saline solution, I was tethered to a device which looks like a rolling coat rack. The nurses call it an IV pole. I do not know whether it has a more formal name. I do know that many of my fellow patients on the floor had their own names for the device. The pole, which can be adjusted to variable heights from about 5 to 8 feet, has four wheels on bottom to allow it to roll freely. Unfortunately, my first pole had considerable friction in the wheels and was difficult to push comfortably. One day, while in the hallway outside my room, I swapped it for a new one left standing unattended.

At the top of the pole, there are four curled hooks from which the IV bags are hung. Clear plastic tubing carrying the IV solution runs from the bags to a flow control device. Mine was labeled "Quest 2001, Intelligent Infusor." Actually it was not so intelligent. A more fitting name would have been the "Confusing Infusing Machine," but I suspect that this would have created marketing problems for the manufacturer.

I had two Infusors, one for each IV. Since both were electrically powered, they had to be plugged into a wall outlet when bedside. Whenever I wanted to leave the immediate vicinity of the bed, I had to unplug the electrical cords (which were about 8 feet long), wrap the cord in loops around the back of the Infusors, and proceed to my destination, whether it be the bathroom or a stroll in the hall. The Infusor can continue to function on its internal battery for several hours, but if it begins to run out of power, it emits a piercing screech to warn anyone within five miles. Even if the Infusor is immediately rescued by plugging it into an electrical outlet, it continues to wail for several minutes as if it were a spoiled child.

The plastic tubing which carries the IV solution from the Infusor to my Groshong was only about 6 feet long, so I always had to push the pole in front of me wherever I went. This became a routine procedure, demonstrating that the spirit of Sisyphus was alive and well in the halls of Fairfax. On several occasions, particularly as I attempted to maneuver at night with the lights out in the room, the plastic tubing would become tangled around the pole, or me, or both. I would like to see a video of how I extricated myself from this mess, but somehow I always managed to correct the problem. Perhaps it was the experience which I gained during childhood untangling yo-yo string that carried me through these silly situations.

During my initial days at the top of the transplant list, I had been wildly optimistic, and, in retrospect, unrealistic. I had based my hopes on the fact that there had been three heart transplants at Fairfax Hospital in a single 24 hour period a week before I was placed on the list. Surely my wait would be a few weeks at worst. Unfortunately, I had forgotten all the lessons I had learned from courses in Probability and Statistics during my college days.

My close friend, John Schrader, with whom I had been in a football pool for the past ten years, was teaching a Statistics course each semester at George Mason University. After approximately six weeks had passed with no action, I decided to obtain data from the transplant coordinator, Linda Ohler, to learn how many O+ hearts of my body size had been transplanted during a 12 month period at Fairfax. The initial report which Linda gave me was not exactly cheerful, because the average wait time at Fairfax for an O+ heart was 238 days. For the entire Washington, D.C. area, the news was even worse - a wait of 456 days for those who had received hearts in calendar year 1993, and 300 days for 1994.

After thinking about this data, I realized that it was interesting, but not necessarily applicable to my situation. The "average wait time" was based on **all** those who had received transplants, both Category 1 and Category 2. Many of the latter had been waiting at home for extended periods of time; in most cases, over a year. One recipient had waited 1,433 days!

The data on which my predicted wait time should be based, John and I decided, was the total number of O+ transplants performed in a year in the entire D.C. area consortium. Since I was at the top of the list, I would automatically receive the next available heart. I was not waiting at home to move up the queue. No one else in Category 1 in any of the local hospitals could jump ahead of me. Thus the important statistic was the mean number of days between O+ transplants in the preceding year, or the preceding 12 months. (It turned out that the two numbers were nearly identical).

The total number of O+ transplants was 16. I made the conservative assumptions that there are essentially three size hearts: small, medium, and large, and that there was an equal distribution of each. In a typical year, therefore, an average 5.33 transplants of my size heart would be performed. This number translates to a mean number of days between transplants of 68.4 days.

I passed this new information to John. He performed the calculations and informed me that I seemed to be headed toward the "unlucky" area, at least from a statistical perspective. After a one month wait at the top of the list, a patient should have received a new heart 35 times out of 100. At two months, the new heart comes 58 percent of the time. By the 75th day on the list, 2 out of 3 O+ patients have had a donor. John's calculations did not make me feel better.

Bear in mind that Dr. Rogan had told me initially that a four month wait was "about the average." Of course, I had dismissed that as obviously impossible, since O+ is the most common blood type and my body size was average. I assumed that he had said four months rather than the real, much smaller, number because he did not want to crush my spirits when that shorter period had passed by with no action. Unfortunately Rogan's estimate was far closer to the actual value for me. So much for statistics.

At first I discounted John's analysis. This was the same guy who used copious quantities of data, analyzed and computed, and still could not beat most of us in picking NFL football winners against the spread. Soon, however, I realized that his numbers were correct, statistically speaking. My reaction to this reality check was not acceptance, but the thought that, being a close friend, he should have lied to me!

From Day 1 on the list, I had written "Day ___ of 180 ±" on the large wall calendar labeled "Today Is" opposite my bed. Each morning I would fill in the ___with the actual number of days that I had been at the top of the transplant list. For example, on the calendar date for Saturday, August 20, 1994, I had written "Day 60 of 180 ±" in a green magic marker shortly after arising that morning.

I was mimicking the same practice I had used as a teacher when I would enter my classroom each morning. Our school year was mandated by the state to have at least 180 days of class in order to receive certification. In order to ensure that this minimum number would be met, our district schedules five additional "snow days" in each year's school calendar. I always told my students that it was foolhardy to count down the number of days until graduation or the end of the school year, because we had no knowledge of exactly how many snow days, if any, would be used. We could go the full 185 days, or as few as 180 days. What we did know for *certain* was the actual number of days that we had been together that school year. For example, on the blackboard I would put up the following:

> **Good Morning!**
> **Wednesday, October 12, 1994**
> **Day 37 of 180 +**
> **Objective:** _____

The + sign was an indication that we could have school for at least 180 days, but perhaps 185, if we were "unlucky." I would then encourage my students to start praying immediately for big-time snow.

I continued to explain, "I love teaching dearly, and being around you in particular, but you are all going to receive the same credit for this school year whether you have 180 or 185 days of class. I myself will be paid the same no matter how many class days we have. So what are we, a bunch of stupid-faces? Bring on the snow! I am holding each of you personally accountable."

This approach was always a big seller, although I suspect that more than a few parents called the principal to express their concern over this subversive teacher. I always felt particularly elated when something totally unexpected would occur, such as the "hurricane" day in early October one year. My students had willed it in here. What was really warming was the fact that the hurricane veered course at the last minute, and our entire area suffered no damage whatsoever. Another classic "snow day" situation resulted from an incident one year when a disgruntled student attempted to burn down the school. Apparently he had not received the part in a school play which he wanted, so he came in that evening with gasoline and set fire to the auditorium. His arson attempt was only mildly successful, but we did not have school for two days afterwards while the smoke damage was cleaned.

So I was accustomed to counting up, vice counting down. This turned out to be a very useful skill during THE WAIT.

After Day 60, I found myself taking no consolation from the fact that I might be on the way to setting a local or national record. In my initial days I had perked up with hope whenever I heard one of the hospital helicopters landing or an ambulance arriving to take a patient to the emergency room. Surely that must be my heart! Each time I was wrong. Following an extended series of such disappointments I began to disregard emergency vehicles coming and going. They had been of no help, so why should I take any further interest in their chopper sounds and wailing sirens?

Major holidays involving heavy traffic on the interstate highways were also duds. Although I had been on the list for just over ten days, I had developed big hopes for action over the Fourth of July weekend. It turned out to be a total bust. Labor Day weekend was also a major disappointment. I found myself in the perverse state of mind hoping for an auto accident involving massive head injuries, so that I might receive a donor heart. At first, I felt guilty about this. Soon I began to rationalize that accidents were going to occur with, or without, my being in the hospital. So why should I not benefit?

I even reached the point where I started to form conspiracy theories. It turned out, in my mind, that the **real** reason that car seats and air bags had become mandatory devices in cars was that they tended to offer effective protection against head injuries in an accident. These safety guys had been scheming against me for several years. Now their perfidy was striking my life directly. It had all been a plot. Another group of anti-Linz people were the ones who promoted safety helmet legislation for motorcyclists. Wild and crazy bikers could now hit a tree head on and still have a reasonably sound brain. "I need brain-dead, not just a mangled body," I complained to myself during one of these irrational periods.

Another group who hated me in my conspiracy theories was the drug dealers. They would get people hooked on drugs, a drive-by shooting in the head would occur as the result of a drug-related dispute, but the heart would not be available because the victim had become an IV drug abuser and was now HIV positive or a Hepatitis B carrier.

Of course, these conspiracies theories were all very sick responses to feeling sorry for myself. Although I openly kidded with close friends about these feelings, I found myself being drawn further each day into believing many of these crazy things. Too much time alone with your own thoughts, particularly at night just before falling asleep, does this to you.

What did keep me going was a self discipline to keep very busy every day. To do this I developed a daily routine. I believe that I adopted this procedure based upon my experience making extended submarine patrols during my Navy days. The ship would leave port, soon submerge, and remain underwater for over two months. Each man on board had his own means of avoiding insanity during these stressful periods of isolation. My technique was to create a daily routine which would keep me busy. It was a mixture of work and leisure which could be adjusted to the requirements of the patrol. If we were actively chasing Soviet submarines, I would sleep little for days on end. Even during these extremely dangerous and stressful periods, I would find time to do my daily activities, such as reading 50 pages of a novel, or working out by running in place for 30 minutes continuously.

My daily hospital routine evolved rather quickly. At no time did I allow myself to lie around bemoaning my fate. I established certain "must be done daily" activities. I believe that I accomplished each one every day during THE WAIT. Well, maybe once or twice I was bad, surely no more.

My day starts at 7:55 AM when the food handler brings in breakfast in a covered tray. I am still in bed, but I always awaken. I request, "Please put it on the chair. Leave the lid on, please."

The rest of the day begins on a sour note - literally. After making it through the night with two doses of Procan (generic: procainamide) at 10 PM and 6 AM, my mouth tastes and smells like bile. It is always touch and go as to whether I will throw up or not. I usually try to grab a quick, but small, mouthful of water. I do not swallow, but swirl it around in my mouth as I race toward the bathroom. "Race" is the wrong word, because I must first unplug my IV monitors, ensure that I am not tangled up, and then shuffle quickly to the other side of the room. At this time I either spit in the sink or throw up. It is impossible to predict which will occur.

Assuming that all goes well, I take one of my approximately ten urinations daily due to the effective action of the two diuretics, Lasix (furosemide) and Zaroxolyn (metolazone). I then brush my teeth and tongue vigorously to try to rid my mouth of the incredibly acrid taste, use mouth wash, and plunk in a stick of Spearmint gum. I soak my face in a hot wash cloth and am ready to meet the world.

I return to my bedside to open the blinds. Since I have so many things (photos, books, a basket of fruit, a Washington Redskins piggy bank, a Korean doll set (given to me by a former student, Irene Oh), personal diaries from 1988 to present, at least three small containers of fruit juice, and considerable research material) piled on the window ledge I have to carefully adjust each so that I can open the pull blinds without a disaster. One morning I tried to do this too carelessly and my prized Redskins bank fell off onto the floor, breaking in the process. My friend "CG" Caruthers made me a replacement within a week. He had made the original, and he was totally sporting about producing another.

My next event is morning prayer. I always silently thank the Lord that he has brought me safely through another night. Then I read the appropriate daily devotion from *Portals of Prayer*, a small quarterly paperback of prayers for each day. It had been sent to me by my cousin, Carole Ulmer. I found the thoughts to be mixed in inspirational impact, but always reassuring. The prayer session helped me to keep my situation in perspective. Whenever I began to feel sorry for myself, I found that this religious moment was a quick tonic to put me back into the real world of universal suffering. Compared to many others, I had it easy. The Lord was indeed watching over me. My day would come. Even if things did not work out with the transplant, I felt ready to face the joy of the afterlife.

As I enter the hallway I begin my daily "laps." I had designated a round-trip walk of the length of the hall as one lap. My goal is to do at least ten laps daily. One day during the 60's (of the 180±) I met a fellow patient named John. He also was a walker, and together we calibrated our respective paces to determine the length of the hall. There was a marked 100 foot section on the wall. We counted our paces to cover this 100 feet several times until we had a consistent value. We then slowly walked the entire length counting our footsteps along the way. Although we had different length and styles of stride, we came to nearly the exact number on the length. We agreed that my lap was 260 feet in one direction, and his longer version was 305. We checked each other and were able to determine that we were both walking (shuffling along is a more accurate descriptor) approximately one mile each day. Not bad, considering that I was also pushing the IV pole with its lines going into my chest during these "walks." I was sorry to see John leave because he was a great walking partner.

At some time during my morning laps I encounter my nurse for the day. It is part of my treatment plan to be weighed each morning before I eat. The concern is that I might be suddenly putting on weight due to water retention, and the amount of diuretics would have to be increased. Fairfax uses beam balance scales, and the nurses soon learned to indulge me by allowing me to go through a weighing ritual. I check the balance of the beam with no weight on the scale, then move the large weight to 200 pounds. I put my robe on the counter near the scale, ask the nurse to hold the telemetry transmitter device which is kept in the front pocket of my hospital gown box (so that the 1/4 pound device is not considered as part of me) and step on confidently. If the beam stays in the lowered position, I exclaim, "Yes!!"

Of course, I know that I no longer weigh 200 pounds, but I did when I came into the hospital in early June. So it is already a moral victory. Then I move the large weight to 150 pounds while sliding the smaller weight to 50 pounds so that the combined effect is still 200 pounds. I slowly edge the smaller weight to the left, saying "Yes!" several more times along the way.

For the first several weeks I was in the 190's. Soon I broke through the 190 plateau, and started to reach regions that no scale had known with respect to my body for at least four years. I slowly edge the weight further to the left until the beam starts to balance. With obvious pride I step off the scale and ask the nurse to announce the result. (I would read the result myself, but my glasses are back in the room - another part of the ritual).

I then go directly to the room, exchange flip flops for a pair of Thorlo padded socks, and ease into my daytime slippers. Upon entering the room I usually exchange pleasantries with my roommate of the day, as he has always completed his breakfast by then. It is approximately 8:30 AM. I am not sure just how some of these roommates manage to eat their breakfast after hearing my gagging and/or throwing up, but they do. This is either a strong testimonial to Fairfax Hospital breakfast food, or an indication of just how hungry they are. I would guess the latter.

I am still not interested in eating at this time. I begin to write letters and thank you notes for yesterday's get well cards and visitors. At **exactly** 9 AM I dial 3351 to the Volunteer office to request a copy of both *The Washington Post* and *The Washington Times*. I have tried 3351 slightly before 9, but there is no answer. Those volunteers are more disciplined than I. They do not answer anyone until 9 or after. After 60 days of 180 ±, I begin to notice that many of the volunteers who answer the phones know me well enough to respond to my, "Hello, this is Ed Linz in 277," by interrupting me and saying, "It's a *Post* and a *Times*. Right, Mr. Linz?" This always depresses me. There are at least 20 different volunteers (mostly senior citizens, one an 82 year old lady who looks no older than 60). If I have been here long enough that they all know me, I indeed have a problem.

My daily routine continues with breakfast at around 9:15 AM. After becoming quickly disenchanted with "cholesterol-free" eggs and hospital pancakes, I had learned to order dry cereal. This entrée could handle the wait indefinitely, and was always satisfactory for my morning tastes.

On more than one occasion I telephoned the hospital dietitian to launch a petty complaint about the food service. Most of my gripes were silly, such as one concerning the substitution of All-Bran for the Cheerios which I had ordered. "Have you ever **tasted** All-Bran?" I yelled.

Apparently the dietitian was accustomed to receiving such calls, or she was an honors graduate of a Dale Carnegie course, because she chose not to respond to the bait. She simply replied, "I'll see what I can do."

My battles with the dietitian had absolutely nothing to do with either her personally or the food. I had decided that I needed a villain during my stay, someone on whom I could blame all of my woes. All the nursing staff and doctors were far too nice to use as targets of wrath. Besides, I learned long ago never to pick a fight with people who can hurt you at a moment of their choosing. I had learned this lesson the hard way as a junior officer in the Navy when I had sharply criticized one of the mess stewards for his delivery of food to the wardroom table. Within a week, guess who had "accidentally" received a bowl of hot soup in his lap?

Early on during my work-up to be placed on the transplant list, the transplant dietitian had decided (unilaterally) that my weight was too high. She promised, "I will help you fix it." Her solution was a very low calorie diet, around 1500 each day. Since I was approximately 200 pounds at the time, I agreed that I could lose some weight. At this time, however, my ankles were swollen from excessive fluid retention due to right side heart failure. My hospital diet, I decided, was not a big player in this issue, particularly since the menu for all of us on the cardiac floor was already devoid of any fat (or taste). So while I said, "Sure," to the dietitian's analysis, I was already plotting how to circumvent her plan.

Within a few days I had lost five pounds of water weight due to the action of the diuretics. After three weeks I was down to 193 pounds. I was also going crazy. I had now become intimate with the repetitive hospital menu. I knew to avoid the beef in any form. The chicken was pleasant enough if one does not mind meat with absolutely no moisture. The baked fish was indeed baked, perhaps three times too long. The bright note was the pasta, which was always rather tasty, if one is a fan of non-cheese cheese. The salad plates were very good.

Based upon this in-depth analysis I asked Dr. Matthews if Sharry could bring me some "real" food in the evenings. To my surprise and delight, he gave me an enthusiastic "Of course." I was now free! The first night we had a steak sandwich, fries, and onion rings from Fuddruckers, a chain restaurant not known for a heart-friendly menu. It was naughty, but it was also a symbol of some degree of freedom.

From that night on, Sharry and I always had dinner together, either in my room when I had no roommate, or in a small closed consultation room a short distance down the hall from my room. Ninety percent of our meals were actually better nutritionally than the hospital fare. Both Sharry and our daughter, Emily, are excellent cooks in terms of low calorie, low salt meals. We always had several fresh vegetables, and I was very conscientious about consuming moderate quantities. During the day I would eat the cereal for breakfast, a hospital deli sandwich for lunch, and our real meal together at night. Under this rational plan I lost additional weight and plateaued at 185-187 pounds for the next several weeks.

I chose not to share my new, enhanced diet with the dietitian. Instead, I silently declared war. Each day I would order a full meal, although I ate little of it. I would scan each tray as it was delivered to see if any mistakes or omissions had been made. She made the first strike. A breakfast at about Day 30 had my order of skim milk crossed out with "half cup only" written next to it. I could have received some additional milk from the nurses on the floor, but I decided to try to make it through a bowl of Raisin Bran on the "dietetically correct" amount of milk. By the time I finished the cereal enhanced with a scent of milk, I was sufficiently steamed to deliver a real blast to my foe. I wrote her a caustic note asking if she had ever eaten *dry* Raisin Bran. She telephoned back later in the day capitulating on the milk ration.

Now that I had the dietitian on the defensive, I went after her on the lunch menu on the "Or Choose From The Deli" section. The daily selections for fillings on the sandwich are "Lean Roast Beef,

Turkey, Special Tuna Salad, and Special Chicken Salad." I have already discussed the beef and poultry problem. The tuna and chicken salads sounded great, but the betrayal came with the word "special." Special, I decided based on personal experience, meant "no resemblance in taste, smell, or texture to the real thing." Just to see what would happen, one day when ordering, I wrote in "Ham." To my surprise, a ham sandwich on rye arrived the next day, with the dietitian's handwritten "OK" next to my ham request. A few days later I decided to push the menu envelope further in my favor. I wrote in "Egg Salad," and much to my astonishment I received an actual egg salad deli roll with chunks of egg white showing. Along with the egg salad, I was on a roll, so to speak.

It was not very long until the dietitian counter-attacked. She began inserting "DIET" next to the gelatin cube selection that I frequently ordered. The regular stuff came in somewhat pleasing cubes, but this diet variant was in a small dish and had absolutely no taste. It was somewhat as I imagined a colorized gel of newspaper might taste. I ultimately won that one also, but only after further negotiation.

As the days of THE WAIT dragged on throughout the summer, I found myself becoming increasingly petty about the food. Any error or deviation from what I had ordered made my day. "Is there a shortage of lettuce and tomato in the area?" I asked sarcastically one day, in what had become my frequent telephone calls to the dietitian. "Can I perhaps help you to have some shipped in from the West Coast? And when was the last time you reviewed the quality control procedures in your department?" I could almost hear her teeth clench.

I realized that my behavior was totally unnecessary, unprofessional, and un....everything. But I also knew that this phony war was helping to keep me going during THE WAIT. I desperately needed someone/something as an anger and frustration outlet. Prisoners on Death Row have natural objects on which to focus their wrath - guards, wardens, lawyers, juries, society itself, etc. While on Life Row, I had to invent something, and, the dietitian became my foil.

During the remainder of my morning I complete several additional letters and thank you notes. I also stuff several envelopes of clipped newspaper articles to send to my friend, Spurway. Most of these stories involved mutual financial woes (such as our investment in an electronic company named Proteon, whose stock had gone south since we bought it) or ads and news with a certain sexual innuendo, such as the Wonderbra ads which flooded the local papers that summer when it made its debut.

The next big deal of the morning is bathing. Since I am unable to shower due to my IV, I have to wash myself using a washcloth in the sink. I tried to turn this into a pleasant ritual, something to look forward to each day. I go out to the clean laundry cart in the hallway, pick up three washcloths and five towels, and return to begin 20 minutes of relative bliss. I drag a chair from the room, place it in front of the sink, and begin by shaving. All of the towels and washcloths later, I finish and put on new pajama bottoms and socks.

This washing thing is not without risk. Before I wash my chest I must remove the five monitor leads attached to that area of my body. Thus I am totally unmonitored and unprotected by the technician at the nurse's main station during this period. Every day I wonder if I will have a dangerous arrhythmia while I am not being monitored and be found on the bathroom floor after sudden death. It is a definite risk, but the doctors know about it, the nursing staff is well aware, and I am certainly more than aware. Life is a series of trade-offs, even on Life Row.

After the bath, I apply large quantities of lotion to my chest, which has become mildly allergic to the ointment and moisture under the monitoring leads. I then return to my bedside, buzz the nurse on the call button, and proudly announce, "I am ready to be re-wired."

The nurse arrives relatively soon, I am wired up, and I eat the deli sandwich which has been sitting untouched with the rest of my lunch for the past 20-30 minutes. I also drink the fruit juice, but everything else on the tray goes back to its home in the hospital food preparation area.

The afternoons are less structured. Phone calls and visitors inevitably come. I enjoy both very much. Former students and athletes were superb "uppers" for my spirits. A few close friends, such as my neighbor, Hugh Boyd, and John Schrader, the discredited statistician, saw me frequently. Several colleagues from Wood-bridge High came on a regular basis. Bill Carreiro, Tom Cindric and Mike Pallo visited weekly to share their latest lies about success on the golf course and the most recent faculty gossip from school. Jessica, Lindy, Krissy, Dave, Nancy and several other of my AP physics students who recently graduated stopped by with flowers and gifts. One of my former students, Regina, brought her new two month old son, Adam, to see me. Several of my West Springfield athletes, such as Meredith Carter, also stopped by.

Emily came **every** afternoon during her summer vacation to cheer me up. She would bring the daily mail, various toiletries and postage stamps, e-mail messages printed out at home, and always a big smile. She was very proud on the day in which she first wore her contact lenses - I thought that she looked great. Because she was still 16, driving by herself was a big deal, and she loved the freedom of the road. Many days she would drive home around 5 PM and then return in her car at 7 PM when Sharry also drove her car. If you are having trouble motivating a child to visit you in the hospital, give her the keys! I am certain that Emily would have been here each evening, with or without her driving, but it certainly took a considerable load off Sharry to have Emily be such an efficient courier service.

I also used the afternoons to make telephone calls of my own, particularly if there was an 800 toll free number available. I called a realtor at Ocean Isle Beach in North Carolina to argue over a beach cottage deposit which they would not return (they finally did). It took at least ten calls, but, what the hey, they had an 800 number. I also fought a telephone battle with United Airlines over two non-refundable round-trip tickets which we had purchased in early spring for Emily and me to fly to Spokane to visit Spurway and his wife, Coco.

I lost this one. United proved to be absolutely inflexible, even at corporate headquarters in Chicago. The response was, "We have empathy for your situation, Mr. Linz, but you have to understand the importance of no exceptions to our refund rule, *unless the prospective passenger dies.*" Someone actually said this! Hospitalization for a heart transplant did not apply. They did give me credit on a future use of the value of the tickets ($804), if I paid a $35 service charge for each ticket. So much for the "Friendly Skies" of United.

I also used our credit card number to order some foolish and unneeded products from catalogs. I actually spent very little. The psychic return was great, and I felt less trapped. One evening just before midnight when I had no roommate, I was sufficiently bored to try something I had never done before. I turned on Home Shopper's Club! Now here was a true narcotic for the bored. Sharry's youngest sister, Mary Ann Madigan, had recently taken a position with the parent company, Home Shopper's Network, in cable affiliation sales and marketing in their Denver office. Sharry and I had frequently kidded about who in the world ever buys any of the HSC "bargains." Now I know. After only 15 minutes a man's gold watch with a flexible band was shown **for only $19.95**! I **had** to have it. And there were only three minutes to call. I grabbed the phone at bedside, called the HSC 800 number and got one of those babies just in time. Shipping and sales tax were added, but who cared? It was still a "bargain" at under 25 bucks. At least, that is what I am telling myself for the rest of my life.

Receiving phone calls from friends around the country was a special treat. I particularly enjoyed hearing monthly from Annie and Charlie Arnest, who were currently living in Oregon. I had served with Charlie on USS NATHANAEL GREENE back in the 70's and we had stayed at each other's homes as our paths subsequently crossed during numerous military moves. Because Charlie had survived some serious medical problems of his own, their advice to "hang in there" carried considerable weight and always cheered me.

In late afternoon I treat myself to a bag of Fritos from the vending machine down the hall. I generally eat these while writing. It is a snack to carry me over until early evening when Sharry arrives with some dinner from home. One day I found myself in a fight with the man who fills the vending machines on the second floor. I had politely asked him if he could place some Ruger chocolate wafers as one of the choices, since I had really enjoyed the taste when they had been there earlier. He must have been having a bad day, because his response was, "I'll put what I want in here."

I responded, "Oh, then you must be the same guy who puts only Barbecue Fritos in this machine instead of Regular Fritos."

His anger level visibly rose. He excitedly pulled open the Frito line in the machine and said, "Look for yourself. There **are** some Regulars in here!"

I was not impressed. There were indeed a few bags of Regulars, but they were being overwhelmed by the number of Barbecues. I could see that I was getting nowhere trying to reason with this guy. He was obviously a Barbecue aficionado. I tried to think of a clever closing line to this dialogue, something that the character George from Seinfeld would say, but all I could come up with was, "Have a nice day." There was a touch of sarcasm in my voice, but I think that it went unnoticed. My only satisfaction out of this encounter came about two weeks later when the machine gave Emily and me two bags of Peanut M&Ms for the price of one. I was tempted to leave a note for the vending machine guy saying, "Gotcha!"

Late afternoons are spent doing work on my laptop computer. We had rented one for a month and found it to be very useful and convenient for the limited space in a double room in a hospital. Emily and I kept a sharp lookout daily in the newspapers for ads for new laptops. When Aaron would arrive on weekends from North Carolina, he would go to the stores which we had selected to check out the merchandise. We were looking for an inexpensive laptop, which had a nice-feeling keyboard, an acceptable black and white screen, and an internal modem. The best price we were able to find was $1399, and that was without a modem. I wanted to write, but not that badly. One Friday morning, when we were ready to give up, Emily telephoned excitedly to tell me that she had seen a laptop with a modem advertised for only $999. Aaron went to inspect it the following day. He reported that it was better than any of the others he had seen. We purchased it immediately. It proved to be great therapy for me throughout the remainder of THE WAIT.

The reason why I had insisted on a modem for the laptop is that the drug of choice for today's college students is e-mail on the Internet. For most students it is a free service. Nelle, at Indiana University, sends out and receives at least five messages each day to various parts of the country. She even sends messages back and forth to her professors on campus. If I wanted to stay in frequent contact with Nelle, I needed a modem. This also provided me with the means to communicate at a very low cost with many of my friends and former students across the country. By the time my 1994 graduates were beginning studies at their universities in late August, I was in correspondence with over 15 on e-mail. I could also zing Spurway and Schrader on their lousy football picks each week and keep in touch with some of my roommates from earlier times in my Navy career, such as Mark Davis in San Diego.

My hospital evening meal goes essentially untouched. It does not even smell good. I do take the fruit juice off the tray for later consumption. I also set aside carrot and celery sticks to snack on. I then take the tray outside the room to eliminate the food odor from the room.

The highlight of my daily ritual is Sharry's arrival around 7:30 PM. She has finished her 10 hour day with the Health Department, has gone home to take care of our dog, Sydney, has packaged up dinner (which Emily has often prepared), and has driven over to visit for the next three hours.

The meals always taste sensational. Not only are both Sharry and Emily very good cooks, they vary the menu wonderfully. Basil chicken over rice is one of my favorites. On some evenings when Sharry is dead tired or Emily is not home to fix a dinner, we eat carry out. Pizza, Chinese, submarine sandwiches, steaks, fries and even French fried onion rings are typical fare. I not only enjoy this food because of the non-hospital taste, but also because I know that the dietitian would have a stroke if she were to find out!

We sometimes eat dinner together in my room, but generally when I have a roommate, we go to an empty conference room and pretend that we are in an elegant French restaurant. Some nights this is something of a stretch, for example, the evening when we had chili dogs.

One of these meals was particularly memorable. Kathleen Kimberlin, the nurse who had treated me three years earlier during my hospitalization for the Amiodarone load-up, arranged with Sharry to have a surprise crab feast for us one evening. Kathleen had talked to my arrhythmia doctor, Ted Friehling, and received his permission to bring a six pack of beer and a load of fresh steamed crabs into the hospital for a private party. They completely surprised me. Kathleen's mother came along to join us. The party consisted of Kathleen, her mother, Sharry, Emily and myself. Sharry brought salad and small wooden hammers to break open the crabs.

Eating fresh Chesapeake Bay crabs is one of life's small pleasures. Over the next two hours, we had an absolute blast talking, gossiping and generally forgetting about my medical predicament. Although we did not keep score, I believe that Emily consumed the most crabs. She just sat there pounding away. Kathleen had also brought along a portable "boom box" with a few good tapes for background music. The effect was as if we were in a crab house on the eastern shore of the Chesapeake Bay rather than on a floor full of seriously ill patients. By the time we finished the feast, the entire hallway smelled like crabs! It is not possible to over-emphasize how much Kathleen's generosity and creativity meant to us. It was events such as this which enabled me to survive psychologically.

After most dinners, Sharry goes over the day's mail and bills with me. Mostly, we just enjoy each other's company and relax.

Around Day 10 of THE WAIT we had received permission from my doctors to leave the second floor where I am being continuously monitored by computer and technicians, as long as Sharry is with me and we stay no longer than 15-20 minutes. We use this respite each evening to feed the goldfish in the small pond in the cardiac garden on the ground floor level just outside the Cardiac Intensive Care Unit (where patients are taken immediately following transplant). We had put nine goldfish into the pond the day after our first visit there. The previous goldfish, we were told, had frozen during the past winter, so we decided that the pond could use some live action. We came to love this daily ritual. Apparently the goldfish did too, because they quickly developed a Pavlovian response to the vibration of my IV pole on the walkway leading to the pond. They would come to the surface on the side where we fed them.

The garden itself is beautiful with several different types of flowering plants, such as impatiens, roses, black-eyed Susans, and clematis - to name only a few. Whenever the weather was nice, Sharry and I would sit on a bench in the garden, breathe in the fresh air, and pretend that this nightmare was all over. One day we released a helium filled balloon with the caption, "If found, please send O+ heart to Fairfax Hospital c/o Ed Linz." It floated away beautifully, but we never received a reply.

Around 10 PM, I walk Sharry to the steps to leave for the evening. Frequently she is nearly asleep on her feet. We kiss goodnight, give each other a prolonged hug, and worry about the other. Sharry takes mail and dirty laundry home for me. I always find myself pushing the IV pole back to the room trying to understand how she is surviving all of this.

Upon returning to the room I take the last Procainamide for the evening, write or read for an hour, listen to the 11 PM news, and try to sleep. If all is well, I am asleep in 30 minutes. On some occasions (about once a week) I finally call my nurse and request that she give me a Valium. The drug almost always works.

Before actually getting into bed, I say a short evening prayer of thanks that the Lord has taken me safely through another day. I then do a ritual of arranging items on my bedside table in a certain manner. Everything has its place, so that when I awake at night, the Kleenex, the water, the pretzels, and my diary are always in the same place. I check that both of my IV bags have sufficient quantity to make it through the night and that the telephone and Walkman are in their assigned locations.

During the night I always awake at least twice to go to the bathroom. This is not a simple process. I must get out of bed without tangling my legs in the IV tubing going to the Groshong, unplug the IV monitors from the electrical outlet, and try to shuffle to the bathroom in the dark without banging into the chairs and other bed in the room. My motivation is not necessarily to be quiet, particularly if my roommate is a monster snorer in the middle of his act. I am simply trying not to hurt myself.

At 6 AM the nurse awakens me to receive the remaining dose of Procainamide. By this time my mouth already has the incredibly acrid taste from the 10 PM dosage and I am generally nauseous. In order to keep the medicine down, I eat three mini pretzels both before and after the pill. Selecting pretzels had been an iterative process. Graham crackers had been a total bust (I threw up almost immediately). Saltines were marginally better, but pretzels seemed to work well.

I then always seem to go back to sleep quickly and enjoy some sound sleep for the next two hours until the routine for the new day begins again.

The importance of following this type of schedule was critical to my sanity. Although it contained many eccentric elements, it helped me to complete each day of THE WAIT without going crazy. There was, of course, always an undercurrent of fear just below the surface. I was continuously aware that I was hospitalized because of a very dangerous condition. Just when I would be enjoying a period of "normal activity," the thought would bounce to the surface that I could have a life-ending arrhythmia at any moment. My defibrillator would fire as designed, but my heart would not convert to a normal rhythm, and I would die.

These concerns were reinforced periodically when I would have a brief period of tachycardia. From mid-to-late August, I had nine separate incidents. The AICD did not shock me, but on several occasions I was removed from danger only by its pacing function which caused the heart to revert to a normal rhythm before the device could charge its capacitor to deliver the dreaded bolt of electricity. Eight of these incidents occurred early in the morning (usually around 6 AM) while I was still asleep. The nurse would run into the room and say, "Are you OK?"

I had learned that this question, when asked by a nurse in a rather stressed voice, meant only one thing: I was not OK.

After waking thoroughly I would answer, "I think so. Why? What has happened?"

The nurse would explain that an alarm had gone off at the monitoring station and that a printout had automatically recorded the "event." Always they would add, "It seems to be normal now."

I also learned to dread the sound of running footsteps in the hallway. This sound was always associated with a life-threatening situation in some patient's room. The procedure is similar in every hospital and is referred to as a "code." Sometimes different colors are attached to the code meaning different types of emergencies, such as "code yellow." The running footsteps were always the give-away for me. Whenever I heard this sound, I would hold my breath and pray that they would continue past my room. One day the action was in the next room, and a lady patient had died. It was not a trivial worry.

My strategy for survival during the hospitalization was simple. I always told my doctors, "You keep me alive physically, and I will handle the mental side of the house." These arrhythmia episodes cast doubt on the credibility of both phases of my plan. Maybe the sarcoidosis was causing the heart to degrade further. Maybe the combination of drugs which I was receiving was no longer effective in keeping me stable. Maybe I had run out of waiting time before the replacement heart could be found.

The major impact of these thoughts was always greatest at night just as I was trying to go to sleep. My mind would lock in on these questions. I would find myself worrying that this might be the night of ultimate bad luck. I tried praying, thinking of other topics, planning the next day's events, almost anything, but the worries continued to dominate. The only effective antidote to this syndrome was to call the nurse and to request a Valium. The pill always served to relax me. I would fall asleep shortly.

If I were awake when an actual arrhythmia took place, I would immediately try to lie down so that I could be perfectly still, just as I had done after receiving shocks early in my hospitalization. This made little medical sense, but it did make me feel as if I were doing something to help. I would remain in this position for nearly an hour, afraid to move anything. These were periods of terror. Fortunately, it was an infrequent occurrence.

On day 30 of THE WAIT, Ted Friehling invited me to come to the EP lab to observe him and Al Del Negro perform an ablation and pacemaker insertion on one of their patients. I readily accepted the offer, if only to provide a break in my normal routine. In order to enter the lab (which is really a mini operating room), I had to "dress out" in a lead apron, jacket, and neck guard due to the radiation danger posed by the frequent use of an x-ray machine during the procedure. Ted and Al like to work with music in the background, so a nurse threw a tape into a small boom box and the show began. The patient was under anesthesia. There were four nurses assisting. A pacemaker specialist, Roger Lambert, from the manufacturer, Siemens, was also present to provide advice on settings and equipment capabilities. Both Ted and Al are exceptionally knowledgeable about the devices which they install, but there are several different brands on the market, and it is helpful to have someone present who is intimately familiar all of the details of each device. It was approximately 4:30 in the afternoon as the procedure began.

The patient had multiple IV lines with bags of solutions in several locations. All were labeled and closely monitored by Patricia, one of the nurses. At any given time there were numerous wire leads inside the patient's heart. One lead had four wires inside it. Two were used for pacing, and the other two provided information for recording onto the computer screens. All had been inserted by Ted using standard heart catheterization techniques. The large x-ray machine, called the fluoroscope, is positioned over the patient's chest and is turned off and on by Ted's foot. Al was standing directly next to Ted providing advice and assistance. Neither seemed to be in charge of the other. They truly worked as a team. My reaction was awe. This was the best example of "Poetry in Motion" that I had witnessed since seeing Willie Mays play against the Cincinnati Reds at the old Crosley Field in Cincinnati 40 years earlier. Having been through numerous EP studies myself over the past three years, it was refreshing not to be on the receiving end for a change.

After approximately one hour of placing the leads in the appropriate locations (the placement is truly an art based upon the experience and expertise of the cardiologist), both Ted and Al removed their scrubs and went to work at the computers. Two of the nurses, Rebecca and Michelle, took data as the doctors worked together on the computers to pace the atrium until heart block occurred. Al was doing measurements on a trace on one monitor while Ted created changes inside the heart with his computer. The purpose of this part of the procedure was to map the electrical system of the patient's heart so that corrective action could be taken in the appropriate area.

Everyone on the EP team had coffee or sodas available. I had no idea that the procedure would take so long. After another hour the two doctors decided that they had sufficient data to make a decision about what to do to correct the patient's underlying condition of frequent dangerous heart palpitation and tachycardia. After several minutes of discussion, they agreed that a partial ablation (removal) of the AV node would not be sufficient and that a full ablation was required.

Ted quickly left the computer area, put on another set of sterile covering and inserted the ablation catheter through the patient's groin area into an artery and then into the heart. When properly positioned in the location mapped by the computer data, Al energized the catheter to "burn" the AV node so that it would no longer be functional. A temperature of at least 55 degrees Celsius (131 degrees Fahrenheit) is required for a successful burn. Obviously this entire procedure is dangerous.

Al now dressed out to perform the surgical insertion of the pacemaker. He introduced a wire into the subclavian vein in the upper chest area through which the actual pacemaker wire is inserted. Incredible quantities of sterile supplies were being used. I now began to understand why surgery costs so much. The remaining nurse, Debbie, assisted throughout the entire procedure and appeared to be the lead nurse. It was now 7 PM. An incision was made in the upper chest area to form a pocket into which the pacemaker could be implanted. This particular model carried a warranty of 7 1/2 years and would be good, according to Roger, the tech rep, for at least 12 years.

The placement of the atrium lead for the pacemaker was not proceeding well, and it had to be relocated several times. Then there was difficulty in screwing the lead into the heart tissue. Everyone in the room was now very quiet. It was at this moment when one of my IV "Intelligent Infusor" alarms went off. I had forgotten to plug it into an electrical outlet when I entered the lab, and the battery was now nearly depleted. I had never reset the dying battery alarm, but I got lucky and hit the correct buttons to silence the wailing alarm. I wondered what my friends would have done if I had been unable to silence the alarm. I was rescued from the focal point of attention by the telephone. The caller was Al's wife, who wanted to know what to do about dinner. Would he soon be home? Debbie took the call and relayed to her that she should go ahead and eat.

After considerably more testing, it was decided that the wires were correctly positioned and that the pacemaker was operating correctly.   Roger was frequently calling out settings, such as "Sensing, 3.3, 3.6, 3.4, 3.3, OK?" I had no idea of the significance of the numbers, but Al would respond, "OK, good R wave."

By 8 PM the procedure was completed except for closing the incision made for the pacemaker and removing the catheter lines. Since I was expecting Sharry to arrive shortly with dinner, I decided to return to my room. Ted and Al had performed four separate procedures in the EP lab that day, beginning at 7:30 AM. I do not know when they got home that evening. During the brief periods when they were not at work in the lab, they were making rounds to visit their other patients in the hospital. I am still not sure how they (and their nursing assistants) keep going.

The next morning I awoke to two separate impressions. The first was mental, that is, a lasting impression of the incredible skill level of the two arrhythmia specialists, Al and Ted. The other was physical. My entire chest area had an intense pain. I did not panic or even call the nurse. I immediately theorized that the 4 hours of wearing the lead apron had strained my chest muscles and that I would have to live with the pain for several days. It turned out that this self diagnosis was correct. In four days, my chest was back to normal.

Each evening during THE WAIT I experienced weird dreams. None could be put into the category of a nightmare, but all had some crazy connection to receiving a new heart. One, in particular, stands out as an example.

In the dream, I was riding on a school bus. I was on the list for a heart transplant. Suddenly the guy in front of me turned around and said, "Hey, they have a new heart for you over at Georgetown University Hospital." I yelled to the bus driver to speed up and to head to Georgetown Hospital (which is located in D.C.).

Unfortunately, the bus was headed downhill on a narrow, winding road with steep drop-offs on the right side of the bus. The road reminded me of some of the more exciting country lanes which we had used at high speeds at night on liberty in Sardinia when I was in the Navy on USS TINOSA. The bus nearly went over the cliff several times. When the bus next stopped to pick up passengers, I hopped off. I did not have an IV pole to slow me down!

I then stole a bicycle which was lying on the ground near the bus stop and continued down the hill at a dangerous speed. I was worried that someone else would get the heart before I arrived at the hospital. I quickly learned that the reason the bike had been abandoned was that its front rim was badly misshapen, making control nearly impossible. But I kept pedaling. Eventually the front wheel flew off the bike, but I leapt off at the last minute and was not injured.

I began to run at a sprint toward the hospital, which by now was only a few blocks away. Apparently the dream did not consider my condition and my AICD, because I was able to run rather fast, and the device, if present, did not fire.

When I reached the hospital, there was a rock concert going on in the large lobby area where I had entered. Everyone was seated on folding chairs. I saw Ted Friehling and his teenage son, Matty. I asked Ted where my heart transplant would be performed. He said that he did not know. I became angry because he was obviously far more interested in the concert than in my condition.

A young woman with a small child in her lap spoke up, "I know where you should go. I will take you if you find someone to baby-sit my daughter."

I began to desperately look around the room to see if I could find some teenage girl to help me meet this woman's offer. I asked several girls that I did not know. Each acted as if I was trying to pick her up and turned my request down, often with a nasty comment. This must have been my mind wondering back to those not-so-glorious teenage days of my youth when I was routinely rebuffed by girls when asking them for a date. However, just as I did in those days, I did not give up. I suddenly spotted one of my former students, Jessica, sitting at least ten chairs from the aisle where I had been searching. (Perhaps the reason my mind flashed up Jessica in this role is that she had visited me several times during THE WAIT).

I yelled to Jessica to ask her to help, but she could not understand me due to the deafening noise of the concert. In desperation, I climbed over the laps of all the people between the aisle and Jessica to ask her to baby-sit. She said, "Sure."

I then ran to an elevator and asked someone in a blue hospital gown, "Where do they do transplants here?" Without answering, this person threw me onto a gurney, pushed me onto the elevator, pushed the button for the basement, and left me for the ride downstairs by myself. When the door opened two nurses grabbed the gurney and started to push me along a long, dark hallway. We arrived at another elevator, boarded it, and went upstairs. The nurses then pushed me out, leaving me to fend for myself. Now I saw the initial person in the blue hospital gown, and the same process began all over again. I yelled out, "I can't believe this! I'm stuck in an infinite 'do loop' in a hospital and somebody else is getting my heart!" (A "do loop" is a term from the early days of computer programming in which the instructions given to the computer cause it to repeat the same process or calculation forever).

Then I woke up. I was not startled or frightened as when waking from a nightmare. Frustrated, or perplexed, would be a better description. These dreams, always with a totally different plot, occurred every night. I did not look forward to them, because there was **never** a happy ending.

As the long days of THE WAIT continued to mount, I became increasingly concerned. I was receiving numerous visitors and well-wishers daily, but each day was also increasing the tension as to whether my diseased heart would continue to function. Two months had passed. Soon the first day of school for teachers began at Woodbridge; I did not feel guilty about not being there. In fact, my main emotion was far more self-centered: where was my new heart?

September arrived on Day 72 with nothing new on the heart front. When the long Labor Day weekend passed with no automobile accidents to provide a possible donor, I began to feel very depressed. "I'm not going to make it," I worried frequently to myself.

Classes began at Woodbridge High on September 7, Day 78. During the past few weeks I had conducted several lengthy tutorial sessions in my hospital room with Tom Cindric. I offered him some final tips on how to teach the Advanced Placement Physics course. Tom was his usual enthusiastic self, but also a sufficiently realistic teacher to understand the challenge of teaching this college level course for the first time. He had taught only one year of "regular" Physics, but he was far and away the best person to take my teaching schedule for the year because of his exceptional motivation, intelligence and work ethic.

Around 9 that evening, my crab feast buddy and "super nurse," Kathleen Kimberlin, surprised me by bringing me a copy of Volume 1.1 of the *PCCU GAZETTE*. It was a newspaper formatted flyer which she had prepared on her day off using the new computer system in her office. The headline, "**Ed Linz Gets A Heart !!!!!!!**" certainly grabbed my attention. The first paragraph read, " A local Physics teacher has waited 79 days while hospitalized at Fairfax Hospital. Ed Linz is now the proud owner of an O + medium size heart. Following his transplant, Mr. Linz was quoted as saying 'Life is good.' Mr. Linz was described by the nursing staff as a strong willed, pleasant, funny, and, even therapeutic (at times) man."

Kathleen's newspaper went on to discuss Sharry's reaction and to take a few humorous potshots at the PCCU nurses in general. We laughed together and I thanked her for thinking of me. She had obviously spent considerable time on this project. "If only Kathleen were clairvoyant..." I mused, as I fell asleep that night.

The next evening, September 8, I had dozed off after dinner while waiting for Sharry to arrive from her day at work. Suddenly, I felt my arm being shaken by my day nurse, Ila, who said excitedly, "Mr. Linz, you're getting a heart!" It was exactly 7:15 PM. I had been waiting 79 days at the top of the transplant list. I immediately thought of Kathleen's prophetic newsletter. Was she some type of psychic? Was I dreaming?

As Ila's words sunk in, I was in disbelief. I said, "Ila, are you sure?" She hugged me. This was the actual confirmation, because Ila was not a hugger.

We both started to cry. Almost immediately, Linda Ohler, the transplant coordinator, ran into the room and said, "Ed, it's a great heart. You will be going to surgery at 11:30 this evening!" Then she hugged me.

Taia, the evening nurse, rushed into the room and ran to me. She was crying, and she hugged me. Taia was an accomplished hugger, and I loved it. Soon almost every nurse on the floor came in crying with their own hugs and congratulations.

By this time I also was bawling. I was definitely in a state of gleeful shock. Soon, however, I became apprehensive that there would be some last minute glitch which would cancel the operation and leave me emotionally devastated. This was not a particularly paranoid feeling, because it is not unusual in the organ transplant field for last minute problems to develop with the donor organs precluding their use.

I crossed my fingers that I would not be involved in one of these "dry runs."

As I tried to force my mind to focus on the positive, I realized that Sharry did not know the good news. Reaching her immediately might be a problem, because she had gone to a local park after work to watch Emily run in her first cross country race of the season. The race should have been over by now, but I suspected that they would not yet be home. Actually this cheered me, because I would be able to beep Sharry on her pager with the special code which we had established to indicate "new heart." I did so.

Within two minutes Sharry was back to me on her portable flip phone. Both of our voices were choked with emotion as I told her the good news. We decided that she should take Emily home, grab some fast food for the two of them, and then come immediately to the hospital. She was at my bedside within 45 minutes. I suspect that a few speed limits were exceeded on her way to the hospital!

After talking to Sharry on the phone, I suddenly realized that, in my excitement, I had neglected to pause to thank the Lord. I reflected quietly for at least five minutes over my good fortune. Literally hundreds of friends had been praying for me. I was on numerous prayer lists. My own congregation at Abiding Presence Lutheran Church, led by Pastor Tom Bailey, had been praying for me throughout the summer. I regarded my own daily prayers as but a minuscule contribution to the process. Many friends of other faiths had also been praying for me. It certainly had not been a one denominational effort.

Soon events started to unfold rapidly. People started showing up in the room to conduct numerous pre-transplant tests. I had two separate urine collections, and at least six blood samples were drawn through the Groshong. A technician brought in a portable machine for a chest x-ray (this was one time in which I did not complain about being radiated!) My blood pressure was monitored every 20 minutes, and a determination of bleeding time was conducted by a nurse from the IV team. There were probably other tests, but I was too excited to remember each of them. Taia came back into the room and asked me to take an extensive and very thorough bath using Betadine (the bright orange-looking disinfectant soap). It was one of the more joyous baths of my life.

By now it was still only 9:30 PM. I had two hours more to wait. I decided to throw caution to the winds. I picked up the phone and began calling friends to tell them the good news. All were excited. I do not recall feeling better about making phone calls other than when our children had been born and I could report that both Sharry and the baby were doing well. Siobhan and her mother came to the room for a few minutes to offer their congratulations. Both were crying. From 10 PM on, Sharry and I sat by ourselves holding hands and occasionally hugging and crying together. It was one of the most precious times of our 24 years of marriage.

At almost exactly 11:30 PM, a nurse arrived from the operating room to transport me to the pre-op room. I still had to be monitored for heart rate due to the chance of a last minute arrhythmia, so a portable device was attached. It had a loud beeping noise which I really liked. Each new beep meant that I was closer to making it on my old, diseased heart. In the pre-op area I was greeted by the anesthesiologist who explained what he would be doing. Several new IV lines were started. Sharry was allowed to remain at my side, and we quietly held hands. We were told that the actual transplant would probably not begin until 1:30 AM. There were still no last minute problems - everything was on track for the transplant. The doctor explained that several organs were being removed from the donor, and that this process had to be conducted in a specific order.

Around 12:30 AM, I received medication to sedate me until the transplant would begin. I have no idea what it was. Although I recall nothing more, I am certain that I fell asleep with a huge smile on my face. THE WAIT was over.

Chapter 13

KRISTI

As the anesthesia started to take effect, my mind began, for the first time, to try to focus on the surgery immediately ahead. I was not frightened. I had complete confidence in the heart transplant team. I was at peace with God, I understood the risk, and I knew that I had no other choice. My last thoughts were of Kristi.

Kristi Lynne Brown had been the donor for the fifth heart transplant recipient at Fairfax Hospital nearly eight years earlier; if all went well, I was about to become the 97th. Kristi had also been the 19 year old daughter of our neighbors, Bill and Karen Brown, who lived directly across the street from us at the time.

Kristi was born in Shreveport, Louisiana on March 16, 1968. Bill was in the Air Force, and over the next several years, his family moved with him to Alaska, Virginia, Michigan, Utah, and California before settling in Springfield in 1979. Throughout this period Kristi, her older sister, Kim, and her younger brother, Allen, had experienced the challenging life of a military family during the Vietnam War era. Their father was gone for a year during a tour in Vietnam, and there was the ever-present concern that he might not return. Every few years, the family had to pack up and move to a new location for Bill's next duty assignment. As Sharry and I knew from our own experience, these moves are stressful for adults, but there is frequently a more profound impact on the children. They must leave their playmates and friends from school, travel to an entirely new (and often strange) area, and try to pick up life as if nothing had happened. Making friends at a new school is often difficult, particularly as the student reaches junior and senior high school. Some children of military families simply give up trying to "fit in" because they know that they will be leaving the area in a short time, so why try?

It is necessary to understand this background in order to fully appreciate how special Kristi Brown was. When she arrived in Springfield, she was a 6th grader. She immediately became involved in a variety of activities. She was a particularly skilled soccer player and quickly became a key member of one of the most successful youth teams in the state. Kristi was outgoing and her enthusiasm was contagious. Everyone liked her.

I had met the Browns shortly after we moved to the Winston Knolls area of Springfield in 1982. They were the type of neighbors who exude hospitality. Karen made us cookies shortly after our arrival, and Bill was always available with tools which I did not have. Even though she had known us for a very short time, Kristi would always, as she bounded out their front door and saw me, wave and yell across the street, "Hi, Mr. Linz, how are you?"

Over the next several years, I learned that Kristi "bounded" everywhere. She was a total bundle of energy. In high school, she was a cheerleader and varsity soccer player all four years. She was chosen as a co-captain for both during her junior and senior years. Kristi also participated in a variety of school clubs and still found time for church and community activities. Her youth soccer team won the state and East Coast Regional championship and finished second in the country in her age group. She was a true student-athlete who excelled both in the classroom and on the playing fields. Her teachers and coaches respected her, her classmates enjoyed being around her, and we certainly loved having her as a neighbor. She was a genuinely popular young lady.

In her senior year, Kristi visited Duke, Penn State, and several other universities before deciding to study architecture at the University of Virginia in Charlottesville. She was awarded two scholarships and began studies there in the fall of 1986.

While at the university, Kristi maintained close contact with her friends from high school, but also joined ΣΣΣ sorority and developed new friendships at UVA. She completed her freshman year having excelled academically and socially. Making the transition from high school to college had been no problem for Kristi.

In May of 1987, Kristi came home to live with her family for the summer. Her summer job required that she commute daily to various locations in the northern Virginia and D.C. area. While driving home from work on June 24, 1987, Kristi was savagely taken from us.

Kristi was heading south on the outer loop of the D.C. Beltway just before 4 PM. Her car was a large, older model, a '77 Oldsmobile. Knowing Kristi, I imagine that she was probably listening to music on the radio and planning her evening ahead. As she was approaching the halfway point home, nearing the Tyson's Corner area in Virginia, a driver on the inner loop of the Beltway lost control of his station wagon, swerved into the guard rail on his right, and rebounded back into the traffic. He crashed into a Subaru station wagon, locking bumpers in the process. The two joined cars then together crossed three lanes of traffic, raced out of control up a grassy embankment separating the opposite sides of the Beltway before becoming airborne as they flew more than five feet above the ground directly toward Kristi's Oldsmobile. The driver of the Subaru told police, "I heard the impact, and the next thing I knew we were in the air."

It is doubtful that Kristi knew what hit her. Following the collision, the Oldsmobile landed upside down on its top. Kristi's injuries were massive. She was airlifted to nearby Fairfax Hospital and taken immediately to surgery by a team of neurosurgeons.

Bill and Karen were both home when a phone call came to them nearly two hours later. Karen answered and was told by a police spokesman, "There is reason to believe that your daughter is in Fairfax Hospital. She was in an automobile accident on the Beltway." Because Kristi's purse and identification had been left behind in the Oldsmobile, her identity was initially unknown. She had been admitted to the hospital as a Jane Doe. It was only later that a positive identification was made.

Karen had heard an earlier traffic report on the radio describing the Beltway accident and was worrying that Kristi might have been held up by the associated tie-up. As time passed and Kristi did not arrive home, Karen became even further worried. The phone call confirmed her worst fears.

When Bill and Karen arrived at the hospital, they learned that Kristi had suffered major head injuries. The prognosis was not good. When the surgeons spoke with the Browns after surgery, they said that they felt that there was no hope that Kristi might live.

After the initial shock, Bill asked the doctors about possible organ donation. He was told that two neurosurgeons would have to independently examine Kristi and declare her to be brain dead. The older doctor added that a representative of the local organ transplant group would arrive shortly to discuss options and procedures.

The wait for the neurosurgeons to complete their examinations was excruciating for both Bill and Karen. At 9:57 PM the Browns were told that Kristi had officially been declared brain dead.

Unlike many other families, the Browns knew exactly how Kristi felt about organ transplants. Bill recalled that she had expressed her feelings on at least three separate occasions. In each case she had stated emphatically that she could not understand why someone would not donate and that, if the situation ever arose, she wished that all of her organs would be made available for transplant. She had also indicated on her driver's license her desire to donate. (Although it is a good idea to indicate one's preference concerning organ donation on the driver's license, it is not a sufficient criteria in most states. Nearly all U.S. transplant centers require explicit written approval of the next-of-kin before transplant procedures can begin. This is why it is so important to discuss this issue with your family).

As Bill and Karen struggled with the shock that their younger daughter was no longer with them, they took some solace in the fact that Kristi would now be able to continue in death to do what she had so consistently done in life: provide joy to others.

Because of their certainty of Kristi's wishes and their own positive feelings with respect to transplant operations, Bill and Karen did not hesitate to agree when the transplant representative arrived to explain the program and to request their approval to proceed. They indicated their intentions to both Kim and Allen, but both were in such total shock over the loss of their sister that they could not talk.

The transplant representative was a Registered Nurse. As he talked with the Browns, he used a checklist to go over the procedures involved in organ donation. He also discussed the consent forms which had to be signed prior to beginning the transplant process. Karen and Bill listened patiently and, upon learning that Kristi had been declared brain dead, consented to the transplant of her heart, kidneys and cornea. (Kristi's liver had been seriously damaged in the accident and was not suitable for transplantation).

The Browns were told that medical information concerning Kristi would be immediately placed into the national computer system for organ donation. As soon as a potential recipient was identified based on an appropriate match of blood type, heart size and other parameters including location, transplant procedures could begin. Coincidentally, a patient there at Fairfax Hospital, a man in his 30's, was suffering from a very serious cardiac condition and was selected to be the recipient of Kristi's heart the following morning. The transplant surgeons for each organ were then notified. They, in turn, continued the process by giving appropriate instructions for the hospital to proceed.

Karen asked how Kristi's body would be affected by the transplantation process. The RN told her that the donor would be treated with dignity. The Browns later learned that Kristi had been placed under anesthesia for the removal of her organs. It was not until several years later, however, that Bill and Karen learned that an open casket funeral is possible following most transplant procedures. In view of Kristi's serious head injuries from the accident, they had decided to have a closed casket so that Kristi would be remembered as the bouncy girl with the perpetual smile.

Still devastated by the loss of their daughter, the Browns returned home. They could not sleep, but there was some comfort in their knowledge that Kristi's organs would soon be providing new life to others.

Procedures to facilitate transplant operations have been refined and improved in most locales in the seven years since Kristi's accident. Here in the Washington, D.C. metropolitan area there is now a formal organization, the Washington Regional Transplant Consortium (WRTC), which coordinates transplants for the 43 hospitals and 7 transplant centers in the area. The WRTC is a non-profit organization which provides services for all types of organ and tissue transplants (heart, liver, kidneys, pancreas, corneas, bone, skin, heart valves, blood vessels, etc). It serves as a link between the local community and the national organization, the United Network for Organ Sharing (UNOS), to ensure equal access for all patients awaiting an operation at the nearly 300 transplant centers in the United States.

UNOS, as mandated by the National Transplant Act, maintains a computerized list of all patients who are waiting for an organ transplant. Priorities are determined based on specific rules applicable to the entire nation. It does not matter where in the U.S. a potential donor or recipient is located. Everyone must follow the same rules based on need and availability.

When a donor in the Washington, D.C. area is identified, all appropriate medical data (blood group, age, height, weight, etc.) is gathered by the WRTC and transmitted electronically to the UNOS computer system. UNOS then immediately initiates procedures to determine the best possible match between the donor and those waiting for various organs. It is not always a simple process. For example, although a person with A + blood type in California may have a higher priority than a patient in North Carolina, the organ involved may be able to tolerate only a short interval between removal and implantation, precluding the availability of its use in California if the transportation time is too great. There are different maximum time intervals for different organs. Hearts, for example, can usually be "out of body" a maximum of approximately four to six hours using current techniques; kidneys can tolerant considerably longer periods (24 to 36 hours). In general, the shorter the time between removal and implantation, the better the chance for success. It is not unusual, therefore, for organs from the same donor to be routed to recipients in different parts of the country.

In spite of the tremendous ethical, religious, legal and logistic pressures involved in organ transplantation, the operation of UNOS nationally, and the WRTC locally, is generally regarded as a major success story. As with any national program, there have undoubtedly been a few instances in which rules were bent or circumvented, but, on the whole, there have been a tremendous number of "happy endings" due to the efforts of UNOS and local organizations such as the WRTC. I certainly was comfortable with their work.

Although the transplant procedures did not delay or alter preparations for the funeral, the Browns still had to confront the difficult process of making arrangements while in the midst of shock and grief. A memorial service was held the following Saturday at Grace

Presbyterian Church in Springfield and was attended by over 500. Many of Kristi's friends, including her high school principal, shared their memories of her during the service. Several described her as "everyone's best friend." Karen brought photos and several of the poems which Kristi had written to pass around. As her favorite song, "You've got a Friend," was sung, many of us in attendance openly wept. The lyrics had a particular significance and poignancy for those of us who were aware that Kristi's organs were giving life to others.

Kristi was buried two days later at Arlington National Cemetery. Her grave site was on a quiet hill, under trees fresh with new leaves. Coincidentally, two other University of Virginia students were buried next to her just a few months later. The service included no gun salutes or bugles as typically heard during burials at Arlington, but rather only the quiet remarks of her soccer coach and pastor. Several friends came forward to place flowers on the coffin. When the headstone was later put in place, Bill and Karen chose to have the words of Peter Marshall inscribed: "The measure of a life is not its duration, but its donation."

Kristi's organs continue to provide life to others. The recipient of her heart, a man then 31 years old (with a three year old daughter), is enjoying a full and active life today. He later wrote to the Browns, "Thank God for people like you who realize just how precious human life is that at the most painful time of your life, you have the compassion to give that gift to someone who would otherwise lose it. You have given my family and me that gift.... Because of your complete and unselfish generosity, my own daughter will not have to grow up without her Daddy."

Both of Kristi's kidneys were also successfully transplanted. One was given to a 57 year old woman, and the other to a woman of 50. Her corneas restored the gift of sight to two others, a 25 year old man and a 60 year old woman.

In conversations over the next several years, Bill told me that he never had second thoughts about their decision to donate Kristi's organs. The easiest part, he told me, was the decision itself. The difficulty was in burying her.

Karen became involved in several activities to continue Kristi's legacy of assisting others. A fund was established in conjunction with the local Rotary Club and K-Mart for an annual Christmas event, "Kristi's Christmas," in which underprivileged children were given the opportunity to receive toys and clothing. Each December the front windows of the K-Mart in downtown Springfield are covered with red paper hearts containing the names of hundreds who have donated to Kristi's Christmas. Karen also established links with the Transplant Consortium to speak before various organizations providing her perspective as the parent of an organ donor.

I had thought of Kristi often during THE WAIT. I knew that my only hope for survival would be the untimely death of someone like her. I knew that a family, such as the Browns, would have to confront the same terrible decision which they had faced. There would be no time for lengthy discussion or gathering of views. My fate lay in the hands of a grief-stricken family who did not know me and a God in whom I had placed my faith and trust.

As I passed into unconsciousness on my way to receive a new heart, I knew that some family had given such a gift for me. I knew nothing about them or the actual donor. It gave me considerable comfort, however, that I had known Kristi and her family. Kristi would always be my "spiritual donor," that is, a face and a personality that I could associate with my actual donor. Her joy had been contagious, her life had been an exclamation point. I was determined that, God willing, I would use my new heart to follow her example of trying to make life just a little better for those around me.

In one of her last writings, Kristi composed the following poem, which was found after her death in a journal next to her bed:

LIFE

Life is not long enough to accomplish all your goals.
Life is too short to waste a minute of.
Life always has to end sometime or another.
It ends when you least expect it.

Life ends instantaneously for some,
Life's end is long and painful for others.

Life's end is known by some, but for others,
It ends when you least expect it.

Life is good to most people for a long time,
Life takes some people very early on.
Life fights with death for the cream of the crop.
It ends when you least expect it.

Life is taken advantage of by some, others live life one
Day at a time, and cross bridges when they come to them.
Life usually ends for the careful ones, not the careless.
It ends when you least expect it.

Life's end is welcomed by those who are suffering.
Life's end is not welcomed for those who are not.
Life is hard after a loved one dies, but
It ends when you least expect it.

Life is a terrible thing to waste.

Kristi Lynne Brown, March 16, 1968 - June 24, 1987

Chapter 14

THE ORDEAL

At Fairfax Hospital there are three surgeons who perform heart transplant operations. Although all three ultimately were involved in my care, Dr. Paul Massimiano, the same doctor who had performed my AICD open heart surgery in 1992, was the one on call on the morning of September 9, 1994. He led the preparations for me to receive the new heart. Throughout the entire transplant process, a specially trained Physician's Assistant, Mechelle Fleischer, and a team of nurses, worked closely with him. There were no last minute problems, and surgery began at 1:30 AM.

At the same time that Massimiano was opening my chest, his colleague, Dr. Nelson Burton, was already in an adjacent operating room at Fairfax with the donor, a 34 year old woman who had suffered a brain aneurysm. When it was determined that her condition was terminal, her family had agreed to donate her organs for transplant. Neither Sharry nor I knew anything else about my benefactor. [Our family subsequently learned the identity of my donor. We later had the opportunity to meet her wonderful family whose donation of their daughter's heart gave me the gift of life. This book is dedicated to her.] Several times during the final hours prior to my surgery we found ourselves wondering how we would react if we were to face a similar decision concerning one of our children. Our dominant reaction was relief that we had not had to confront the issue. Mostly we were grateful, very grateful.

The stress which accompanies such a critical decision by a family with regard to organ donation is probably understandable only to those who have had to make such a decision. In the years since Bill and Karen Brown had to agonize over Kristi, the procedures followed by local transplant agencies have been improved and standardized to minimize emotional trauma for the families.

Upon receiving information from UNOS that an organ is available for a transplant center in the Washington area, the WRTC transplant coordinator telephones the appropriate doctor's group (in my case, Dr. Edward Lefrak's heart surgical team of himself, Burton, and Massimiano). A doctor on the team then evaluates the available information and makes the decision as to whether or not to proceed. I was told that two hearts had been rejected for me during THE WAIT because the surgeons did not want to implant an older heart due to my relatively young age and otherwise healthy condition. I did not know this at the time.

Once the heart surgeon decides to proceed with the transplant, arrangements are made by the WRTC for a member of the team to travel to the donor to retrieve the heart. Sometimes, after inspecting the condition of the organ on site, the doctor decides that it is not suitable for transplant and calls off the entire operation. Although this "dry run" scenario is psychologically traumatic for the potential recipient (who has generally been notified of the possibility of a transplant by this time), it is critical to the success of the transplant that the organ involved be carefully evaluated by the surgical team which will be performing the procedure.

Several of my recipient colleagues, such as Trudi Anderson and Benno Duykers, had two such dry runs before receiving a donor organ. I visited with Trudi after both of hers. She had been able to rationalize the first rather well, but was quite shaken and disappointed following the second. As with most transplant candidates, her condition was worsening while she waited. It was not at all certain that she would live much longer. In fact, another patient at Fairfax waiting for a new heart at the same time as Trudi had passed away before a suitable donor could be found. She knew that her time was limited and was beginning to seriously wonder if she would make it. Our visits to her, she later told us, were a significant factor in keeping Trudi reasonably sane during these disappointments. The fact that someone else that you can see and talk to had been through the same stress provides comfort.

This type of emotional support, that is, facilitating those who have received organs meeting those who are still waiting, is one of the main goals of TRIO, Transplant Recipients International Organization, which has its headquarters across the Potomac River in

Washington, D.C. Our local TRIO group, "The Nations Capital Area Chapter," is particularly good in promoting this interchange. On several occasions during my lengthy stays at Fairfax Hospital, I had been visited by TRIO members, whose own transplant experiences provided such encouragement and hope for me. Just seeing them in such obviously good health and spirits was a major factor in strengthening my resolve to proceed with the transplant operation.

Once the surgeon inspects the heart and gives a "go" for the transplant, events take place quickly at the hospital where the operation will take place. The recipient receives final preparations, such as a thorough scrubbing of affected portions of the body with an antibacterial soap. Sterile draping is then placed over all of the body except the planned incision area on the chest. In my case, Dr. Massimiano began the transplant surgery by opening my chest. He performed a medial sternotomy, that is, a vertical incision beginning approximately two inches down from the Adam's apple to a location on my abdomen ten inches below. The sternum (breast bone) was cut open with a Sarnes saw, a special tool frequently used in open heart operations. (For those interested in tools, it is essentially a medical version of a small, portable, hand-held jig saw).

The chest opening proceeded quickly. The phase involving the saw, for example, was completed in less than 15 seconds. Massimiano then applied a special type of wax, "Bone Wax," to the edges of the sternum to reduce bleeding. (This stuff has the same color and consistency as the white cork grease which is used by my daughter, Emily, on her soprano sax). It was then time for the rib spreader. This piece of hardware has been cleverly designed to fit into the narrow opening in the sternum created by the surgeon's saw. One side rests against the right edge of the open breast bone, the other against the left. The surgeon then turns a small hand crank on the side of the spreader to adjust and maintain an appropriate amount of access during the operation. (When I later saw one of these ribs spreaders, it reminded me of the set of parallel rulers which we used for navigation aboard submarines).

Because of the previous surgery to insert the AICD and to sew its patches and leads onto the sides of my heart, Dr. Massimiano had considerable difficulty separating the lateral wall of my heart from the pericardium, the membranous sac enclosing the heart.

During the nearly three years since the AICD was implanted, numerous adhesions and scar tissue had formed on the sides of my heart where the patches and wires were located. Massimiano later told me that he had to pull, tug, and even punch the "old" heart to separate it from the pericardium.

Steps were then taken to prepare to place me on extracorporeal circulation, that is, a heart lung-machine. Obviously, during the time my heart was being physically removed and the new one transplanted into its location, the rest of my body still had a continuing need for blood flow and oxygen. The heart-lung machine provided both. First, plastic tubes, called cannulae, were inserted into various locations leading to and from my heart. A "24 French arterial" cannula was placed high in the ascending aorta, the main trunk line carrying blood to all of my body except the lungs. A right angle cannula was inserted into the superior (upper) vena cava and a regular venous cannula was used on the inferior (lower) vena cava. (The vena cava are the large veins which discharge blood from the body into the right atrium of the heart to begin the pumping action through the lungs). Snares, sort of a medical equivalent of a noose, were placed to encircle the cava so that blood flow could be redirected at the appropriate time in the procedure. Instead of going to the heart, the blood would be redirected through the cannula into plastic, wire-reinforced tubing going to the heart-lung machine. With all of the cannulae in place, an alternate blood flow path had been established so that the heart could be safely removed. Heparin was injected to prevent coagulation of my blood during the period I was on the heart-lung machine.

At the same time that Dr. Massimiano's team was preparing me to receive a new heart, Dr. Burton was surgically removing the heart from the donor in an adjacent operating room. Obviously the work done by Dr. Burton's team was of equal importance to that of Massimiano's group. The goal is to obtain the optimum amount of donor heart so that transplantation onto that section of the recipient heart which remains is quickly and easily achieved. Because some of the upper sections of my heart were retained, only approximately the lower 7/8 of the donor heart was removed by Burton. The surgeon removing the donor heart must be intimately familiar with the technique used by the surgeon performing the transplant so that there are no matchup and alignment problems with the two hearts. It is for this reason that most transplant teams insist that only a surgeon from their team remove the donor organ.

The heart transplant procedure is basically a plumbing problem. The heart is a pump which receives blood from multiple intake piping (veins) and sends the fluid through the lungs and then back to the body through outlet piping (arteries). Rather than cutting all of the lines entering and exiting the heart, the surgeon severs only the two largest, the aorta and the pulmonary artery. By retaining that section of the heart to which smaller piping (e.g., the four pulmonary veins at both vena cava) is connected, unnecessary and time-consuming re-connection problems are avoided when the donor heart is attached to the recipient heart.

My temperature had been lowered 12 degrees from 98 to 86 degrees Fahrenheit (30 degrees Celsius) by chilling my blood as it passed through the heart-lung machine. The temperature of the operating room was lowered to 60 degrees Fahrenheit to further cool my body. In addition, a cold solution of saline slush was dumped into my chest cavity after it had been opened. The phrase, "Chill out!" used by some of my students would have been appropriate to describe my condition.

The reason for all of this effort to cool heart transplant patients is that, at the lower temperature, all bodily functions are slowed, giving the surgeon increased time to work while the patient is on the heart-lung machine. This concept is related to the situation in which a person who falls into icy water can often be successfully resuscitated after relatively long periods without breathing due to the slower metabolism caused by the cold temperature. During the earlier days of transplant operations, patients were literally put on ice to gain this advantage. I, however, received slightly higher-tech chilling. There is even a slush machine in the operating room at Fairfax for the specific purpose of making the icy solution. (I think of this whenever I see the Slurpee machine in a 7-11). The donor heart is also transported in an icy saline solution. The "Igloo" cooler frequently seen on television portrayals of transplant operations really does exist; a friend of mine recently saw an organ being transferred through the Atlanta airport in such a cooler.

As soon as Dr. Burton entered the operating room with the donor heart, I was placed on total cardiopulmonary bypass. My blood now bypassed the heart and lungs completely by flowing through the cannulae and external tubing into a complex heart-lung machine about the size of a large office copier. All of the blood which ordinarily returned from its flow path in my body to the right atrium of my heart was now being diverted to this device.

The heart-lung machine is just that: it performs the function of the heart by using a series of roller pumps to transport blood, and it replicates lung action by simultaneously removing carbon dioxide and adding oxygen to the blood as it passes through an oxygenator. The freshly oxygenated blood is then returned through the cannulae into my aorta. The machine is operated by a "perfusionist," a specially trained technician whose sole responsibility is to ensure that the machine keeps the patient alive while the patient is on the bypass. The perfusionist not only controls the pumping operation, but also maintains blood temperature, adds medications when necessary, and follows the patient's vital signs.

I subsequently learned that there are several "Perfusion Schools" where perfusionists receive their training. The Cleveland Clinic, St. Louis University, and the New England Medical Center in Boston are some of the locations in the eastern half of the U.S. Perfusionists may well be the least known subset of medical professionals. I have never heard anyone answer, "What do you want to be when you grow up?" with, "A perfusionist!" At any rate, this perfusionist person did his part to keep Ed Linz afloat during the transplant, and I am grateful.

Once it was determined that I was stable on the heart-lung device, my heart was quickly removed. Dr. Massimiano made a cut across both atria and severed the aorta and pulmonary artery. All of the wires from the pacemaker and AICD were cut in locations close to the heart. The devices themselves were not removed until later in the procedure. Once again the adhesions from the prior operation were a problem, but Massimiano managed to work the heart loose and pull it from its nest of 50 years. The image of a surgeon yanking, prodding and muscling my heart out of my body still causes me to take a very deep breath.

The new heart was carefully positioned for attachment. The left atrium was sutured first using a needle pre-attached to 3-0 Prolene thread, a blue, sterile, monofilament line made of polypropylene. (It looks like thin fishing line). Then the right atrium was sewn together with the same type of suture. Next the pulmonary arteries were joined with 4-0 Prolene (a suture of a smaller diameter). Finally the aorta were brought together, also with 4-0 Prolene. The skill of the heart surgeon is paramount during this phase. The ability to place the sutures sufficiently close and neat is an art which few possess. Although the stitches are placed very closely together, there is sometimes excessive bleeding which requires the use of a type of medical adhesive (thrombin glue) to supplement the sutures. I doubt that Super Glue would work, in spite of its advertising claims.

The attachment of the donor heart took approximately 50 minutes. It was not yet beating, but I was about to be re-born. My donor's heart was now part of me!

My body was re-warmed to normal body temperature of 98.6 degrees Fahrenheit using the heat exchanger in the heart-lung machine. Dr. Massimiano and the Physician's Assistant closely examined each of the connections (called anastomoses) for hemostasis, that is, no bleeding. I did not require the glue. In order to ensure that no air would enter my arterial system (a serious problem if it occurs), extensive de-airing maneuvers were performed before I was removed from the heart-lung machine.

Two sets of wires were placed on the outer side of the right atrium and right ventricle of the heart to provide pacing as the new heart started to beat. As my body was warmed, the heart began on its own, but there was some initial (not unexpected) atrioventricular (AV) disassociation, that is, the body's natural electrical signal for the heart to pump was erratic. However, after several minutes of pacing, the heart reverted to a normal sinus rhythm. The pacing leads were kept in as a precaution for a period of time following the transplant operation. Because the vagus nerve which helps to control heart rate has to be severed during the surgery (and cannot be re-joined), some patients require permanent post-transplant pacing. I was fortunate; my new heart beat nicely on its own.

I was removed from the heart-lung machine without difficulty. The perfusionist slowly re-directed blood to the new heart while my blood pressure was closely monitored. Surprisingly (to me) I required only two units (about two pints) of replacement blood during the transplant. The cannulae were removed and their entry sites were sewn together with 4-0 Prolene. The pericardium was kept open for drainage, and two chest tubes were inserted and connected to external suction for the removal of fluids from the area.

As soon as Dr. Massimiano determined that I was stable on my new heart, he made an incision in my left abdomen region to remove the AICD and its four leads. Once the cavity was opened, the AICD box was simply lifted free, but its wires had to be pulled downward under the skin from where they had been severed near the heart earlier in the procedure. As soon as they were clear of my body, the area was thoroughly cleaned and then closed in normal surgical fashion with Vicryl suture. The pacemaker pocket in my upper chest area was similarly opened so that the pacemaker and its leads could also be removed. The Groshong catheter had been removed prior to the initial opening of my chest, so I now was, for the first time in nearly three years, free of internal hardware.

Several members of the transplant team made a final inspection of the heart to ensure that it was functioning well and that bleeding was not a problem. I had been given protamine sulfate to reverse the anti-coagulation of the heparin received at the beginning of the operation. The entire area was irrigated with the antibiotic, Bacitracin. My chest was then closed by wiring the sternum together with stainless steel wires. The Physician's Assistant, Mechelle, and one of the nurses closed the incision with running PDS and subcuticular Vicryl.

The transplant operation was truly a team effort. In addition to the two cardiac surgeons, the Physician's Assistant, and the perfusionist, there was an anesthesiologist, a nurse anesthetist, and several staff nurses who scrubbed, circulated and directly assisted the surgeons. Throughout the procedure the team was serenaded by light rock music coming from a CD player behind the perfusionist. Each of the three heart transplant surgeons at Fairfax has his own favorite music. I would have voted for Jethro Tull's *Teacher*, but no one asked for my input.

All had gone remarkably well. I arrived in the recovery room less than five hours after the transplant operation had begun. The final sentence of the Operative Report was the standard "good news" summary: "The patient tolerated the procedure well and left the operating room in stable condition."

Unfortunately, this was not the end of the story.

During the operation Sharry went to the front lobby of the hospital to wait it out. She had obtained blankets and a pillow from our nurse friends on 2 East and actually slept off and on for a few hours. Around 5:30 AM, one of the transplant coordinators, Mary Beth, came by to recommend that she move to the Intensive Care Unit (ICU) waiting room. There Sharry received word that my new heart had been started and was beating fine. The surgeons would close my chest when the blood seepage stopped. In approximately one hour I was transferred to the ICU.

Kim Hill and Ted Friehling, our arrhythmia friends, had heard that I was having the transplant and had remained in the hospital overnight to follow my progress. When they saw Sharry in the waiting room, they came to her and reported that the new heart "looked good." Sharry's two public health nurse colleagues, Kathy and Peggy (who are assigned by the county to maternal and child health at Fairfax Hospital) stopped by to see her first thing in the morning and stayed for support. Around 7 AM Dr. Massimiano came to see Sharry and said, "The two hearts - what a perfect match! He is going to be fine."

Just after 8 AM, Sharry was allowed to come into my room in ICU. She ran to the bed and squeezed my hand in relief. Since I was still unconscious and all looked well, she went home to check on Emily and to telephone Nelle that I was OK. Aaron did not yet know that I had received a new heart because he was camping overnight somewhere in southern Virginia. Ironically, this was the first time in at least a year that Aaron was incommunicado for an extended period of time. He did not learn of my medical situation until he pulled into our driveway later that afternoon. Sharry greeted him with, in a rather nonchalant manner, "Oh, Aaron, your father got a new heart last night." I think that Sharry was (1) exhausted by this time, and (2) my nominee for Person Making **THE** Understatement of the Year!

Sharry returned to the hospital twice more on the 9th of September. I continued to look "normal." I was now conscious and talking, my dressings were fine, and the doctors were pleased with my progress. The device to aid my breathing, a respirator (or ventilator), had been removed in mid-afternoon. Everyone was optimistic that I would have a quick recovery.

The weekend was pleasant and encouraging. My new heart was working so well that Sharry swore that the bed was shaking with each beat. I was moved from my bed to a sitting position in a chair in the ICU unit. My spirits were high. Although I felt as if I had been hit by a big truck, I knew from my previous heart surgery two years earlier that this pain was to be expected and that I would soon feel better. I ate potato soup and had some fat free pudding. Aaron visited me each day of the weekend. "How soon are you going to start running, Dad?" he asked.

"Quite frankly, Son, I haven't thought about it much. I've been busy concentrating on breathing," I explained as we laughed together.

On Sunday, I was able to make some telephone calls to Spurway and a few other close friends. I began to count the days until I would be home. Perhaps I could set a new Fairfax Hospital record for the shortest post-transplant period of hospitalization for a new heart.

Unfortunately, things began quickly to go wrong early the next day. It was Monday, September 12. I began to develop breathing problems. The oxygen level in my blood started to decrease to unacceptable levels. The nurses kept encouraging me to take deeper breaths. I replied that I was breathing as deeply as I could. I felt as if I were doing heavy labor. Maybe I was not going to set a record.

By the following morning, my condition had further deteriorated. The nurses were now threatening me, "Mr. Linz, if you don't keep taking deep breaths, we're going to have to put the ventilator back in."

Since I felt that I was already doing as much as I possibly could to take deep breaths, I lost my temper and yelled, "If you have to put it back in, then put the [obscenity] back in. Just quit bothering me!" I remember nothing else that took place during the following two weeks.

My breathing continued to worsen and, shortly after my outburst, the ventilator was re-inserted. In the next few hours all hell broke loose. THE ORDEAL had begun.

I was not responding to the assistance being provided by the ventilator. My vital signs worsened. I was rapidly going downhill. A decision was made by two of my doctors for me to be placed under anesthesia so that a central line could be surgically inserted through my chest into the superior vena cava, a major artery. Following this procedure (which was similar to that in which the Groshong catheter had been inserted), I was able to receive medication, food, and all types of IV solutions quickly and directly into my blood stream. The Groshong had two lumen (lines), but had been removed during the transplant along with the AICD and the pacemaker. This new central line had three lumen so that multiple medications could be inserted simultaneously.

Soon a Foley catheter was inserted through my penis to allow the release of urine. I regard myself as being extremely fortunate that I was never conscious when a Foley was inserted. As a guy, I have a real psychological problem with respect to this procedure, or anything in that immediate area of my body.

When Sharry arrived at the hospital from her work at a Health Department clinic late that morning, she was not allowed to see me due to the seriousness of my condition and the fact that a crowd of medical personnel were working on me. She went down to the cafeteria in shock, alone and frightened. After all that we had been through, it appeared for the first time that I might not make it.

As Sharry was sitting with her head in her hands, she saw Kim Hill and Al Del Negro at a nearby table. After regaining some level of composure, she went to them to say hello. Both were very serious and obviously concerned. They told Sharry that they "had heard" and would find out exactly what was going on. When they returned a short time later, Dr. Del Negro was extremely somber as he reported, "they say it looks like ARDS."

Although Sharry had heard of ARDS, she looked puzzled. Al quickly added, "It's Adult Respiratory Distress Syndrome. It is very dangerous. It may be due to the long time he was on Amiodarone."

Kim explained to Sharry that ARDS was sometimes a side effect of lengthy periods of taking Amiodarone. Since I had been on a significant dose of the drug for the past three years, it was likely that my lungs had been damaged. The strain following the transplant had been too great for the weakened condition of my lungs, and they had essentially failed. I was being kept alive by the ventilator, which was doing my breathing for me.

Not knowing exactly what to do and feeling very alone, Sharry went back to the ICU waiting room. As she reviewed the situation, she became increasingly upset that no one had contacted her to inform her of my worsening condition.

"Exactly what **do** they call you for?" she thought. "Why wasn't I notified?"

Exasperated, Sharry telephoned the Health Department to say that she would not be returning to work that afternoon. The clerk at her office said that there had been a telephone message to her from Dr. Massimiano. Apparently he had attempted to reach her at the Health Department while, unknown to him, she was at the hospital. He wanted her to call him.

Sharry's anger at not being notified diminished. Just as she was about to have Massimiano paged, she saw the head of the transplant team, Dr. Lefrak, as he walked toward the ICU.

"Dr. Lefrak!" she yelled. "I'm Sharon Linz. What can you tell me about my husband?"

Lefrak spoke in a quiet monotone. "Your husband has developed a serious case of ARDS. His kidneys are also failing. Overall, his condition is critical. We think that the kidney problem can probably be eventually alleviated by dialysis. We've already started that. The lungs are the more serious problem at the moment. We're doing everything that we can. It's too early to tell..." His voice trailed off.

Sharry was somewhat surprised by Dr. Lefrak's compassion and concern. Although he was recognized as one of the top transplant surgeons in the country, the "conventional wisdom" around the hospital was that he was difficult to communicate with. "Thank you, Doctor, for all that you are doing," Sharry responded as he walked back into the ICU. Still, she was not being allowed to see me due to the ongoing efforts to save me.

One of the ICU nurses, Ann Marie, noticed Sharry's obvious chagrin. She came over to her and had what probably should be termed, "a nurse-to-nurse heart-to-hearter."

"You really need to talk more to these doctors," Ann Marie said. "They're busy, but every one of them will take the time to talk. I know them. They are really good. Don't be so timid. They will understand." She squeezed Sharry's hand and smiled. Money cannot buy this type of advice.

Although nothing had changed to improve my condition, Sharry felt encouraged. Everyone was not against her. Ann Marie had put the situation in perspective.

Sharry was not permitted to see me until later in the evening, but she was able to speak with many of the doctors. She stayed until midnight and received frequent updates from the nurses and doctors. There was nothing that she herself could do except pray. Emily was home studying for school the next day, Aaron had returned to his classes at Chapel Hill, and Nelle was back at Indiana University. Sharry felt very alone and helpless. She finally went home, but could not sleep. The ICU nurse had told Sharry to telephone at any time during the night for an update. She did call several times, but there was no good news. I was not worse, but there was not any improvement. After calling at 5:30 AM, she decided to go to work, if only to try to take her mind off the situation.

It was now Wednesday, September 14. By 10:30 AM Sharry had become so concerned that she could no longer stay at work. She drove to the hospital and went directly to the ICU. Ann Marie was one of the nurses on duty. She was once again helpful in bringing Sharry up to date on my condition. It was not good. My kidneys and lungs were in bad shape.

The nephrology (kidney) specialist, Dr. Geoly, spoke with Sharry later in the morning after he examined the latest test results. He told her, "The numbers are quite bad, but not unusual. We will keep him continuously on dialysis for a week and watch the numbers. If all goes well, we will then shift him to dialysis every other day. He may need some more blood transfusions."

My room in the ICU had a large matrix of lab test results and applicable medical information posted on the wall so that the doctors and nurses could track my progress (or lack thereof) as they entered the room. Each piece of data since my arrival in the ICU was available so that trends could be easily detected. Since there were several different teams of doctors monitoring my condition, this chart was particularly handy. It reminded me of the "log sheets" which we kept on the submarines to record the temperatures and pressures associated with the nuclear reactor plant so that we could determine its status. Later, when I was conscious and recovering in the ICU, I was always impressed by how much time each doctor would take analyzing these results before physically examining me. Linda Ohler, the transplant coordinator, had recommended to Sharry that she scan the data chart daily, not only to gather information for questioning the doctors and nurses, but also to act as yet another backup in the event some developing trend was not noted.

During the afternoon I received some of the transfusions ordered by Dr. Geoly. These units of "packed cells" were blood with the liquid removed. My hemoglobin was dropping, there was no desire to increase the already high fluid levels in my body, and I needed red blood cells. The units of packed cells were given intravenously. There was no immediate improvement, but I was stabilized.

During the early afternoon, Sharry spoke with Dr. Lo Russo, a pulmonary (lung) specialist. He said that the ARDS was "a problem." There was no additional medication to help. The only thing to do for my lungs was to keep me sedated with medication, such as Versed (midazolam hydrochloride), and to let the current medications being received with the respirator keep me breathing. The lungs were the primary concern. Everything else would probably resolve itself or respond to treatment.

During his daily visit to see me, the heart surgeon, Paul Massimiano, encouraged Sharry by telling her, "His new heart is doing great. It is not part of the problem. It's been my experience that as long as the new heart continues to function well, everything else will eventually resolve itself."

During this dangerous phase of my transplant recovery, each of the three heart surgeons, Massimiano, Burton and Lefrak, saw me daily. On any one given day I was being cared for by an incredible amount of medical talent and expertise. Most of the specialists worked in teams. The immunologists, for example, had a group practice consisting of four doctors. At least one would see me daily. They were all impressive. In addition to these teams of doctors, the nursing staff in the Fairfax Hospital ICU was exceptional. These professionals were with me around the clock and made frequent decisions on their own to improve my condition or to respond to emergencies. If I did not make it through this, it was not going to be due to a lack of attention or effort by my medical team.

In the evening Sharry called Aaron in North Carolina to give him the bad news about my condition. It was a difficult conversation. How does a mother tell her son that his father may be dying? Aaron had long since rationalized the seriousness of my original medical condition, but the transplant had given renewed hope that all would now be well. The lung and kidney complications were a terrible psychological blow to everyone. He and Sharry agreed that he should drive from North Carolina to see me following classes the next day unless conditions suddenly worsened.

Sharry then telephoned Nelle at Indiana University. Nelle was terrified and wanted to come to Virginia immediately. Sharry insisted that she continue her classes through the week as previously planned and then fly back on Friday evening. Prior to the transplant we had discussed options regarding school for Nelle and Aaron. Sharry and I had decided that it was important to us that both of our "university types" complete as much of their semesters as possible, regardless of my condition. Having them home was a luxury that would not necessarily translate into direct help for either Sharry or myself. We wanted them in college.

There was no improvement in my condition on Thursday. In fact, I was actually worse. I had become psychotic, or, as one of the nurses put it, "wild and crazy." My arms had been placed in restraints for my own protection. Sharry later told me that I was "totally out of it." She said that whenever I was awake, my eyes were pleading. In view of the fact that I had over ten different lines going in and out of my body and was thoroughly drugged, I am sure that I was looking for help wherever I could get it.

By late afternoon I took my matters into my own hands - literally. I wriggled my one hand sufficiently free from its restraint and, somehow or other, managed to reach down to my groin area and disconnect the luer-lock connector leading to the dialysis unit. How I was able to do this with one hand remains a mystery. To be successful, I had to line up notches on both sides of the connector and then pull the two lines of plastic tubing apart. Never underestimate a wild man!

I was now bleeding directly onto the bed. As soon as I disconnected the luer-lock, blood started shooting out of the line coming from my artery. When the two nurses who were in the room saw the sheets soaked with blood, they reacted quickly to restore the connection and called for additional assistance. By the time the team was able to correct my irrational antics, I had lost well over a unit of blood.

The next day, Friday, September 16, was no better. I was fighting and pleading most of the day. Whenever I was awake, I was thrashing about, pulling at my restraints and yelling. Aaron had called Nelle the previous night to compare what Sharry had told each of them. By the time Nelle arrived on Friday evening, she was terrified. Seeing me did not help, because I presented a totally frightening sight. Watching her father tossing about pleading for help was too much. Sharry could not offer much hope to the children. Her most recent conversations with the doctors had not been encouraging. Everything possible was being done. The plan was to continue to support my lungs with the ventilator and to hope that I would somehow pull through the ARDS.

According to Sharry, the weekend was not a happy one. I continued to show no improvement. Sunday, September 18, was my 51st birthday. The nurses had encouraged her to bring in balloons to celebrate the occasion. Unfortunately I was still out of it and was fighting at every opportunity. If I was aware of my birthday, there was no indication of it. I do remember seeing Nelle sometime over the weekend, because I later recalled her telling me that she had obtained a job with the Indiana University Chemistry Department doing research for $6/hr. Apparently I smiled when she told me this. There was quite an emotional scene when Nelle had to leave the hospital to go to the airport for her return to Bloomington. Because of the seriousness of my condition and the total uncertainty that I would survive, Nelle did not want to leave. She and

Sharry broke down crying and hugged each other for several minutes. I was aware of none of this. What a birthday for my family!

At Sharry's insistence, Aaron returned to his studies at Chapel Hill the following morning. My condition had not improved, but I was well enough to be taken to the cath lab for a heart biopsy which was an important part of the post-transplant protocol. Four small samples of heart tissue were obtained by entering my heart with a small instrument inserted into the jugular vein in my neck. The samples were then stained and analyzed in the laboratory to determine how much, if any, rejection of the new organ is taking place. The body's natural immune system had long been the major barrier to successful transplant operations. Surgical techniques to transplant organs presented no serious obstacles; heart tranplantation has been surgically feasible since the early 1960's when the procedure was initially developed by Dr. Christian Barnard in South Africa. However, most early transplant patients died soon after the operation because the immune system saw the new organ as an invader and attacked it. This process of rejection can now be controlled in most patients by administering doses of powerful immunosuppressant drugs, such as Imuran, Cyclosporine, and my old friend, Prednisone. I had been receiving each of these since my transplant.

The one (and only) source of good news during this period came from the biopsy. It indicated that the immunosuppressants were doing their job. My body was not trying to reject the new heart. The laboratory results were recorded as a "one" on a scale of zero to ten. Zero is no rejection, ten is maximum rejection. A "one" was definitely OK! At least my new heart was continuing to function satisfactorily.

One area of my body which was not working well was the digestive system. By this time I had a Nasal Gastric (NG) tube threaded through my nose into my stomach, but little or none of the liquid food was being absorbed. An alternative method of feeding, TPN (Total Parenteral Nutrition), was rejected by the heart surgeons, because they were concerned that the highly caustic solution which would have to be fed directly into the aorta through the central line would be potentially dangerous for my new heart. There were no immediate plans to remedy the food absorption problem other than to continue with the NG tube and to hope for improvement.

The daily test results provided both good and bad news. The good news was that creatinine levels (a measure of kidney function) were beginning to decrease as the result of the dialysis. My kidneys appeared to be mending. Another positive development was that stool, urine and sputum samples indicated that I had not developed an infection. If I were to have an area become infected, the consequences could be serious due to the high levels of immunosuppressant drugs which I was receiving to keep my body from rejecting the new organ. The bad news came from the chest x-rays. My lungs were still in a dangerous condition and not showing improvement.

Sharry had spent several hours in the hospital library trying to learn more about ARDS. Her research was not reassuring. According to the literature which she read, ARDS was a killer. Over 50 percent of ARDS patients died from the condition. It was definitely a dangerous situation. In somewhat of a panic, she telephoned Dr. John Cleary, one of the pulmonary specialists who had been seeing me daily. Sharry asked Cleary to "be straight with me." He replied that she should not make herself crazy by reading statistics which may not be applicable to my case. Although ARDS was a very serious condition carrying the possibility of fatality, there was no reason, he said, to believe that her husband was in immediate danger.

"The respirator is doing its job," Cleary explained. "It's impossible to predict what might happen, but our best ally is a tincture of time."

Although this was not a totally reassuring conversation, Sharry did feel better. After several more conversations with Dr. Cleary over the next few days, she learned that patience and prayer were her best options and that Cleary's favorite phrase was "a tincture of time."

By all accounts, Thursday, September 22, was the low point of THE ORDEAL. The day had begun on an optimistic note. The doctors had decided to see how well my lungs would function on their own, so the respirator was removed in the morning. I was struggling to breathe, but was, in Sharry's words, "making it."

Hoping that I was now finally on the road to recovery, Sharry went home to take a nap. She was exhausted. She slept all afternoon until Aaron arrived from Chapel Hill. They ate a quick meal together with Emily and then came to the hospital. When they arrived in the ICU, Sharry immediately began to cry. Although I was sitting up in the bed, I looked terrible. I was unshaven and spitting up blood, which was now all over my clothing. The respirator was removed, but I was struggling desperately for each breath, even with an oxygen mask on. The NG tube in my nose was apparently as ineffective as ever in providing nourishment. I was still on dialysis, and the steady noise from the machine served as a constant reminder that I was in big trouble. There was little cause for optimism. Things definitely did not look good at this point.

Sharry bathed me so that I at least looked better. Aaron remained in the room with his mother. Few words were spoken. The gloom was heavy. Around 1 AM, Aaron convinced Sharry that she should go home to rest. She reluctantly left, but telephoned Louise, my nurse that evening, several times during the night to receive an update on my condition. During a call around 4:30 AM, Sharry learned that I had told Louise that I could not make it on the oxygen and had pleaded to be put back on the respirator. In view of how much I hated (and feared) this tube down my throat, I must have felt that I was going to die without it.

Morning brought the two week anniversary of my transplant. I was not able to celebrate because I was unconscious during most of the day. In fact, even if awake, there was nothing to celebrate. The ventilator was back in, I still had tubes going in and out in all directions, and my arms were tied down. I was also having incredibly intense nightmares, the worst imaginable.

Occasionally I would awaken, my mind racing in total fear, only to discover a real life scenario comparable to the nightmare. I was soaked with sweat, and in incredible pain and confusion. I would scream and try to move my arms, but to no avail - those restraints really did work! As my anxiety level rose, this vicious cycle repeated itself. The more I struggled, the more I became terrified. **Reality was far worse than the nightmares!**

I found myself wanting to return to the nightmares - at least they were different each time.

Aaron spent the day studying in the cafeteria. Every few hours he would take a break and come to the ICU to check on me. It must have been very depressing for him, because my condition was frightening. The hemoglobin levels kept dropping, indicating the need for another unit of blood. I was back on the ventilator due to my lungs not working, my digestive system was not operating properly, I was throwing up a combination of blood and thick green mucous, and my mind was delirious. What more could go wrong?

Plenty!

During his morning rounds, Dr. Lefrak had noticed that the color and thickness of the sputum being suctioned out of my lungs was different from that which he was accustomed to seeing. He ordered a culture of the sputum and directed that the infectious disease team be summoned. The results of the culture indicated that I had developed a serious infection in my lungs. Dr. Mary Schmidt, an infectious disease specialist, arrived shortly. She determined that an unusual bacteria was involved and started heavy doses of antibiotics to combat it. Many of the doctors and nurses involved in my care said how much they were impressed that Lefrak, a heart surgeon, had been the first one to pick up that I might have an infection. I was not impressed. I was too scared to be passing out "atta-boys."

Fortunately, the antibiotics were successful in combating the infection. It had been a strange situation. My temperature had not increased noticeably during the entire episode. I cannot say that I felt worse during the infection. Of course, I continuously felt lousy, so the infection was a minor blip on my radar screen. I still had other problems, such as the food absorption problem.

Jerry, who was my evening nurse, believed that the reason that the NG tube was not working effectively was that my stomach was not functioning properly. He decided on his own to advance the tube directly into my small intestine. This move proved to be inspired. I began to digest the liquid food being fed into me by the NG tube and to gain strength. Jerry's actions reflected the exceptional nursing care which I had received from my first day at Fairfax Hospital. The nurses were truly a key ingredient in my successful stint on LIFE ROW. On several occasions their observation and judgment were the difference between severe consequences and an improved condition. If nurses are replaced from their current role in primary care by the use of "nursing assistants," i.e. nurses aides, in the name of economy, I believe that there will be an inevitable decline in the quality of care received by patients. Nurses are keen observers and are most effective when they see their patients face-to-face several times each shift. Jerry's actions were another example of just how vital a good nurse is to a speedy recovery.

By the weekend (September 24), I was beginning to show some improvement. Breathing was still a major problem, but I was now sufficiently "with it" to want to communicate with anyone who would listen. Actually "listen" is not the correct term, because I could not speak intelligibly with the respirator down my throat. I began to use my hands to signal that I would like to write a note. Sharry found some paper and a pencil. I was on line!

Actually, I was not totally "with it," because in my first note I wrote, in barely legible script, "DEAD HORSES UNDER BED." As Sharry read the note, she said, "Dead horses under bed?" I enthusiastically nodded, "Yes!" Aaron thought that this was the funniest thing he had heard, and, for the first time in several weeks, laughed loudly. Sharry kept a straight face and said, "You may be right. We will check."

With considerable drama, they carefully bent over and slowly looked under the bed. Sharry stood back up and gave me her report, "No, I don't see any horses under there."

Aaron chimed in, "Dad, I don't see anything either. There are **no** horses under there."

I felt reassured, - and not the slightest bit embarrassed.

When Sharry left the room in the early afternoon, I found the nurse call button and, when Ann Marie entered the room, went through rather elaborate hand and arms signals to ask for another pad of paper. She left without granting my request, but soon returned with a white board and several dry markers. I have no idea where she so rapidly procured these items, but I was grateful. I could now communicate. My first note was, "Need to talk to my wife." Because my handwriting was so shaky, interpretation required an iterative process similar to charades. The nurse would look at my scribbles and then guess what I had written. I would shake my head with a disappointed "no" or an enthusiastic "yes."

This process would continue until we had connected. Sometimes I simply could not be understood no matter how long we tried. It was an incredibly frustrating situation, because after two weeks of silence, I wanted desperately to communicate.

Actually both Sharry and I had considerable experience in communication deprivation. A career in submarines will give that to you. During our 70 day submerged patrols, U.S. submarines could routinely receive messages, but we were prohibited from transmitting. Any radio signals coming from a ship at sea can be easily triangulated by opposing forces providing information concerning its location and movement. Because the primary mission of American submarines during the Cold War was to remain undetected at sea, there were strict rules against sending any message once the ship had cleared port unless there was a dire emergency affecting the mission. Thus when Sharry and I waved good-bye as the submarine departed the pier, we really were waving **good-bye**. There would be no communication for the next two months.

Well, not exactly, because there were "Familygrams" - at least when I was assigned to a ballistic missile submarine. These ships (called SSBNs) were the ones which carried missiles with multiple nuclear warheads continuously aimed at the Soviet Union. USS KAMEHAMEHA, for example, the ship which I commanded, had 16 Poseidon missiles, each loaded with 10 hydrogen bomb warheads. These 160 warheads could by themselves destroy a sizable amount of the USSR. Remaining undetected was the essential element of our mission of deterring a nuclear war between us and the Soviets. So long as the Russians did not know where we were at any given moment, they had to assume that we were fully prepared, and capable, to blow them away if so directed by the U.S. command authority. If they had some way of knowing the location of the U.S. SSBNs, the Soviets could launch a pre-emptive strike to destroy this threat, and then be in a position to dictate whatever they wished to the world. [I am not including the other elements of the U.S. strategic forces, our bombers and land based missiles, in this discussion. They would also have to be countered in any pre-emptive move by the Russians.]

In addition to remaining undetected, our missile submarines remained in constant reception of radio messages from our commanders. Our opponents had to assume, therefore, that we were always capable of receiving a message to launch our missiles at short notice. Both the Russians and ourselves had radio systems which allowed submarines to receive messages while submerged, so long as the ship was moving slowly at a modest depth under the ocean surface. The messages received by the submarine are diverse and continuous so that there is no noticeable increase in communications traffic in a time of crisis. Tactical messages concerning nuclear weapons or the suspected whereabouts of enemy forces, administrative information (such as a change in duty station for a crew member), and personal messages all flow through the same circuit into the SSBN radio room. These personal messages were called "Familygrams."

Each member of a SSBN crew (there were roughly 110-130 men aboard) could receive five such messages of up to 20 words each during the 70 day patrol. These brief bursts of communication from home were essentially filler when the ship was not receiving operational messages. A typical Familygram from Sharry was, "All OK here, new tires on VW, garden great, miss you like crazy, have special treat for you, Love, Sharry." As one can imagine, these personal messages had to be screened for taste and content prior to transmission. Although the messages were encrypted exactly the same as the operational ones, they could be (and were) read by sailors in every U.S. submarine radio room. Imagine the reaction, both on his own ship and throughout the fleet, if Seaman Jones at sea aboard the KAMEHAMEHA received the following Familygram, "Fallen out of love with you, love Joe better, your parents ill, dog died, taking car, leaving you, bye, Rhonda."

Maybe you can receive a lot of information in 20 words. But it did not seem that way to most of us. Even the newest crewmembers quickly calculated that Familygrams amounted to just over one word per day from home. Crews on the other type of submarines, SSNs, attack submarines, were not so lucky: they received nothing. And no submarine, SSBN or SSN, was permitted to send an outgoing message when on patrol. Even if Seaman Jones had received the above message, he would not be able respond to Rhonda to find out more about "Joe," his parents, the dog or the car. (It would be interesting to know which he would ask about first!)

Even though Sharry and I, having spent many years separated by my assignments aboard both SSBNs and SSNs, were accustomed to lengthy periods of minimal communication, we were still frustrated by the difficulties as I came out of the depths of THE ORDEAL. I wanted to shout to the world, " I'm back!!" And I wanted very much to tell Sharry that I loved her. Unfortunately, I could not yet do either.

By Sunday, September 25, I was definitely showing improvement. The nurses were able to get me up into a chair for a brief period of sitting. I was so weak that this evolution was essentially a dead lift on their part. But I was out of bed! The dialysis shunts were still in my body, but they were not being used on a daily basis. The dreaded ventilator, however, was still required because my lungs were too weak to function on their own. The NG tube was providing nourishment. If someone were to assess my condition based on the number of tubes and lines running in and out of my body, the only conclusion would have to be that I was still in deep trouble.

I decided to take matters into my own hands. When I was by myself, I found the pad of paper and a pencil and proceeded to draft a game plan to get out of ICU. I wrote:

> MON　　VENTILATOR OUT
> TUE　　EVERYTHING ELSE OUT
> WED　　REST UP
> THU　　GET OUT OF ICU

When Ann Marie came into the room, I proudly showed her "the plan." She laughed, but did not tell me that I was crazy. Sharry was not so charitable when she came in. She said, "Well, let's take this one day at a time. Maybe you can get out of here by the end of the week. First you have to breath on your own."

"Details, details!" I muttered to myself.

On Monday, as the various doctors came in to see me, I held up "the plan" for their inspection. None said, "No way." In fact, the pulmonary guy, Dr. DiCicco, said, "OK, Ed, let's see what you can do off the ventilator."

Around 11 in the morning one of the Physician Assistants came to remove the ventilator. There is nothing terribly sophisticated about this procedure. It is the basic, "One, two three, pull," technique, with the hose flying out of your throat on "pull." In the removal process the patient's throat receives what amounts to a wire-brush treatment and remains sore for several days. Ann Marie had promised earlier in the morning that she would give me a cherry popsicle as soon as the ventilator was removed. I held her to her promise. In fact, it was the only thing I could think about all morning.

The popsicle was soft when it arrived. I was able immediately to take small bites and to allow the cool fluid to dissolve in my throat. I do not know of any taste sensation which has ever been so pleasant! I told myself that "the plan" was working. Later in the day, Ann Marie brought me some ice chips and another cherry popsicle. I took as long as possible in savoring these frozen delights, because my throat was killing me whenever I did not have some soothing coolness on it. I felt so good about my progress that I started to refer to Monday, September 26, 1994 as "The First Day in the Rest of My Life."

Now that I could communicate orally, I talked quite a lot to Sharry. I learned that another successful heart transplant, number 99 at Fairfax, had been done three days earlier and that the recipient, a man my age named Ron, was recovering in a room in ICU next to me. Knowing that I had been number 97, I asked Sharry what happened to number 98. She paused for a brief moment and then said, "I think that he died." It took me a few minutes to digest this sobering news. I became very aware of how lucky I had been. I also realized that I had not thanked the Lord since learning that I was about to receive a new heart over two weeks earlier. I immediately corrected this oversight.

The x-rays of my chest remained much the same. Sharry was not particularly confident that my lungs were strong enough for me to make it without the respirator. However, I was determined to proceed with "the plan," and the respirator definitely had no continuing role in my script. Oxygen levels in my blood stream were being monitored by a device that clipped onto the end of one of my fingers. I am uncertain how it works, but the readings were remaining above 90 percent, a level judged to be acceptable. Although there was nothing which I could do myself to improve the oxygen level, I spent considerable time praying for an increase. My worst fear was that a decrease would require the reinsertion of that miserable ventilator.

On Tuesday, the NG feeding tube was removed. I was feeling much better, particularly after I was able to enjoy some warm soup for lunch. I was back on real food! Surely a Big Mac was just around the corner. The nurses, with Sharry's help, moved me to a comfortable chair. I remained out of bed for two hours, basking in a sense of freedom. However, I could achieve little movement myself because I was so incredibly weak.

I awoke early the next morning. Jerry had the night shift. After he weighed me and took vital signs, I asked if he could help me with "the plan." Jerry agreed. Together we completed my bathing. He helped me to shave. My hands were so shaky that I probably would have bled to death from razor cuts if I had to do this by myself. He put a clean hospital gown on me, and, when we were finished, I looked pretty good - if I must say so myself.

The next step was to move to a reclining chair next to the bed. We managed this, although there were a few difficult moments in the transition. By the time the doctors arrived, I was projecting an image of total health (Well, at least I did not appear to be dying!).

The first doctor in was Lefrak, the senior heart surgeon on the transplant team. He was his usual methodical self. Suddenly he turned to me from observing the data chart and announced, "I'm moving you up to the 3rd floor today. You don't need to be here any longer. As soon as a bed becomes available up there, they will come to get you." He then turned and left the room with no further comment.

I was dumbfounded. This was better than my wildest dreams. Even the most optimistic versions of "the plan" had not anticipated leaving the ICU this soon. I certainly was not arguing. After three weeks, I was ready.

In order to ensure that no one was going to counter Lefrak's order, I decided to remain in the chair rather than return to the bed. I was determined to stay there, "looking good," all day, if necessary. I telephoned Sharry with the good news. Her reply was more pragmatic, "Right. In your dreams."

I reassured her that I was moving out of ICU today. My exact words were, "No, seriously, Lefrak said I could go. I'm out of here." I felt like I was a grade school kid telling my Mom that the teacher said that we didn't have any homework over the weekend!

Sharry has never admitted this to me, but I am certain that she immediately called the daytime nurse in ICU to confirm the news. After all, I had been totally delirious just a few days before. I was also the guy with the dead horse under the bed.

Lunch came. I was beginning to become more than a little paranoid. Surely a bed should have become free by now. At 2:30 PM Louise came in and said, "They will be here in five minutes. You're headed to the 3rd floor." In spite of my fondness for the ICU nurses, I was not sorry to leave. Maybe THE ORDEAL would soon be over.

All Fairfax Hospital heart transplant patients are transferred from ICU to the 3rd floor in preparation for discharge. There is no set time table involved. The length of the stay is dependent on the patient's recovery progress and how soon the patient can learn to administer the large quantity of drugs required to suppress the body's immune system. In order to minimize the chance of infection or the transfer of a virus, each patient has his own room. If I were to hear a snorer, it could only have been an imaginary flashback to my roommates of THE WAIT. Anyone entering the room - nurse, doctor, cleaning personnel, visitor - was required to wash hands before coming near my bed. Surprisingly, face masks were not routinely required, unless the visitor to the room had a cold or a virus. I had face masks available for my own use when I was transported from the room to another part of the hospital (for example, when I was taken down to x-ray).

My first night on the 3rd floor was uncomfortable, but I was smiling the entire time. The problem was my extreme weakness. During the nearly three weeks in ICU, my muscle tone had evaporated. My lower extremities now resembled chicken legs. I had virtually no upper body strength. Whenever I attempted to move or to reach something on the table next to the bed, it was a major effort. My overall mood, however, was ecstatic.

The following morning rehabilitation began in earnest. Shortly after breakfast, my nurse informed me that she was ready to help me walk to the bathroom. Since I could barely stand, I thought that this might be a bit ambitious. Although it took over five minutes each way, we made the trip. I was exhausted physically, but elated mentally. After resting for thirty minutes, I soon set up shop, returning to many of the habits and routine of THE WAIT. I read the *Post* and the *Times* and wrote several letters and thank you notes.

After lunch, Sophie arrived. She was young and cheerful and was my Occupational Therapist. Sophie was responsible for preparing me to gain sufficient strength to be able to go home. Each day she would arrive to supervise me while I attempted ten separate exercises from a sheet which she had prepared. Some of the movements were relatively easy. Others were initially impossible, given my incredibly low level of strength. One day, after Sophie had been rather brutal in putting me through her paces, I said to her, "Sophie, your problem is that you were born too late. You would have made a great boot camp sergeant in World War II." She laughed as she promised, "Wait until tomorrow, Private Linz!"

It was due to Sophie's no-nonsense approach that I was able to gain hope that perhaps I could soon go home. I became determined to try to outdo her expectations. One day I went through all of the exercises before she arrived, and then, without telling her what I had done, performed everything she asked. This was not a particularly brilliant plan, because, although I was thoroughly exhausted by early afternoon, I did not take a nap and was like a limp wash cloth by evening.

I was also able now to receive visitors. Our friends, Kathy and "CG" Caruthers, were the first to come by, followed shortly by my teaching buddies, Bill Carreiro, Mike Pallo and Tom Cindric. I also started to receive phone calls from other friends at the high school, such as Pattie Hutchinson and Don Maeyer. Sharry told me that Siobhan had been discharged from the hospital while I was in ICU and had written me a letter. Apparently I had read it sometime during THE ORDEAL, but I had no memory of it. I telephoned her to thank her and to ask how she was doing. She came to visit later that afternoon. She looked great and said that she was "doing reasonably well." She had not yet developed noticeable side effects from the Amiodarone. Of course, she now had yet another boy friend. After all, it had been four weeks since I had last inquired.

By the weekend, I was walking better and was able to stand alone, unsupported, for three minutes. My handwriting was somewhat illegible because my hands were still extremely shaky, but most of those to whom I wrote were polite and did not complain. Saturday was Sharry's birthday (the big "five O"). Emily was in Williamsburg, Virginia for a cross country race with her team, so Aaron and I decided to have a mini-celebration with a surprise birthday dinner in the hospital room. He baked a great cake, using our favorite recipe for "best of the best" chocolate. The rest of the menu consisted of a Caesar salad which he made at home and spinach lasagna, which he purchased in a gourmet food section of a local supermarket. It was wonderful.

I had telephoned the volunteer office earlier in the week to request assistance in purchasing a birthday card from the hospital gift shop, so I was able to give Sharry something. We promised each other that we would have a "real" birthday celebration to make up for mine in the ICU and hers here in the hospital when we were home, perhaps at the same time we celebrated our 24th wedding anniversary on Halloween.

On Monday morning I was taken down to the cath lab and received my second heart biopsy. Dr. Rogan performed the procedure. The good news was that it was another "one," indicating no rejection so far. The immunosuppressant medications were working. There was no bad news. My new heart and I were getting along fabulously.

One of the heart transplant coordinators would come to see me daily to quiz me on the types and amounts of medications which I would be taking when I left the hospital. This was not a problem for me because I was already taking the medications by myself at the appropriate intervals. The floor nurse would come to the room to check to see that I had taken the correct amounts on time throughout the day, but I was essentially on my own.

The only new medical problem which I had was that my fingers were disintegrating. For some unknown reason, the skin on the tips of my fingers had begun to peel away, making touch a very sensitive issue. It hurt. A dermatologist was brought in. After determining that this was probably not a life threatening situation, he prescribed a lotion (LacHydrine) which "fixed it" in two days.

I also had a very sore throat. It was at this time that one of my favorite nurses, Tony Chan, came to my rescue. Tony worked the night shift and dedicated himself to keeping me supplied with the only medication which actually worked: popsicles. Several times during the night Tony would appear bearing the wonder drug. Because my feet and ankles were swelling each evening, I kept them raised on a pillow at night. Tony would bring in lotion and popsicles. As I savored each bite of popsicle, allowing it to trickle slowly down my throat, Tony would massage my feet and ankles with the lotion. We would talk about our wives and our children during this process, and after about 15 minutes of this heaven on earth, I would go back to sleep for a few more hours.

On Thursday, October 6, Dr. John Miller, the immunologist who was now the lead doctor for me, walked into the room and, with no advance warning, said, "You're going home today. There is no reason for you to stay here. You need to be home so that you can really recover." I liked this guy.

There were several details to be completed before I could leave. The floor nurse arrived shortly to provide me with discharge instructions, i.e., what I should, and should not, be doing at home. I telephoned Sharry at her office at the Health Department to relay the news and to see when she could come to pick me up. Much to my disappointment, she did not say, "I'll be there right away." Since she had no idea that I might be discharged before the weekend, she was in the midst of a clinic and also had a full schedule of clients to see during the afternoon. Her supervisors and colleagues had been incredibly flexible and kind to us throughout my entire illness and hospitalization, so we decided to wait a few extra hours until she completed her work. It turned out that this was not a problem because I had to wait until late afternoon to receive the handful of prescriptions to be filled for my medications at home. It was an exceptionally long afternoon for me. I kept looking at the clock on the wall while worrying that someone would suddenly decide that I should not go home.

Sharry arrived at 5:30 PM. Within 20 minutes we were out the front door of the hospital. THE ORDEAL was history.

Chapter 15

HOME

Sharry drove our van to the front entrance of the hospital. She had "borrowed" a small stool from the third floor, and she placed it near the open door of the van. With her help, I took one step onto the stool. Then I was able to maneuver my bottom onto the van seat, swing my legs into position, and eagerly await our departure.

The drive home was during maximum rush hour traffic, but I did not care. For the first time in four months I felt free. It was warm enough to roll the windows down part way, and the early October evening breeze was a total tonic. One tends to forget life's small pleasures.

We had decided not to telephone ahead from the car to tell Emily that I had been discharged and was on the way home. She would just be arriving from cross country practice, and we thought that it would make a great surprise for her to see Dad when she was not expecting him. Based on the daily assessments from the doctors, the earliest that any of us thought I could come home was late the next day or the day after.

We achieved total surprise. When Emily saw me in the van, she waved and came running. Emily had always put on a brave, silent front with respect to my illness and hospitalization, but she was obviously overwhelmed to see me. She gave me a huge hug as I maneuvered myself out of the van with the small, portable step and my cane.

After hugging Emily for an extended period and saying how great it was to be home, I immediately noticed how the grass was still very green due to the unusually wet summer and warm fall. The flowers were in full bloom, and the yard looked wonderful. I had forgotten how many different types of flowers I had planted in the spring. They all seemed to be saying "Welcome Home!"

Once I was out of the van I was able to walk assisted only by the cane. I slowly made my way up the short grassy incline to the front porch. Here I required Sharry's assistance to go up the one step. I was still very weak. We then took the final step up through the front door into the living room. Now I did start to cry. Everything inside the house looked so "non-hospital." I felt as if I had been liberated from a concentration camp or some other unspeakable horror.

Our dog, Sydney, proceeded to go wild. She had seen me once in the past four months. It was uncertain whether she remembered me as the guy who would periodically give her pieces of hot dog, or as a new target on which to jump and seek attention. I did not care about her motives. I was just glad to see her. We did have to restrain her so that she would not jump up onto me and accidentally scratch my skin. I did not need an open wound which might become easily infected due to the immunosuppressant drugs I was taking. After about 30 minutes of sniffing while restrained on her leash near me, Sydney was released on her honor. She did not jump up and contented herself with wagging her entire rear end while she rubbed against me as much as possible. At dinner she assumed her usual pre-hospital position directly under my legs waiting for any possible handout. She seemed to remember that I was a total pushover in this regard.

Sharry fixed a great dinner of grilled salmon steaks, fresh green beans and a salad. This was not hospital food! The irony was that it not only tasted like "real food," but it was also probably better for me. It was at this moment that I sensed that my recuperation had truly begun.

Our great neighbor, Hugh Boyd, came over at Sharry's request, to help her move Aaron's bed from upstairs to the living room on the first floor where I would be sleeping. There was no way that I was yet ready to go up steps. The main floor of the house became my turf. I had everything necessary for my recovery within walking distance. There was a bathroom, the kitchen, the dining room table (which became my desk), and the family room whenever I wanted to watch the weekly professional football games on television.

I quickly became fairly independent, - even on the first night home. I learned that it was helpful to sit on a pillow whenever I was in a chair. From this higher position, I could better use the small amount of arm strength which I had remaining to push on my cane. Together with a simultaneous push from my leg muscles, I would usually be able to rise to a vertical, although shaky, position. Then with the assistance of the cane I could take steps to a new location, typically stopping to catch my breath several times along the way.

By early evening I was exhausted. Bed was calling for me. I felt fine with respect to my heart, my incisions, and the entire surgery. Unfortunately, what was not fine was my throat. I began to notice shortly before bedtime that I could swallow only with an incredible amount of pain. Every time I swallowed anything, even the excess moisture in my mouth, my entire throat felt as if it was being reamed out with a wire brush (like the type we used to scrape old paint off metal surfaces on ships). Sucking on Popsicles and frozen fruit bars helped somewhat while I was awake, but night was genuine hell in this regard. When I did finally fall asleep, I found that every time I woke up, I would be in total agony due to the swallowing problem. The situation had not improved by morning.

Sharry had gone to the local pharmacy the evening I had arrived home to pick up all of the medicines which I was required to take. One of the transplant coordinators, Paige, had given us a handful of prescriptions and a schedule to follow throughout the day for taking the required post-transplant medicines. In addition to the three immunosuppressants (Cyclosporine, Imuran and Prednisone), there were several other drugs in the daily regimen. These included some over the counter items, such as aspirin, iron supplements and Tums.

Four times each day I also inserted a white, rather chalky tasting pill, Mycelex Troche, to dissolve under my tongue. The purpose of this annoyance was to counter *Candida albicans,* the organism which can cause the disease, thrush. Apparently we all have bad guys throughout our bodies just aching to start thrush if given an opportunity. Frankly, I had never heard of the disease. Sharry, my on-scene medical encyclopedia, informed me that thrush typically occurs in infants and young children and is characterized by whitish patches and ulcers on the membranes of the mouth. "I saw a premature baby just last week that had it all over the inside of her mouth," she said. "You are at risk because your immune system is being compromised by the daily steroids which you have to take to prevent rejection."

I winced as I formed an image of the baby's mouth. I resolved to take my Troche, like a good boy. As a result, the inside of my mouth often looked as if I had just chewed several pieces of classroom chalk.

I also was taking the diuretic, Lasix, to aid in removing fluids. Due to a steady buildup of fluid in my ankles during the first week home, we called the hospital for advice. After discussing the situation with me, one of the doctors at the transplant clinic added Aldactone to the Lasix. When little, if any improvement was observed when I came to the clinic for my regular appointment, he decided to stop the Aldactone. Initially I had also been taking Theo-Dur, a medication typically prescribed for bronchial asthma. Its purpose was to help to elevate my heart rate. When my resting pulse stabilized between 70 and 80, the Theo-Dur was immediately discontinued. I was always pleased that none of my doctors seemed to be prone to over-medicating me.

In order to insure that I did not miss or err in my administration of all of the drugs, I initially used a chart which listed each medication with an "x" marked on the appropriate hour. I became meticulous in checking each medication twice so that the chances of error would be slight. Even in the hospital there were at least three occasions in which I "caught" a nurse trying to give me either the wrong medicine or an incorrect amount of the right medicine in spite of their own detailed procedures (as developed by the hospital's "Risk Management" team, i.e., lawyers).

When Paige telephoned me at home to set a new dose level of Cyclosporine (based on the previous day's blood work at the hospital), she also told me that the swipe taken earlier from a blister on my lip had been cultured and was definitely herpes. She said that she had discussed the situation with the immunologists and had already telephoned in a prescription to our pharmacy for Zovirax to help to combat this virus. I was to take it five times a day for the next five days. I added it to my already lengthy list of medications.

The news about the herpes was actually good, because I now had an explanation why my throat was killing me when I swallowed. I also began to notice soreness in other locations in my mouth. Sharry picked up the Zovirax within the hour. Contrary to the stated directions, I immediately took a double dose to try to load up my system to fight the virus. It turned out that we also had a few pills remaining from a previous herpes problem in my mouth which Robin Merlino had diagnosed sometime during the past year. With the new prescription I had plenty of the anti-herpes pills so there was no danger of running out before the five days were up. Actually, Sharry's advice to load up on the drug was based not only upon her own experience with the health department, but also Robin's previous directions to me with her original prescription. Neither Sharry nor I free lance on medications. In fact, I always describe myself to the doctors and nurses as "Mr. Compliance."

I had one more bad night with the swallowing before the Zovirax began to provide relief. Since I was having no other problems, I felt genuinely on the road to recovery.

Everything was not totally rosy. I was still too weak to do several typical household actions, such as lifting myself up from a sitting position. Once again Sharry was my savior, as she had been in a thousand ways for the past several years. Whenever I would become "stuck" in a low chair because of insufficient strength to lift myself out, she would assist me. Sometimes when I was particularly weak by the end of the day, my body became almost a total dead lift for her. In most cases, however, I was able to extricate myself from low sitting positions due to prior planning (such as the pillow technique). I found that it was also helpful to have arms on the chair or a railing nearby so that I could lift up easier.

The toilet presented a unique situation, because (1) sitting on a pillow was obviously not in the cards, and (2) our bathrooms at home were not rigged with those "handicapped" rails found in public restrooms. The cane was some help, but, more than once, I found myself stuck and had to wait for assistance from Sharry. I thought of this often when she went to work and I was "home alone." I **always** ensured that there was at least 8 hours of reading material in the bathroom - just in case I had to pass a few hours until she returned home!

Emily was a huge help during these first days home. She did countless chores around the house and ran numerous errands for me. Due to my poor mobility I had many requests, and she fulfilled every one in a cheery manner. She raced around the house getting me various drinks (I preferred warm drinks due to my sore throat). She found all of the writing items which I required to keep up a steady stream of correspondence. Emily would even dial numbers for me from the kitchen telephone, then hand me the phone. At the end of the conversation, she would hang up the phone and ask if there were any other numbers which I wanted to be dialed. This period of "Emily's Help Service" lasted several days. Her attitude was always positive and cheerful. My love and admiration for her was reinforced daily. She had a full school schedule, daily cross country practice, and Spanish tutoring lessons. Add to these items her normal desire for socialization with high school friends, and this was one busy teenager. I was impressed, and proud.

My first clinic visit back at the hospital was the following Monday. We had to be at the lab at 7 AM for blood and urine samples. Sharry took along our borrowed wheel chair so that I could travel the long distances in the hospital with little effort on my part. After the lab work, we went to the transplant clinic on the 10th floor to receive a thorough evaluation by one of the transplant coordinators (usually Paige or Mary Beth) and then Dr. John Miller, an immunologist, who would now be in charge of my recovery, essentially forever.

Miller is an outgoing, very likable person. While he was examining me, we compared our picks for the football games the coming weekend. Occasionally we would bet a buck or two. I always won. This bothered me a little, because I do not like to collect money from someone in a position to hurt me. What if Miller suddenly decided to get even? Fortunately, I was not betting against Paige, who was a major football fan. She knew more about the teams than Miller and I combined.

Everything went well at the clinic. They were pleased with my healing and progress and told me to keep working on regaining my strength. Miller recommended that we obtain a stationary exercise bicycle to aid in my rehabilitation. We took his advice and found a good used one later that afternoon for $99. Sharry and I were very pleased with the first clinic visit. There had been no bad news, and whatever we were doing at home seemed to be working.

While at the clinic I met several other heart transplant patients. All were men. They ranged in age from the early 20's to late 60's. I quickly observed that, compared to most of the others, I seemed to be doing well. One of the main advantages which I enjoyed was that my donor heart had been such an excellent match. Apparently 30 to 80 percent of the public is positive for cytomegalovirus (CMV), a condition which is not dangerous to the normal person, but which can be very serious in a transplanted patient. Neither my donor nor myself had this virus present. In view of the high incidence of CMV in the general population, the odds are high that a transplant patient may have problems with this virus, so I had been extremely fortunate in this regard. I certainly did not feel guilty about this good luck. After being incredibly unlucky statistically with respect to sarcoidosis and the extremely lengthy duration of THE WAIT, I felt that it was my turn for some good luck.

Several of my fellow patients at the transplant clinic had not been so fortunate with respect to CMV. The transplanted patient with CMV (either from the original heart or the donor) can develop symptoms involving fever, malaise, nausea, and even flu like conditions. To attempt to prevent these from developing, the patient must receive ganciclovir, intravenously, twice a day for 14 days following transplant, and then a different drug, immune globulin, also intravenously once a week for the next 8 weeks. Several transplant recipients at the clinic were required to sit for two additional hours receiving this IV therapy. This was obviously not an enjoyable experience for them.

The CMV problem does not end there. Acyclovir pills must then be taken 3 times a day for the next three months. If the symptoms of CMV do appear, it is back to IV therapy involving ganciclovir twice a day for the next two weeks - a distinctly unwelcome and psychologically disturbing development.

There were some other apparent problems involving patients at the clinic. A few seemed to be having emotional problems dealing with their new situation. In each case these were recent transplants who were discouraged by their drug regimen, the lack of a rapid recovery, or, in one case, an unrelated condition which had pre-existed before the transplant. I do not wish to give a negative impression. Overall most of us were very happy to be alive, and were doing whatever was necessary to achieve total recovery.

My own drug regimen at home was not proving to be difficult or burdensome, but it did involve paying close attention to the daily schedule of medications. The daily dose of cyclosporine (initially Sandimmune and then Neoral) was adjusted based on a weekly blood test [as I progressed further from the transplant, the frequency of this test was decreased to a monthly basis]. The target level for cyclosporine in the blood was set by the immunologist, Miller, or one of his partners, Dr. Richard Binder or Dr. Gregory Orloff, based on their judgment of the minimum required to prevent my immune system from rejecting the new heart. The daily doses of the two other immunosuppressants, Imuran and Prednisone, were not adjusted depending on blood samples. The goal was to lower the amount of these two as much as possible without initiating a rejection. Setting appropriate levels of these three interacting drugs is an aspect of the transplant process which is continually evolving as doctors gain additional experience.

As with all transplant (heart, lung, liver, kidney, etc.) patients, I am currently required to continue on a combination of immunosuppressant drugs for the rest of my life. Acting together, they minimize the chance of rejection of the new organ by reducing the effectiveness of the body's immune system. This is obviously a desired result with respect to the rejection of the transplanted organ, but it is truly a double-edged sword situation. With the immune system being artificially weakened by the immunosuppressant drugs, the rest of the body is much more susceptible to infections and viruses. Consequently, the transplant patient must take precautions to avoid placing himself in situations in which infection is likely. If circumstances required that I be in a potentially infectious situation (such as the waiting room at a Social Security office), I was instructed to wear a disposable face mask to filter the air and to wash my hands frequently, at least for the first few months post-transplant. [After four months, I was "normal" in all my activities.]

Rather than worry myself to death about exposure to viruses and disease, I decided to make some conscious decisions about reducing infection and to allow nature to take its course in all others. One of my basic principles throughout this ordeal had been not to worry about things which I could not control. The only precautions which I took involved not allowing our dog to jump up and scratch me and avoiding close contact with people having colds and other obviously communicable diseases. If visitors came to the door with a cold, we would politely request that they remain outside or telephone me. Everyone proved to be very understanding in this regard.

I had been told at the clinic to avoid other high risk situations for infections and viruses such as movie theaters, malls, crowded restaurants and the like. Discharge instructions from the hospital also recommended not taking airplane trips for at least four months afterwards due to the recycled atmosphere in the plane. Based on previous flights from Washington to Spokane to visit Spurway, I knew that the chances were at least 50-50 that I would pick up a bad cold anytime I took a lengthy airline flight, - and that was when I had a fully operational immune system. John Schrader, my football pool buddy, always had a particularly bad time with cross country airplane trips. He never failed to pick up a cold or some other virus during his frequent trips back and forth to the West Coast. I also knew from personal experience that, because of the recirculated air in a totally enclosed environment, nearly everyone aboard our submarine would come down with a virus within five days after we left port. With 110 men aboard, someone would bring something for all of us to share - and we had healthy immune systems.

None of these restrictions proved to be bothersome, particularly when I thought about the alternative. Without the transplant, I would have been dead. These small inconveniences were but a minor blip on the radar screen of my new life!

During my first full week at home, I showed daily progress in regaining a portion of my strength. It was a difficult, and sometimes frustrating process, because I had lost so much muscle tone and strength during my ordeal in the ICU. I was incredibly weak. I could not even open a window by myself. I could lift virtually nothing. Getting up from a chair was always an adventure. Would I make it vertical, or would I fall back into the chair? Even Sydney could pull me around.

I did the recommended exercises daily, spent additional time on the exercise bike, and forced myself to walk around the house.

With Sharry's constant encouragement, I began to try the steps to our second floor, and on my 6th day home, I made it upstairs, although it took me at least 10 minutes to ascend the 14 steps. I still operated on the ground floor for several more days. The stair climb had been strictly a confidence builder. By afternoon I was always bushed and required a nap. Some days I would try to do too much. These days were usually counter-productive because I would feel so worn out by evening that it was difficult to get out of a chair by myself.

In fact, any low chair continued to be a challenge. For example, I still could not raise myself from the toilet without Sharry's assistance until we purchased a toilet bowl height extender. This device, which probably has some more glamorous marketing name (such as, "Lift It Up" or "Tall Johnny"), is a plastic device which sits on top of a regular toilet to raise the sitting height about eight inches. Even if this new addition to our home looked goofy, it did give me a feeling of independence. I could now feel reasonably comfortable being home by myself knowing that I would not become stuck on the toilet unable to get up! Of course, none of these problems are mentioned in the discharge instructions from the hospital. All are learned through the school of hard knocks, and I was, like it or not, becoming an honor student.

My new heart also brought with it some new jewelry. While I had been busy in the hospital using the Home Shoppers Club to buy items for which we had absolutely no need, Sharry had the foresight to order something which would be useful. It came in the mail about a week after I arrived home. She handed me the mailing package and said, "This is not for you. It's for your new heart."

I have always loved to open anything which comes in the mail, particularly unexpected packages, such as those free samples of a new brand of dish washing detergent. I even enjoy ripping open the "You may have won ten million dollars" envelopes. As I took this small package apart (it gave no hint of what was inside), I first noticed that it was some type of jewelry. My new heart now had its own "Medic Alert" necklace with a circular silver pendant approximately the size of a quarter with the inscription:

HEART TRANSPLANT
IMMUNOSUPPRESSED

It also contained a serial number and more information, "CALL COLLECT 209-634-4817 USA." The front of the pendant had gold lettering on the silver background saying:

M	A
E	L
D	E
I	R
C	T

Between these words was a Caduceus, the emblem of the medical profession. I have long been intrigued why doctors continue to use a mean-looking snake entwined about a staff as a symbol of their profession. If lawyers (or medical insurance companies) were the ones who displayed a Caduceus, I could **readily** understand the connection.

Apparently the Caduceus did not always have the snake. It began, with the ancient Greeks, as a herald's wand indicating that that person holding it was sacred and not to be molested. The wand was thought to be nothing more than a straight branch with two twigs on the top pulled back and twisted around the branch. At some later date, the twigs were replaced by snakes. This snake version became the symbol of the physician, Hermes, who also carried a magic wand. "With all of this hardware," I thought, "Just where did Hermes carry his stethoscope?" At any rate, I now had a gold snake hanging from a silver necklace around my neck.

My second clinic visit was one week after I had come home from the hospital. It went just as well as the first. The following day Sharry drove me to an appointment with the pulmonary specialist, Dr. Lo Russo, from the transplant team. His office had called to request that we come in so that my lungs could be evaluated. This visit also went well. Although my lungs were nowhere near normal capacity, there were signs of definite improvement. Sharry asked if I would eventually regain "near normal" lung function in view of the extremely bad case of ARDS which I had developed in the ICU following the transplant. Lo Russo responded that he could not be certain, but that he was confident that my lungs would improve steadily over the next year. He told me to return in three months for a complete pulmonary function test.

A major breakthrough for me took place the following morning. I made it up the steps to the second floor by myself using the cane and the banister for support. This short trip up was still a laborious process, but I now had the confidence that, given sufficient time, I could climb all the stairs at home. While upstairs I took my first shower in months. I was able to step into the shower without Sharry's assistance and to savor the refreshing feeling of warm water splashing over my entire body. I had been washing myself in a sink since June, and the shower seemed to be heaven. I remained in the shower for at least twenty minutes (in no way endangering the Linz family time records established by Emily in her daily baths). As I stepped out of the shower, I felt as if I had taken one further step toward a normal life.

The following day I felt strong enough to take another step forward in my recovery. Without assistance I climbed the stairs in the evening and was able to sleep in my own bed. Aaron, who was home for the weekend, moved his bed back to his room upstairs. I was now no longer a first floor person!

While going through some of our previous medical supplies which we had accumulated over the past three years, Sharry discovered the device which Ted Friehling, my arrhythmia specialist, had provided us to monitor the internal defibrillator at home to determine if it was functioning properly with respect to power, etc. We obviously no longer required this device, and it brought back bad memories. I telephoned Kim Hill, Ted's assistant, to ask her if she wanted the testing unit returned.

Kim, whose role within Ted and Al's practice has continuously expanded due to her talent and good judgment, said that we could return the testing device at our convenience, but to please stop by so that everyone in the office could see me and Sharry. That afternoon, on the way to another doctor's appointment, we visited their office. It was an incredibly moving experience for all of us. Kim hugged both of us, and then Ted walked in with his huge and distinct smile to offer congratulations. Ted appeared to be the same as always with his long hair and relaxed, casual manner. This man and his partner, Al Del Negro (who was in China at the moment), had been key players in keeping me alive for the three years preceding the transplant. How does one possibly acknowledge an appropriate level of gratitude and respect for individuals who have saved your life? They had kept me alive on Life Row.

Kim then announced that she had a surprise for us in exchange for the testing device. She went into her office and returned with two clear plastic envelopes. One contained the actual defibrillator and wiring which had been removed from my body during the transplant. The other contained the mesh patches which were sewn onto the sides of my heart in February, 1992, during the open heart surgery inserting and installing the initial AICD. The patches had been the instruments which transmitted the shock from the AICD to my heart during tachycardia episodes.

The AICD was the second one which had been installed in February of 1993 when the original device had become inoperable. I did not know whether to regard the AICDs as old friends or as prior tormentors. No matter my feelings at the moment, these high tech devices had been key to my survival.

As I looked at the AICD and the patches, I was struck by their large size. The AICD was 4 1/2 inches by 3 inches and was 1/2 inch thick. It was also quite heavy - well over a pound. This, and its defective predecessor, had been in a pouch in my upper abdomen for 2 1/2 years. No wonder that I could not get my weight down! The size of the patches was also surprising. They were nearly 5 inches in length and 3 inches wide. I had no idea that something this large could be sewn onto the sides of my heart.

Although both the AICD and the patches had been sterilized following their removal during the transplant, the patches looked dark with several stained areas. The thin wires which transmitted the electrical shock from the AICD to the patches had been snipped about one inch from the bottom of the patches. All of the other wiring was still attached. The AICD itself was a very shiny metallic with a serial number and "Sydney, Australia" etched on one side of it. I immediately sensed the irony of us having unknowingly named our dog after my AICD!

Kim gave the packages to me as a memento of my past three years. She said that we could do whatever we wished with the devices. Rather facetiously, she suggested that we have the AICD enclosed in some clear plastic mounting to place on display in a prominent location in our home. Kim and Ted then laughed. I was not certain how to react, but I took both packages home with us. I doubt that we will ever display them. Perhaps when I return to teach, I will show them to my classes to hear them exclaim either "Wow!" or "Gross!"

As Sharry and I left Ted's office, we both reflected aloud on how different this visit had been from our numerous previous appointments. Assuming that the new heart continued to function properly, I would never again have to sign in with Arrhythmia Associates. On the other hand, I had become close friends with Kim, Ted and Al, and I would miss them. It was their skill, concern and tenacity which had helped tremendously to keep me alive for over three years.

During the period of my recovery at home, I sometimes reflected on how differently I could now carry on daily actions without fear of being shocked. My worse AICD-related fear had always been that the device would shock me repeatedly (as it was designed to do), but with no success in converting my heart rate back to a safe rhythm, causing me to die immediately. Now, however, I could do physical activities which would have certainly set off the AICD prior to the transplant. For example, I could bend over without worry. Basically, I was now free to resume a normal life once I regained my strength. I remained very aware and grateful that I had been fortunate to develop my disease in an era when medical devices such as the AICD were available. Just 10 years earlier I would have not had such an opportunity to "buy time" with an AICD.

As my recovery continued at home, I could see evident progress. Each day I would attempt something slightly more physically challenging. I learned to descend and climb the stairs to our basement where my computers and desk were located. I discontinued use of a urinal at night and walked to the bathroom. I made up my bed in the morning and learned how to pry myself up from low chairs without the benefit of a pillow underneath. Each of these breakthroughs served to encourage me greatly, even though they were minor events.

Near the end of my second week at home, Sharry and I went to the local Social Security office to initiate paperwork for disability payments. To our pleasant surprise, the lady who assisted us, Ms. Crew, was unbelievably helpful and friendly. We had been expecting a DMV type experience. Instead we not only received accurate and valuable advice, but Ms. Crew went far beyond the expected to speed our claim and maximize the payment. She even telephoned us at home twice the following day to ask for additional pieces of information which would speed our application. This wonderful lady gave an entirely positive meaning to the term "civil servant."

In contrast, a few days later, I telephoned the dental clinic at the Veterans Hospital in Washington, D.C. to discuss some needed dental work. It was an entirely unpleasant experience.

While in the Navy I had developed a mysterious erosion problem with most of my teeth. During my retirement physical from the Navy in 1985, the military dentist had recommended to me that I apply for VA dental disability. I would receive no monthly payments, but the VA would pay for any dental work associated with the erosion problem. I decided to do so, but soon learned that nothing is simple with the Veterans Administration.

A three year long paperwork battle with the VA bureaucracy resulted. My initial request was rejected for no stated reason. All subsequent appeals were turned down with the one-liner, "Not service related." Presumably this meant that the cause of the erosion could not be connected to a specific event during my time in the Navy.

Finally I was granted a formal hearing before the Board of Veterans Appeals. This five member group, consisting of an attorney, two VA bureaucrats, a physician and a dentist, heard my case in a wood paneled courtroom in the VA building in D.C. I chose not to be represented by a lawyer. When asked to provide any additional information not included in the stack of correspondence already on file, I walked to the front of the room, bared my teeth, and said, "See for yourself." I noticed that the lawyer on the Board turned his head away and muttered, with apparent distaste, "Wow, that is bad."

With no deliberation other than glancing at each other and nodding, the Board unanimously granted me permanent dental disability on the spot. I was now eligible to receive dental treatment related to the erosion problem for the rest of my life. Using this benefit, I had several additional root canals and crowns over the next few years at a local civilian dentist. The last work was done in 1989.

During THE WAIT, however, I had noticed that three additional teeth were now affected by the erosion problem. During my recovery period at home I telephoned the dental department at the VA in D.C. to make arrangements to have the work performed by my local dentist. The first indication of trouble was that the person who now handled this type of claim would not return any of my calls. Whenever I tried to reach him, I was told that he was "in a meeting" or "away from his desk."

This process went on for two weeks. I then called again and demanded to speak to some human - any human - in the dental department. I was connected to a man who was perhaps the least helpful and most surly bureaucrat I have ever experienced. His first response to me was that as far as the VA was concerned, I did "not exist" because I was not in "the computer." He then stated that it was impossible for me to receive any dental work anyway because "the VA doesn't do that sort of thing." When I offered to send him a copy of the letter from the Board of Appeals granting me the coverage, he snapped, "Don't bother, it will get lost."

By this time I lost it. A shouting match followed. When I asked his name, he refused to tell me. I hung up. All of my previous misgivings about the VA had been reinforced. I pity any veteran who must rely on this organization for medical treatment or any services. I would have been dead long ago if the VA had been my only option for diagnosing or treating the sarcoidosis. It is bad enough for a federal agency to be blazingly incompetent, but all of the personnel I encountered at the VA seemed to go out of their way to be rude and unhelpful. Probably I will eventually win this latest round with them, but only after months of paperwork, additional phone calls and a large investment of my time. If the VA is in any way a model for a national health care system, the US could be in deep doo-doo.

Seventeen days after returning home, I was strong enough to attend church services with our congregation at Abiding Presence. We arrived (as usual) a few minutes after the service had begun.

We sat in the rear so as not to draw attention to ourselves. No one, including the Pastor, knew that we were coming, so our appearance was going to be a total surprise.

It was another emotional experience for me. I cried when we sang my favorite hymn, "This is the Feast." I found myself looking around at other members of the congregation wondering which had been among the 47 who had donated blood for me. As I periodically scanned those worshipping, I realized once again how fortunate I have been to have such giving friends who had prayed for me, sent cards and even visited during my ordeal in the hospital. The sermon was based on Mark 10: 35-45, the Gospel for the day, the 22nd Sunday after Pentacost. As Pastor Bailey spoke, I occasionally drifted from listening to his words and reflected instead about the role which God had played in my physical rebirth. I came to no specific conclusion, but I could not help but believe that a Divine Creator had somehow intervened to give me additional time here on earth.

I sat for most of the service, but I did walk to the front without my cane to receive Communion. While receiving Communion, I asked Pastor Bailey if I could address the congregation near the end of the service. He said, "Sure, I was hoping that you would do so."

When the Pastor announced just prior to the final hymn that Ed Linz wished to make a few remarks, I stood, and much to my surprise, the entire congregation turned toward Sharry and me and began to applaud. I became choked up, but did manage to speak. I first thanked the members who had donated blood in my name during the August Blood Drive. I then thanked everyone, on behalf of my entire family, for their prayers, love and support during our entire ordeal. Following the service many of our long time friends, such as Tom and "El" Porter, Gary and Charlene Traub, and the Pastor's wife, Carol, came over to welcome us and to share their joy that I was back with them. I left the church with more than misty eyes.

By late October my medical news was universally positive. The heart biopsies continued to indicate essentially no rejection of the new organ by my body's immune system. Although a biopsy of the heart tissue sounds as if it is complicated, it is, in fact, a very simple procedure. The entire process takes less than 30 minutes, and the patient is awake throughout. Some patients prefer to receive a Valium to relax during the procedure, but I prefer to skip the medication. At Fairfax Hospital, the biopsy is performed in the heart catheterization lab. The patient lies on a narrow operating table and is "prepped" by a nurse and technician. The prep consists of a thorough cleansing of the neck area where the catheter will be inserted and a draping of sterile gowns and coverings over affected portions of the body.

Dr. Rogan then shows up, exchanges small talk with me, before inserting a numbing agent, such as Lidocaine, into the right side of my neck near the jugular vein. As soon as the area is numbed up, he says, "You will feel some small pressure." He then inserts a small plastic hollow sheath directly into the jugular vein. I have never experienced any serious pain during this process, but some of my transplant colleagues tell me that they hate this part of the procedure. After the sheath is in place, he threads a very thin catheter wire through the hollow portion of the sheath down the vein system into the heart. I am lying on my side during this action and am watching the progress of the wire going into the cavities of my heart on an x-ray machine screen. Rogan is looking at the same image and uses it to position the wire against the inside of the heart. When he is satisfied that it is in a good location, he activates a pair of snips on the end of the catheter to gather a tiny sample of tissue. The only sensation I feel is a skip beat of my heart as the sample is taken (due to the irritation of the wall by the snips). He then quickly withdraws the sample from the sheath and deposits it in a vial for later laboratory staining. This process is repeated until the cardiologist feels that he has sufficient samples. Rogan always takes four from me. After the last sample is taken, the sheath itself is removed, pressure is applied to the insertion area by hand for a few minutes, and a single **Band Aid** (!!) is placed over the incision. I remain in the hospital for about an hour for observation and blood pressure monitoring to ensure that I am OK, and then I head home!

I asked Rogan why blood did not spurt out from this hollow tube sheath thing when it went into the jugular vein. He explained that it has a check valve type opening inside it which allows the wire to be inserted and withdrawn through it, but seals to prevent back flow of blood in the outward direction. I also was curious why I did not bleed from the location in the heart where the sample was taken. He laughed and said, "Of course it bleeds, but where does it bleed to?" He quickly answered his own question, "Into the rest of the blood flow through the heart." He went on to explain that the snipped area heals very rapidly, typically within a few minutes.

The tissue sample is taken to the hospital lab where it is stained to determine a color. This process takes several hours and the results are generally not available until the following day. So the patient sweats it out until receiving a phone call from one of the transplant coordinators who reports the results on a scale from zero to ten. Zero indicates no rejection whatsoever, while ten is an indicator of big time rejection requiring immediate action. Some of my fellow transplant friends become very nervous both before the biopsy and while waiting for the results. They are not concerned as much about the procedure itself, but rather the potentially bad news. If a moderate level of rejection is occurring, the patient is immediately placed on high levels of Prednisone for a five day period and another biopsy is taken in two weeks to assess the effect. If major rejection is taking place, there are specific medications such as OKT-3, manufactured by Ortho Biotech, which can be given. Each of these carry bothersome side effects, but it was always reassuring to me that the drugs did exist if I ever needed them. Perhaps if I receive a higher number from a future biopsy, I also will begin to worry. As of the moment, all of my results have been no problem.

There were some reality checks during the initial stages of my recovery at home. The day after Sharry returned to work, I decided to take our dog, Sydney, for a short walk. I was moving along slowly with my cane in my left hand and Sydney's leash in my right. We had progressed less than a block from the house, when I saw three ladies walking two large dogs toward us. Sensing that this encounter might be a problem, I led Sydney off the sidewalk into a grassy area to allow plenty of room for them to pass. As soon as Sydney went into a crouch/pounce position, I knew that major trouble was ahead. When the ladies and their dogs were exactly perpendicular to Sydney, she pounced. The leash was pulled from my hand, Sydney bounded toward the dogs, and I fell over onto the grass into a kneeling position.

Sydney unwisely jumped into the midst of both dogs, and action followed. Sydney, an Australian cattle dog (a "red heeler") wanted to play. The big dogs wanted to fight. Basically there was a whirl of dogs and leashes with the ladies in the middle of all of it. The one lady without a dog managed to grab Sydney's leash and to yank her away from the other dogs before major damage occurred. I told the ladies thanks and apologized, but immediately saw that I had a new problem: I could not get up.

I was on my knees in soft grass. I tried, but I was still too weak to right myself. I suspect that I also had a rather pleading, "Help me, please" look on my face. The two ladies with the dogs seemed far more interested in getting as far away from Sydney as possible than in providing assistance to her obviously foolish owner. All of the dogs were still barking like crazy.

It was the lady who had grabbed Sydney who showed the first sign of mercy. Maybe she thought that departing would be like leaving the scene of a hit and run. Maybe she was just a nice person. Anyway, she came over to help me get up. Although she grabbed me under my left arm and lifted as I pushed on my cane with my right arm, we were unable to achieve a vertical position. We tried this several times with decreasing success as I became more fatigued. The other ladies had the look of wanting to call 911 for assistance. Fortunately they had no portable flip phone with them. If the EMTs came, I could see the news item in the next day's *Washington Post*, "Healers raise kneeler knocked over by heeler."

I started thinking about other options. I could crawl home. This possibility had certain disadvantages. If I went back via the sidewalk, I would undoubtedly scrape my knees badly risking infection. If I used the grassy strip between the sidewalk and the street, my knees would fare better, but I would reach home covered with dog excrement, because virtually no one in our neighborhood uses a pooper scooper. That grassy strip is a favorite site for all the dogs. It is a dog crap minefield.

Fortunately the lady who was holding Sydney had a better plan. She asked where I lived and volunteered to take the dog to our house so that she could return to use both hands to help me get up. I said, "Great!" When she returned shortly, we tried again, but even with her full strength, I remained stuck on my knees. Now the lady with the big white dog came up with an idea. She tied her dog to a tree and helped to lift my other side. With the three of us lifting together, I managed to finally stand up so that I could walk home. The ladies followed me back to ensure that I made it safely.

I learned some lessons from this "Sydney Incident." I decided not to attempt to walk the dog by myself until I was considerably stronger, and, in more general terms, to think about possible problems before I tried new activities by myself. Sydney seemed unfazed, even when I spoke harshly to her. Those dogs were ancient history in her mind.

Although I continued to gain additional strength with each passing week, my ankles began to swell noticeably more during the last week of October. The extra fluid was not only visibly greater in my ankles and feet, but my weight also went up three pounds in two days. Dr. Miller did not seem terribly concerned. He increased my dosage of Lasix from 20 mg daily to 40mg in the AM and 20mg in the late afternoon. He also decreased the Prednisone from 35 to 30mg daily. After several days there was considerable improvement.

Our 24th wedding anniversary on Halloween was very special. Both Sharry and I realized how fortunate we were to have a 24th - it had been a close call. I sent a floral arrangement to her office and we exchanged cards and small gifts after dinner. As always happens on our anniversary, we were interrupted by several trick-or-treaters at the door. We did not mind. We were happy just to have each other. Once again I began to understand my incredibly good fortune to be blessed with Sharry as my wife.

The next day I received a phone call at home from a lady at the Virginia Heart Center (at Fairfax Hospital). She invited Sharry and me to be their guests at "an evening of cultural heart cuisine" at the Hyatt Regency Hotel in Reston (about 25 miles west of DC in Virginia near Dulles Airport). She explained that there would be food from several area ethnic restaurants and entertainment from 6 to 9 PM.

I talked this over with Sharry and we decided to attend. It would be a good test of my stamina, and I was definitely in the mood to get out for an evening. Although I was supposed to avoid crowded events such as a hotel ballroom filled with people, I decided to risk infection.

The evening turned out to be very enjoyable, in spite of the fact that I ate far too much. The food was sensational, and, true to form, I insisted on trying something of everything. This tendency must be a Linz genetic defect, because all of my relatives do the same thing when tempted with free food. Some of those rather portly folks frequently seen at all-you-can-eat buffet restaurants are probably carrying my blood line. Sharry kept admonishing me, but I was a driven, out-of-control, heart cuisine junkie.

The entire setup had obviously been planned with great care. There was live entertainment, but we preferred to have conversations with several of the doctors who had been such key players in my survival. Nelson Burton, who had performed my transplant with Paul Massimiano, surprised everyone by grabbing the microphone and doing a super Elvis imitation of *Blue Suede Shoes*. He followed this with a modified version of *I Left My Heart in San Francisco*, which, he explained, had become a theme of the cardiac unit at Stanford Hospital when he was there learning cardiac transplant techniques under Dr. Shumway His version was entitled, *I Left My Heart in Palo Alto*. Since Sharry and I had been married in Palo Alto when she had been working at Stanford, we both stopped cold as he sang and thought of the irony. By the time Dr. Burton stopped singing, we were again both in tears. On the way home I began to wonder if my new found tendency to become so emotional was in any way related to the fact that I now have a female heart.

During the evening at the Hyatt, we met several spouses of our Fairfax Hospital friends. For the past three years, Sharry and I had heard Al and Ted, my "rhythm and blues docs," talk about their wives. Now we had faces to put with the names. Mrs. Friehling was actually Doctor Friehling, a pediatrician, and a very interesting one at that. Our conversation with Mrs. Del Negro was equally enjoyable. We also enjoyed visiting with several of the doctors who had worked on me during the period in Intensive Care. Sharry knew most of this group far better than I did, because I had been out on drugs most of that period, while she had daily interaction with most of them. Her memories of THE ORDEAL were still very intense.

Meeting these medical professionals in a social setting underscored the major sacrifices in terms of family which most of them have made to help others. For example, my transplant was performed during the very early morning hours. Yet both of the heart surgeons involved saw me several times throughout the same day. Just when do these doctors go home? Many are essentially tethered to the hospital for incredible amounts of time. Emergency surgeries wait for no one, and the doctors are constantly being paged on their beepers to give instructions or advice to hospital personnel or other colleagues. I now bristle whenever I hear someone complain about the amount of money received by doctors for their work.

I also found considerable empathy for doctors based upon my similar experience with respect to total responsibility and accountability in the Navy as an Executive Officer and then Commanding Officer of a submarine. I had not thought of this correlation in detail before I met some of the families that evening. By the time we reached home I was thanking God that we had settled in an area of the U.S. with so many talented and dedicated professionals who were willing to give so much to save my life. They had kept me on Life Row.

It did not take long for the payback for our evening at the Hyatt to make its presence felt. Two days later I came down with a bad cold. I do not know if the virus came from the evening of cultural heart cuisine or elsewhere (Emily had given a pizza party for about 20 girls on the cross country team at our house the night before). At any rate, I was now entering the uncharted waters of combating a virus while being immunosuppressed.

It turned out that my concerns were premature. Within two days the cold symptoms disappeared. In fact, we then drove, as previously planned, to North Carolina to look at some colleges for Emily to consider. During the trip I encountered no medical problems. I toured the campuses in our wheelchair, but had no difficulty with the long ride in the van.

By mid-November, my blood pressure had been increasing steadily over the past several weeks. It was now consistently in the 150 over 100 range during my twice daily measurements at home. Part of my recovery regimen included keeping a daily record of temperature, weight, pulse, and blood pressure. I would measure these at home in the morning and evening and show the data to Paige and Dr. Miller during my clinic visits each Monday. He initially was reluctant to prescribe medication to lower the blood pressure, because he thought that the lower levels of steroids which I would soon be taking might correct the problem. Eventually, when there had been no improvement, he prescribed Cardizem, which did help to lower my blood pressure to more acceptable levels, although it was still high by pre-transplant standards.

For some unexplained reason, the swelling in my ankles which had been occurring by late afternoon each day for the first six weeks I was at home suddenly decreased markedly several days before I started the Cardizem. The only explanation I had was that I was now considerably more active in terms of walking and movement in general. I was rarely using the cane and had already become very independent. I could now climb one flight of stairs without holding onto the banister, and a slow two mile walk with Sharry and Sydney at one of our local parks posed no problems.

Thanksgiving 1994 was indeed very special for us. Nelle flew home from Indiana and Aaron drove up from North Carolina. For the first time in nearly a year, we were together as a family in our home. And, for the first time in over three years, we did not have the specter of terminal illness confronting us.

Emily and I had decided to make a statement about my medical re-birth. We rose before dawn, dressed quickly, and drove to nearby Centreville. There we participated in an 8 AM road race. She ran the 5000 meters and I walked. We both felt great afterwards and headed home with that major "smug factor" that comes only from doing a strenuous workout before most people have pulled themselves out of bed. We could also now rationalize consuming large quantities of turkey later in the day.

As usual in our family, I alone prepared the Thanksgiving meal. The cooking of the turkey, dressing and all other traditional components of the holiday feast is something which I not only look forward to, but jealously guard. Each year I add some new secret ingredient to the dressing. There is always considerable discussion during the meal as to the identity of the mystery component. This year it was diced green chilis, - not your typical Thanksgiving food. At any rate, the 1994 dressing was declared a hit.

When we sat down for our meal, I think that everyone was expecting a lengthy prayer of Thanksgiving. I found, however, that mere words were not an adequate expression of our sentiment. How does one even scratch the surface of the gratitude which each of us felt for the generosity of the donor's family, for the perseverance and skill of my doctors, for the favors and errands of our neighbors and friends, and for the prayers and support of so many?

Reflecting on all of this, the five of us simply joined hands around the dinner table. We said nothing aloud as we looked each other in the eye. Just as Sharry started to cry, Emily said the only words of our Thanksgiving, "Thank you, Lord." If they could have heard Emily, I am certain that the hundreds, if not thousands, of our friends and medical personnel who had been so integral to the successful ending of my time on Life Row would have joined our family as we all quietly declared, "Amen."

The Linz Family

Ed   Nelle   Aaron   Sharry   Emily

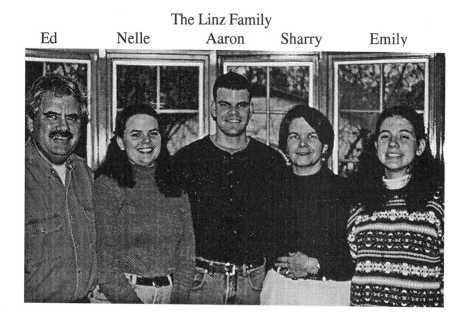

10 STEPS TO SURVIVE
AN EXTENDED MEDICAL CRISIS

Any serious discussion of "survival" must begin with an important, and possibly unpleasant, caveat: we will **all** eventually die. It is essential to state this fact "up front," because the advice which follows is <u>not</u> a magic elixir to provide eternal life or even a fountain of youth.

What these **10 Steps** can do is to provide a framework of ideas which will enable you to fight back when confronted by medical adversity. At the minimum, you will now have a shopping list of specific actions which you can take to improve your life-style as you battle your disease. In some cases, such as mine, you may be fortunate enough to discover an avenue which can lead to complete recovery.

Every situation involving disease of the human body is a unique situation. Because each of us is made up of an incredibly complex structure of billions of cells in constant interaction with each other, there are no two medical scenarios exactly the same. Each person will have his/her own individual response to disease (and also to medication and treatment). There are no two cases of any disease which are identical. No matter whether the problem be the common cold, breast cancer, or AIDS, each victim's body will react in a unique manner. This is the reason why alternative forms of medicine are successful for some people, yet of little value for others. A trip to the cold and flu remedy section of your local pharmacy illustrates this point. Recently I counted at least 25 different products available for treatment of the common cold alone. The lesson is that we are all very different, and that we must keep this in mind when battling a life-threatening disease.

Even though the study of medicine has given us sufficient evidence to be able, in many cases, to predict how the "typical patient" will react to a given disease and various treatments, our knowledge is statistically based and may have little applicability to **your** body's reaction to its disease and the recommended treatments. Your goal should be to take actions which elevate your chances of survival so that you are **not** the "typical patient." This chapter, based upon our experience on Life Row, provides you with a list of those actions.

Now let's talk about those steps which you (and your family) can take when confronted by a medical crisis. I will first list the **10 Steps** which we found to be useful. Then I will expand on each with reference to specific page numbers in **Life Row** (in bold print within parentheses, e.g., (**36-38**)) which contain an illustration of this particular point.

The **10 Steps** are not intended to be followed in sequence, nor are they listed in order of increasing or decreasing importance. My advice is that you consider each of these ideas as candidates to include when developing your own unique plan to confront your medical condition. At one time or another during my four years on Life Row, my family and I used each of these ideas, sometimes individually, but more often in tandem or in combinations. As you have read, we did have setbacks, and we did face extremely dangerous and trying situations. But ultimately we survived, and I am convinced that many of you can do the same.

The important concept is to use these 10 Steps to develop your own plan to survive your medical crisis. Good luck!! And, please, let us know about your success story.

The 10 Steps to Survive

1.   **Know your enemy.**
2.   **Seek professional help.**
3.   **Recruit a support team.**
4.   **Examine all options.**
5.   **Understand yourself.**
6.   **Live for the moment.**
7.   **Develop emotional outlets.**
8.   **Manage your brain.**
9.   **Be aggressive.**
10.   **Have faith.**

Step 1   Know your enemy.

The most effective first step in combating a disease is to learn as much as possible about it. This is not always possible because of the natural human tendency to deny that there is a problem. Learning that one has a dangerous, life-threatening disease will cause most people to become very uneasy, if not absolutely terrified. Because most of us proceed through life assuming that we will live to a ripe old age (and no one seems to define exactly what that may be), we become upset when confronted with "premature death." A very natural reaction is to go into denial. Your first task, therefore, is to recognize your denial, so that you can minimize the time spent in this unproductive state of mind. Every extra day spent in denial robs you of the opportunity to learn about your real enemy, the disease which is threatening your life.

We were very fortunate. The doctor who gave us the bad news that I had a fatal disease immediately suggested that we learn as much as possible about my condition, cardiac sarcoidosis (3). He had even prepared photocopies of journal articles on the subject for us to read at home. Thus, while I was in the midst of some very strong initial denial, Sharry was researching my diagnosed disease and reading every piece of available literature on the subject. Throughout our battle, her knowledge, gained independently of mine (262), often enabled us to work together to make an informed decision on what to do next, and, more importantly, what not to do.

Once I passed through the initial denial phase, I soon realized that if I was to have any chance to overcome this disease, I myself had to learn as much as possible about it (24-32). My background in coaching and in the military certainly reinforced this decision. If one is about to engage in battle, whether it be on the athletic field or against another ship at sea, I had learned that ignorance is not bliss, but deadly. Since we were about to enter the battle of our lives, we decided early on to arm ourselves with as much information as possible about this disease.

Where to start? I recommend asking your doctor for suggested reading materials. In addition to preparing photocopies of relevant articles for us, our cardiologist also recommended that we use the hospital library to search for additional information. As we visited other specialists and medical facilities to obtain second and third opinions, we always asked for their recommendations for further reading.

Do not hesitate to ask every physician you meet, "Doctor, what can you tell me about this disease?" (**15, 43, 64, 118, 152, 262**) You will be surprised how many different responses you will receive concerning the same illness. Include nurses, physician assistants, and other medical professionals in your search. Some of our best information came from nurses who had the patience to thoroughly discuss their experiences with us (**58, 265**).

There are also many computer-accessed resources now available to assist you in knowing your enemy. Rather than giving you a list of current sites on the world wide web, I recommend that you surf the web yourself for answers. Applicable sites for your disease are constantly changing and being updated. Most will have links to other sites. Use as many different search engines as possible. You may wish to print your findings from the computer screen and place them in a folder with notes from your readings and discussions with medical professionals.

While you are searching the internet for additional information, you will undoubtedly have the opportunity to obtain opinions and experiences from non-professionals, such as other patients. My advice is to listen politely and to exchange views, but not to regard everything that you hear (or read) as gospel. This same advice obviously applies to direct conversations with other patients who have a similar condition. My hospital conversation with "Tom", the patient already on Amiodarone (**67-68**), is an excellent example of why one needs to weight anecdotal information very carefully.

The purpose of obtaining as much information as possible from as many different sources as possible is to enable you to make informed decisions, rather than blindly going along with whatever one of your doctors recommends. I found that by the time we had been on Life Row for over a year, Sharry and I were probably two of the more knowledgeable people in our area concerning cardiac sarcoidosis. We knew what symptoms to expect before they occurred, and we understood the known side effects of each of the medications before I took them.

More importantly, we were able to use the experience of others to shape our own life style as we battled the disease. I understood that I could continue to teach and coach with only modest adjustments (**77, 125**). After I had the internal defibrillator (AICD) surgically implanted, our understanding of how the device worked (i.e., how it sensed the dangerous heart rhythm and the exact process it followed before delivering the shock) helped considerably to ease my fear both when I felt my heart going into tachycardia and following the shock (**110-113**). The fact that I knew all the information about the AICD was of direct benefit whenever I had to discuss my situation with doctors who were not specialists in this field. When I went into complete heart block in early 1994, I was able to assist our internal medicine doctor by describing the pacemaker function of my type of AICD to her so that she could decide the best course of corrective action (**147-148**).

Knowing your enemy is a continuous process. Just as conditions change during any prolonged conflict, your disease will typically take many twists throughout its course. It is essential that you adjust to each of these developments by learning as much as possible about the new situation. For example, when we learned that the deterioration of my heart necessitated that I undergo new tests involving nuclear medicine, I tried to obtain as much information as possible, not only about the mechanics of the test, but also concerning exactly what information might be obtained and how that knowledge might help us (**152**). When Sharry learned during "The Ordeal" (when I was unconscious) that I was now suffering from ARDS (**255**), she immediately asked both nurses and doctors to explain this condition to her (**256**). She then spent several hours in the hospital library learning more about this new condition (**262**). Armed with this knowledge, she then had further discussions with doctors enabling her to ultimately achieve a "comfort zone." She was no longer in a helpless battle against a mysterious enemy. The situation was dangerous, but she felt increased resolve to fight back due to her improved understanding of the disease.

Once you are on the road to recovery, you must continue to seek as much information as possible about your condition. If you are fortunate enough to see your cancer go into remission, to have your HIV status improve, to receive a donor organ, or to have a cardiac condition reversed through surgery or treatment - whatever the mechanism for improvement of your condition - now, more than ever, you need to learn exactly what dangers remain and how respond to them most effectively (**281, 283**).

If you are on medication, you must become knowledgeable about each medicine. Not only should you become familiar with the side effects of the drugs, but you should also know what to do if you accidentally miss taking your medications on schedule. And, most importantly, you must be aware of all known indicators of a relapse or reoccurrence of your disease.

Throughout your battle with your disease, you will occasionally encounter someone who be reluctant to share their knowledge with you (**156**). My advice is to be persistent, and as forceful as necessary. It is your life, or your loved one's, at stake. If you are to be a part of the recovery process, it is imperative that you be able to make informed decisions, based on as much knowledge as possible. The first step is to **know your enemy**.

Step 2　Seek Professional Help.

Most of us, when faced with a leaky roof or a sputtering car engine, know instinctively that the best policy is to look for professional assistance. Strangely, this is not always the case for medical problems. Many times I have encountered the reaction, "Why should I see a doctor? They can't do anything for this."

This method of self-treatment may work for a cold or the flu, but it will undoubtedly place you at a disadvantage when you must confront a deadly disease. I certainly had my own misgivings when Dr. Merlino recommended that I see a cardiologist (**15**) [my exact words were, "Why should I go see some *other* doctor?"]. Fortunately, my wife was more objective. It was her insistence that led me to see a specialist. After performing several diagnostic tests, it was this heart specialist who made the diagnosis which led to my ultimate survival (**16**). By availing myself of the expertise of this physician, I was able to benefit not only from his own experience and talent, but also, through his referrals, from the network of other cardiac experts throughout the country who participated in my recovery (**4, 41-47, 97-99**).

Professional help comes in many forms. Most serious diseases require sophisticated and often expensive tests to refine the diagnosis and to track the progress of your condition. My experience (EKGs, blood tests, MRIs, x-rays, echocardiograms, MUGAs, PFTs, slit lamp exams, etc.) was that they were worth the expense and the effort. This is not to suggest that every recommended test is necessarily one to which you should automatically agree (**108**).

Deciding which tests to have is a matter of your own understanding of the cost-benefit ratio involved. Once again, this becomes a matter of how well you have proceeded on Step 1, knowing your enemy. When a doctor suggests a test, do not hesitate to ask exactly what type of information will be gained by the test, how much it will cost, and what side-effects/dangers are involved. Then you can make an informed decision based on your answer to: "Do the potential benefits of this test outweigh the costs?"

When receiving professional help, Sharry and I always lived by this thumb rule: never accept bad news from a single source. When faced with the initial diagnosis of a potentially fatal disease, we sought out second and even third opinions (**41, 98**). Most doctors are very comfortable with this approach. Anytime a doctor discourages obtaining a second opinion, get a new doctor!

In this era of managed care and HMOs, you may find that the physician who is your primary care provider is reluctant to provide a referral for a specialist. Our advice is to insist on getting a referral for any serious condition. It is your life at stake, and if you do not fight for the right to see an expert in the field, you are entering the fight of your life without all available weapons. Fortunately, we were blessed with the combination of a wonderful internal medicine physician who was intent on obtaining the best available professional assistance possible and insurance companies who did not attempt to limit our referrals (**258-259, 262, 264**). Just in the past two years since I have recovered, there have been major changes in insurance procedures making referrals more difficult to obtain. So be advised, and be prepared to fight, if necessary, to achieve the professional assistance which your case demands.

Your family may find that they are having difficulty coping with your disease and its implications for them. If this is the case, whether the problem be emotional, financial, or otherwise, they should not be reluctant to seek professional assistance also. Most medical centers have resources to assist families in each of these areas. With respect to finances, for example, there are services which can help you to draw up a plan to address your own situation. It is very difficult to find a successful path to recovery in any difficult medical scenario if there are associated problems within the family. If you are going to wage a successful battle against a disease, it is far easier if everyone can concentrate on the disease rather than being distracted by other factors. You need to be on the lookout to detect these situations as they arise and to seek professional assistance to correct them.

In summary, while "going it alone" may be in some sense admirable, it is not smart when you are confronting a dangerous medical condition. Whether it be AIDS, cancer, a cardiac condition, liver failure, or anything serious, you should **seek professional help** if you are to improve your chances to survive.

Step 3   Recruit a support team.

It is virtually impossible to fight a life-threatening challenge by yourself. In any protracted battle there is inevitably a series of "ups and downs" which will sooner or later stress the emotional stability of the best. Our experience certainly confirmed this.

Shortly after being confronted with The Diagnosis (**1-5**), my wife and I discovered that we were very much in need of each other for emotional support. Sometimes this took the form of "tough love," such as when Sharry's strong persistence forced me to overcome my initial denial (**20**). At other times her research and intelligent discussion of the pro's and con's of procedures (**64-74**) allowed us to filter most of the emotions out of the decision-making process. Mostly, however, it was her strong daily presence throughout our 40 month ordeal which kept me going. Whether it was a well-timed smile of support, the management of our family finances, interaction with insurance companies, bringing home-cooked food to my hospital room, or simply a good night kiss, I could not have had a better partner on Life Row. Our final moments together as we waited for my transplant operation to begin (**235**) remains perhaps the defining moment of our marriage.

As you search for a support team to assist you in your battle, I suggest, therefore, that you begin with family. If circumstances do not allow this, then find **someone** who is willing to play a primary role in your struggle. As I observed the series of over 40 roommates pass through my life during The Wait (Chapters 11-12), I noticed that most had some one person who would visit daily. Often it was a family member, but in other cases, such as Bennie the Cabby (**181**), there was a life-long friend who showed up each evening. It is very helpful to have a "lead player" whom you can count on to be there throughout your ordeal. The two saddest situations I saw (one ended in death in the bed next to me, and the other later at his home) were both cases in which the patient had no one to give that daily emotional lift.

I also recommend searching for some "electronic buddies." Although some of my close friends were far away throughout most of my lengthy illness, I was able to communicate with them on a frequent basis via telephone or e-mail. Ensure that you have a telephone next to your bed if you are in the hospital or laid up at home. I looked forward very much to the frequent calls from both local and distant friends (**221**). If you have a hospital roommate, it is important to bear in mind that you are probably sharing a "party line" and that you do not want to hog usage of the phone. I tried to make several short calls each day rather than extended conversations. That policy not only kept peace with my roommates, but also seemed to encourage my callers to continue the process each day since they were not tying up large quantities of their own time. This is an important point to remember if you are in for a "long haul", whether at home or in the hospital. You do not want to burn out your sources of emotional support!

I also found that e-mail is an important connection to other members of your support team (**222**). Most hospitals now do not mind if you bring your own laptop (or even full size computer) into the hospital room. You will need to have an internet provider to which you can connect from the hospital phone line, but this is no longer a difficult problem in most areas. The advantage of internet access for a hospitalized patient is that you can send and receive e-mail messages as **your** schedule dictates (some hospitals will not allow you to receive incoming phone calls after a certain time each evening). My friends on the West Coast could not telephone me on evening rates during the week due to the time difference and the fact that incoming calls were blocked after 10 PM in my hospital. With e-mail, they were able to send messages whenever they wanted throughout the day and I could download them at my convenience. Telephone calls can also come at inopportune moments, such as when your doctor is making his daily visit, or you are receiving a procedure from a nurse. Murphy's Law (what can go wrong, will go wrong, and usually at the worst possible moment) always seemed to dictate that the phone would ring just as I had spent the past 20 minutes maneuvering myself and my IV pole to the bathroom! E-mail just seems to work better.

You can also use the world wide web to further research your disease via libraries, user groups, or bulletin boards and to establish friendships with others in a similar situation. Many medical problems or conditions now have dedicated home pages linked to other resources which you can access. I recently visited several patients who spent hours each day communicating and researching on their computers while they were in the hospital. Once again, you need to remember that if you are sharing a telephone line, you are tying it up by remaining on the computer modem for extended periods of time.

Your support team for an extended illness should have varying levels of participation. Neighbors and friends can easily become burnt out over a long haul, so use their assistance wisely. Every time that I was hospitalized, there would be an initial outpouring of offers of assistance from colleagues at work, folks in the neighborhood, members of our church congregation, and friends in general. Ironically, this can lead to problems when you least need them. For example, one problem that we had not anticipated was that of casserole management. In the first few days after I had entered the hospital Sharry was inundated with so many casseroles and dinner dishes from well-meaning friends that she had no place to put them. Our solution was to ask one of our neighbors to become our "casserole manager." This person would establish a queue for preparing food items so that they were spread out over several weeks. She also ensured that dishes were returned to the correct person. The last thing that a caregiver of a sick person needs is additional worry that someone has been offended because of "casserole slight" or a lost dish!

We found that most folks who initially offered assistance were very understanding when we replied, "We are fine now, but can we get back to you if we need something in the future?" Our experience was that people seemed to be very responsive to this approach, and we did not feel so guilty when we approached them later on for a favor.

It turns out, of course, that the person who really needs the majority of assistance is not the patient, but the caregiver. I had the entire hospital staff available to meet my needs, but there was no one dedicated to helping Sharry try to manage all of our ongoing family matters while trying to take care of my medical condition, holding down her job, visiting me, and trying to keep her own mental stability. A significant effort in recruiting your own support team must be directed at obtaining help for the caregiver. This is particularly important if you are faced with what you know will be a long term fight against your disease, such as with some cancers, AIDS, or other chronic conditions. There are many excellent resources now available to assist you in developing a game plan for this situation, such as the series of books on care giving by James Sherman.

Other key members of your team should include spiritual supporters. Our pastor and members of our congregation were steadfast in their prayers, visits, and assistance throughout our lengthy battle (**234, 290-291**). Whether or not one belongs to an organized religion is not as important as having someone, or group of individuals, pulling for you to succeed. Although I did not personally know the hospital chaplains who would periodically stop by my room to visit, I certainly appreciated their support and encouragement. Two of the ladies who cleaned my hospital room introduced me to their religious beliefs (one a Far Eastern meditation-based process and the other a Pentecostal movement). Both promised to pray for us. My motivation to fight on was strengthened by each of these encounters. I believe that it was a significant ingredient in my recovery (see Step 10).

Some of the key players on your team will be medical professionals. I was blessed with excellent doctors and nurses throughout my illness. I did run into some situations, however, where I saw my roommates saddled with physicians who certainly gave the appearance of either disinterest or incompetence. In the event that you are uncomfortable with your doctor, it is usually best for all concerned that you terminate the relationship early into your treatment. Consider the analogy of you being on death row: would you tolerate an attorney who did not seem up to the job? While on Life Row, I encountered one doctor with whom I had a serious personality conflict. Sharry and I discussed the matter with one of our physician friends and said that we preferred that "Dr. X" no longer treat me. I do not know how our friend handled the situation, but I never saw Dr. X again.

In a long term illness it is inevitable that a close bond develops between patient and doctor. In general, I believe that this is a healthy situation. I always felt as if a friend was entering my room whenever one of my long-standing physicians appeared in the doorway for their daily visit. However, you will also be seen by interns, residents, physician assistants, nurse practitioners, and a host of other "pokers and prodders" who will ask you many of the same questions which you have answered at least one thousand times before. Be patient, if only because you do not know which of these individuals may be an important ingredient in your recovery. Sometimes a slightly new perspective can provide the necessary understanding or idea which will lead to your recovery.

Although I am admittedly biased (Sharry is a RN), your most frequent, and often most effective, professional care provider is the nursing staff. If you are hospitalized, nurses should be the glue which holds your support team together. It was the daily, and sometimes hourly, evaluations of nurses which kept me alive through some of my most difficult moments, particularly during my time in intensive care (**257, 263, 265, 268-270**). Other nurses, such as Teresa (**67**) and Kathleen (**199**), introduced me to patients with similar cardiac conditions so that I could benefit from their perspectives. It was also Kathleen who arranged the surprise in-hospital crab feast (**223-224**) which so lifted our morale when all else was appearing darkest. If you find yourself hospitalized, all members of your family, including yourself, should talk to the nurses as much as possible. Most likely they have seen your situation before and are usually very willing to share their perspective with you.

Another asset to consider adding to your team should be actual support groups dedicated to your disease or condition. I benefited tremendously from the advice, moral support, and wisdom of members of Transplant Recipients International Organization (TRIO). These folks visited and talked with me throughout our long ordeal (**61, 247**). They have also been there during my recovery phase providing wisdom and advice based on their own personal post-transplant experiences. Nearly every major disease now has some form of support group. In our local area, for example, the National Kidney Foundation has a particularly effective program. I urge you to find and join at least one support group.

My final recommendation to round out your support team is optional, and some of you may argue, silly. But I firmly believe that it can be helpful to many. Get a pet. In our case it was a dog. Sydney, our Australian cattle dog, proved to be a most loyal member of our team (**145-146, 170, 223, 276, 283, 293-294**). Pets give unqualified love and expect little in return (other than the occasional hot dog!). When I was ill at home, Sydney was always near me. When I was hospitalized, the mention of the dog always gave us something cheerful to discuss. Obviously this suggestion is not for everyone, but a "pet" can be either animal, plant, or mineral (remember the pet rock craze?). In my mind, no support team is complete without a pet.

In summary, some folks have undoubtedly survived a potentially fatal disease by "going it alone," just as a few people have single-handedly sailed around the world. But I think that, just as in sailing, your chances for success are far better if you make a concerted effort to **recruit a support team**.

Step 4   Examine All Options.

Any serious illness will inevitably present you with several options to consider. At the minimum, you will be faced with the "Do Nothing/Do Something" decision. Don't laugh. This is often a basic, serious issue which will set the course for all future decisions.

When confronted by my internal medicine doctor with the initial finding that something appeared to be abnormal with the EKG during a routine physical (**14**), my initial reaction was "Do Nothing," as in "Maybe if I do nothing, it will go away." It was only through the persistence of Sharry and the doctor that I was ultimately swung over to the "Do Something" school of thought (**15-16**).

As I progressed through the initial phases of my disease, I soon learned that there were to be frequent major decisions which had to be made. The methodology of decision-making which seemed to suit the personality of both Sharry and me was to gather as much information as possible to determine all available options. We would then debate the pro's and con's of each, and try to take the most conservative approach which would yield the highest potential pay-off. We tried to avoid any irreversible action unless all other avenues had been explored. For example, we were first informed in August 1991 during one of my initial hospital stays after having been placed on Life Row that I might be a candidate for a heart transplant operation (**60**). At the time, Sharry and I listened politely and even read all the literature which was left for us, but neither of us had any desire to pursue what we judged to be such a radical, and potentially dangerous, solution (**61-62**). Three years later, after exhausting all other alternatives, we eagerly accepted the opportunity to be placed on the transplant waiting list (**174-176**).

During those three years there were, indeed, many less dramatic alternatives which we explored. Our first action was to pursue a better diagnosis, that is, one which did not condemn me to a certain, and early death. This may sound ridiculous, but it is critically important to be sure in your own mind that you really are facing a potentially fatal disease. Get a second, third, or even fourth opinion. This is not denial. This is making sure. As I said in Step 2, never accept bad news from a single source!

In our case, we did not have to ask for recommendations concerning second opinions - the doctor who made the initial diagnosis gave them to us in his office shortly after he had told us that I had a fatal disease (**4**). You may not be this fortunate and may find yourself searching for an "expert" in your disease. If there are no local assets, you may need to contact a major medical center. Most large metropolitan areas have at least one such center. If receiving a second opinion involves travel, and if you are physically able to do so, I recommend hitting the road. The cost and time involved are usually a wise investment. Be prepared to take all of your records and test results with you (or to forward them ahead) so that you do not have to repeat expensive tests or remain at the new location for an extended period of time.

Although both of our visits to receive other opinions at Johns Hopkins (**41-47**) and Duke (**98-99**) confirmed the bad news in our initial diagnosis, the process increased our confidence that we knew exactly what we were dealing with and gave us additional insight into the latest treatments for the disease. More importantly, it kept us from pursuing fruitless options based on the false hope that I was not suffering from cardiac sarcoidosis.

Most serious diseases have several available treatments. You may face decisions concerning which to choose, or the order in which each will be attempted. AIDS, many types of cancer, kidney and cardiac ailments come immediately to mind. In my situation, we were initially presented with several choices. The first was to attack the disease chemically, that is, through medicine. Although none of the available drugs could cure the disease, some offered the hope that the life-threatening arrhythmias caused by the disease could be eliminated. The next tier of treatment involved surgical insertion of a defibrillator to monitor the arrhythmias, and to provide shock therapy whenever a dangerous condition existed. The ultimate treatment was an organ transplant operation, followed, if successful, by a lifetime of immunosuppressant drug therapy.

As we examined each option, we attempted to weigh the benefits and risks associated with each. Our first decision was to try the chemical route, because it did not involve surgery and was a reversible action. If the drugs did not work or had intolerable side-effects, I could simply stop the medication and try a different approach. The first three medicines attempted did not work, in fact, one exacerbated the condition (**63**). We were then faced with another decision: should we attempt the next level of drugs, which, although more powerful, had potentially dangerous side-effects? (**65**) After considerable research, discussions with patients currently on the medication, and inquiries with other doctors (**66-67**), Sharry and I examined the issue at length and decided to proceed with the new medicine (**74**).

This decision served us well for six months. I was able to return to work and to resume all normal activities. My underlying disease had not been cured, but we were able to enjoy an improved lifestyle.

Our next decision came when the drug therapy was no longer protecting me (**101-107**). At this stage we moved to the next tier. Our remaining options were two: surgery to insert a defibrillator or to try for a heart transplant operation. Both entailed considerable risk. However, by choosing the defibrillator route, we remained more in control. My condition had not yet deteriorated to the point where I would be at the top of the transplant waiting list. Sharry argued that we might be able to do both. Have the defibrillator installed, see how it goes, and then decide if we wanted (or even needed) the ultimate risk, the transplant operation. I was so frightened/discouraged/disheartened that I did not want to do anything. I was ready to give up (**115**). Fortunately, I had a great support team (Step 3) which immediately went to work to force me to make a decision. Their efforts (primarily Sharry and my team of physicians) turned me around (**115-116**).

As you consider each option, make certain that it really is an option. If most of your costs are being covered by insurance, it is vital that you, or someone on your team, determine if your insurance will pay for the option you have in mind. If the answer is no, do not necessarily accept this setback. You may find that the insurance companies will change their decision if you are sufficiently aggressive (Step 9). In our situation, this usually involved Sharry assuming the role of "bad guy" and exercising her considerable powers of persuasion (**115**).

One final thought on options: once you make a decision to pursue a particular strategy, do not look back. You have only a limited number of brain cells. Do not waste them on what might have been if you had chosen Plan B instead of Plan C. Once you make a difficult decision, learn to live with it. If things are not going well, do not look backwards. Instead, concentrate on what you can do to make your decision work, and start searching for new options. The wonderful truth about "modern" medicine is that new developments are taking place almost daily throughout the world. If you can find options to keep you alive long enough, there may well be a breakthrough which will enable you to survive. I have spoken with many AIDS and cancer patients recently who are successfully pursuing this strategy at this very moment. **Examine all options!**

Step 5   Understand yourself.

Who knows you better than you? Probably no one. Some may argue that a spouse or a close personal friend is the best judge of a person due to a greater degree of objectivity. This argument may or may not be correct in some areas, but in the realm of medicine, you alone know where it hurts.

In the case of a serious medical condition, it is particularly important to remember this fact. You should be alert to detect changes in your condition. This information can be critical in determining how your treatment should proceed.

You will have to fight through periods of denial. I delayed reporting my initial symptoms of arrhythmia because I was hoping that I was only imagining the heart perturbations (**38, 53-54**). This was, as Sharry so aptly put it, "Stupid!" Fortunately, I did eventually learn to listen more closely to what my body was telling me, but it was only after I had nearly killed myself through denial in the racquetball court (**100-102**). That episode, and the ensuing out-of-body experience in the E.R., finally convinced me that I had to start taking my responsibilities as "primary reporter" seriously if I was to survive. In fact, my first opportunity to do so occurred in the ambulance as I was being rushed to the E.R. that evening. As the medics in the ambulance received instructions to administer a standard anti-arrhythmic drug to me, I remembered that previous EP studies on me had shown that the drug in question actually made my condition worse. Although my protestations to the EMTs did not deter them from pushing the harmful medicine into my veins, the thought that I was able to participate - even unsuccessfully - seemed to energize me and give me increased will power to fight back. By the time we reached the E.R., I was determined to report everything I felt, as I felt it, to the medical team which was trying to save my life (**104-106**). To this day, I credit the will of God and my understanding of my own body as the key elements in my survival that night.

It is also very useful to know how your body reacts to various medications with which you have had previous encounters. You should, for example, be very knowledgeable about antibiotics - not only which ones you are allergic to, but also how your body reacts to each. This information may help to keep you alive by preventing an intern or resident from prescribing a potentially dangerous drug for you. If you are hospitalized, you will inevitably find yourself in a situation where a resident M.D. will be treating you for a new symptom, such as diarrhea or a rash or......the possibilities are endless (**206**). Many times these doctors-in-training will have only a passing familiarity with your case. You may find that you know more about your disease than they do! Do not be alarmed if this is the case. Simply listen carefully and (this is particularly important if you are a family member who happens to be present) ask questions.

Following my first major surgery, I learned that my body seemed to react very violently to pain medication. The pain would be eased, but I had incredibly frightening nightmares. As I pondered what to do, I recalled that my father had experienced the same reaction when he had received pain medication. Although I doubted that such a tendency had any hereditary component, I requested that a much milder pain reliever be substituted for the narcotic I was receiving. The nightmares disappeared immediately (**121**). Subsequently I was always certain to instruct my doctors and nurses that I wanted to go off heavy pain killers as soon as possible following surgery. I found that I could tolerate any residual pain very easily and that this was an excellent trade-off for me. Obviously, everyone is different, but the point remains the same: know **your** body.

It is also important to learn how you can best "make it through the night." Nights are difficult when you are seriously ill. Your mind will often wander to places you do not want to be (**227**). This can happen both at home and in the hospital. I tried a variety of tricks (several are listed in Chapter 11). You may reach a point, however, where it is prudent to ask for some form of medication to relax you sufficiently to fall asleep (**227**). I have never been a big fan of medication, but sleep is a precious commodity when you are trying to survive a serious medical problem. In my own case, I found that I did not have to take serious "sleeping pills," but simply a relaxant. Once again, you need to learn what works best for your body.

Speaking of sleep, you may find that you have rather dramatic dreams while you are ill. While most of mine could not be classified as nightmares, they were weird, if not bizarre. I did not have anything like this before I became ill, and there has been no repetition since. In Chapter 12, I give a rather detailed example of one of these dreams so that you can understand just how wacky they may be (**230-232**).

If you are facing a period of prolonged illness, you must learn what you have to do to keep yourself sane. I will discuss this at length in Steps 6-10, but it is essential that you understand the importance whether you are the patient or the caregiver. We are not talking about a one week or one month illness. Those are "easy," at least from the mental health perspective. A disease involving a lengthy battle can be unnerving for all concerned. To succeed you must develop a game plan for sanity. It will probably differ for each individual. In my own case, I found that developing a specific daily routine was a tremendous help while I was hospitalized. Most of Chapter 12 deals with this issue, but it is my hope that the details of my daily routine can give you an idea of what you may have to do to maintain your own sanity (**212-227**). As I frequently told my doctors, "You keep me alive physically, and I will handle the mental side of the house."

In designing a daily routine, I recommend that you build your model around the principle of keeping busy. One of the reasons why I disparage television (**180-185**) is that it encourages the viewer to become mentally lazy. Although television can be a useful diversion when you are physically incapacitated, periods of lengthy viewing should not be a regular component of your daily routine. If you are able to work while you are ill, I strongly recommend doing so. If this is not possible, find a hobby. The important thing is to **DO SOMETHING** each day! Having a reason to live is directly related to having something to do.

From the caregiver's perspective, Sharry found that her best technique for survival was to try to keep moving forward at all times. She found that it was best not to dwell on what might happen next, or to grieve over each setback. She simply chose not to consider questions such as, "What's the prognosis?" or "How long do they give him?" or "What are his chances?" She kept busy, mostly by necessity (job, homemaker, parent of three, caregiver, etc.), but she did not allow herself the luxury of worrying. Knowing her own personality, she understood that her best hope was to concentrate on the positive as much as possible.

Each of our three children found their own techniques for survival. None tried to avoid the issue. They knew that their father could die any minute. Yet they also understood themselves and developed, sometimes unconsciously, daily routines which helped them to be effective caregivers when required, while still maintaining their own lives as students (**220, 253, 259**).

What worked for us may not be the correct prescription for you. We were always grateful that we had been blessed with some significant advantages compared to other families confronting life-threatening disease. Only one of us was ill, we had no initial financial problems, excellent medical facilities were nearby, our doctors were superb, and Sharry was a nurse. Your situation will be different (perhaps better, perhaps worse). Rather than fretting about perceived misfortunes, you should try to focus on your strengths. The important thing to remember is that the key to developing a successful plan is to first **understand yourself.**

Step 6   Live for the Moment

Learning that a family member, perhaps yourself, has a potentially fatal disease is obviously a somber moment. You might think that all types of wild thoughts will swirl through your mind as realization of your mortality begins to sink in. However, according to those whose occupation or circumstance dictates that they inform families of such diagnoses, there is no "usual" or "typical" reaction. My wife, Sharon, for example, has the task as a Public Health nurse of informing some of her patients that they are infected with HIV. "It is never the same," she reports. "It is impossible to predict how a given individual will react."

There certainly is not a "correct" way to receive such devastating news. If you weep or scream or wail about the injustice or sit silently and reflect or......., it does not matter. What is important is how you pull yourself together after the initial news has been absorbed. It is our belief that you should try to pass through the inevitable period of denial and proceed on with life. I like to call this "living for the moment."

By this I do not mean cashing in all your savings and heading for a final fling in Vegas. Instead I recommend that you learn to live with your condition as well as possible, and that you take each day one at a time [to paraphrase many of my fellow coaches who, when asked about the remainder of their season, inevitably respond, "We're gonna take the rest of the schedule one game at a time."]

We did not cancel planned family vacations, nor did we sit around bemoaning our bad luck. In fact, less than three months after learning that I had a dangerous cardiac condition, I flew to Arizona to visit relatives and hike part of the Grand Canyon (**51**). This was not a reckless adventure further endangering my life. I took along a unit to monitor my heart, and I was alert to detect any symptoms. What was significant was that I was determined to show myself and my family that I was going to remain in control of my destiny for as long as possible.

In the same vein, as soon as I was released from my first lengthy period of hospitalization, I immediately returned to both teaching and coaching (**78**). I was not going to sit at home waiting to die. I made adjustments, of course, (**88**), but my goal was to attempt to operate as near to normal as possible, for as long as possible.

In the face of setbacks, both personal (my mother's car accident and death (**89-95**)) and physical (the near fatal tachycardia episode in the racquetball court (**100-107**)), I tried to rebound as quickly as possible. It is important to remember that life around you will continue to evolve independently of your illness. Friends and relatives will continue to have both good and bad times. Someone may die, or be seriously injured, or win the lottery. When this happens, you should try to stay focused on your own battle. You must learn to guard your emotional resources. You do not want the reservoir to be empty when you need it the most.

As we sensed the clock ticking away the remaining months of the original prediction that I might have only two years to live, Sharry and I paused one evening to have a detailed discussion about our future (**125**). We decided to do something special together, and Sharry suggested fulfilling our dream to someday visit Alaska. Although there was some risk involved (due to travel in remote areas distant from immediate medical assistance), we decided that the psychological benefits would outweigh the health risk. This proved to be an excellent decision. We returned refreshed and energized to continue our battle versus my disease.

By the following spring my condition had deteriorated, but I was still searching for ways to divert our attention from the death sentence which I had received. On the spur of the moment, I purchased plane tickets to take my older daughter, Nelle, to England for a five day visit of her birthplace. During this trip Nelle did all the driving and helped me to walk, as if we had reversed parent-child roles (**140**). But, once again, the psychological gain was substantial. Although the rigors of the journey made me very aware of my increasing disability, I felt empowered and renewed in my commitment to fight back.

Both of these anecdotes involved travel, and both may have been medically imprudent given the seriousness of my condition. In retrospect, however, I would certainly do both again, because not too long afterwards, I found myself hospitalized and unable to travel. By deciding to live for the moment, we gained confidence as a family that we could somehow survive this ordeal.

Once I received the life-saving transplant operation, we continued to seek every opportunity to savor life. This, we believe, is an important strategy for any long-term condition involving peaks and valleys. Cancer going into remission, AIDS symptoms abating, a heart condition alleviated by a by-pass operation - all may produce a sustained ray of hope. In my own situation, my new heart appears to be fine, but I must live continuously with the awareness that my body will be trying to reject this new organ for the remainder of my life. Our reaction to this is not to remain in a perpetual state of worry that the ax is about to fall, but rather to live life to its fullest. As soon as I returned home following the transplant operation, I vowed to regain my strength so that I could return to the Grand Canyon and hike from the rim to the floor and back. Within seven months we were dipping our toes in the Colorado River at the bottom of the canyon.

The lesson which we have learned from our stay on LIFE ROW is that it is far better to attempt to remain "in control" than to simply react to each new development. Do not allow the disease to control your lives. Search for ways to assert your independence. Find ways to stay mentally in charge. **Live for the moment!**

Step 7 Develop emotional outlets.

Few of us have the ability to remain emotionally stable when confronted with death, particularly if we find ourselves "twisting in the wind" as we await the final moment. Elisabeth Kübler-Ross explored this emotional turmoil thoroughly in her excellent book, *On Death and Dying*. As one typically passes through her five classic stages of denial, anger, bargaining, depression, and acceptance, I believe that there is a need to develop mechanisms to allow venting of emotions before they reach the danger level. At some time during your ordeal, you and each of your loved ones may become very angry. Sustaining this anger can rob you of the energy you need to fight your real enemy, the disease. Thus, it is important to actively seek diversions which will allow you to vent this anger before it harms you.

Once again, because everyone is different, there will likely be a myriad of solutions. What works for Jane, may not be effective for Janice. During my longer periods of hospitalization, I found that it helped me to create "bad guys" who could be the focal point of my anger. I chose the hospital dietitian (**216-218**). I found myself looking forward to my daily battles with this lady (who had done nothing wrong and who was probably totally unaware that she was being so instrumental in maintaining my mental stability!). Later I picked fights with the fellow who filled the vending machine near my hospital room (**221-222**), a realtor in North Carolina (**220**), and even United Airlines (**220-221**). None of these "battles" were of any significance, but they did serve a very useful purpose in allowing me to vent my anger that I was sick and dying.

There were also positive outlets for our emotions. In addition to reading and writing letters daily, I learned to scour the newspapers for situations or news related to my illness. Any article discussing heart diseases or new surgical techniques caught my attention. I would cut out each clipping and discuss it with my doctors. In this way I felt as if I were personally involved in defeating my adversary. In the case of a disease such as AIDS, where new research findings seem to be publicized daily, there would appear to be considerable opportunity for this type of diversion.

Do not be afraid to discuss diet with your doctors. Although your condition may require restriction of various food types, it may be better for your long term survival to occasionally eat a "forbidden fruit" (such as a hamburger or fries) if it brings you a surge of joy in an otherwise dreary situation. When I became thoroughly disheartened by the steady diet of no-salt, low-fat hospital food, we discussed the situation with our cardiologist (**217**). To our surprise he agreed with our request that I have occasional "real food." Given this apparent reprieve from terminal culinary boredom, I actually lost weight and found myself looking forward with eager anticipation to each evening when Sharry or our younger daughter, Emily, would bring me home-cooked food. In fact, less than a week before I received the transplant operation, we had an absolutely joyous crab feast in the hospital arranged for us by Sharry and one of our nurses (**223-224**).

We also sought and received permission to briefly leave the floor of the hospital where my heart was being continuously monitored by special equipment. This was also a trade-off in terms of absolute safety versus improved spirits. Fortunately our doctors had a keen sense of appreciation for this trade-off and made arrangements to allow it to occur. Sharry and I took this opportunity nearly every evening to visit a small garden and goldfish pond on the hospital grounds (**224-225**). This brief respite from reality energized us to face yet another night apart in our terrible struggle.

You may not have access to a garden or some other source of instant joy, and you may have to be creative in developing villains. But you do need to find something which will allow you to level out the almost certain emotional peaks and valleys of an extended illness. There may be trade-offs involved, and you should discuss various possibilities with your medical team. Overall, it was our experience that you will almost certainly benefit if you **develop emotional outlets.**

Step 8   Manage your brain.

One of my more frequent requests to my team of doctors and nurses was "You keep me alive physically, and I will handle the mental side of the house." I mentioned this in Step 5, but the concept is so important that we should discuss it further.

At sometime during your illness, you may find yourself on the verge of death. To most of us, this is very frightening. No one knows what lies on the other sides of human life, both birth and death. Many of us rely on faith in God to provide an answer, but there is no certainty even in the strongest among us. It is this inherent ambiguity of the human condition which plays upon the mind during these darkest moments. Managing such moments will be one of your greatest challenges.

I found that nights were the worst times for me. During the day I always kept busy. My day was designed so that I would not have time to worry. But as I lay in bed trying to fall asleep, my mind would inevitably wander to the unthinkable: if I fall asleep, maybe I will not wake up (**158, 166**). I do not know how many of these terrible nights I had throughout my illness. I am certain that my wife had at least as many, if not more. Unfortunately, I know of no foolproof remedy for these moments of severe depression. Perhaps the best antidote is the realization that you **will** have moments such as this.

Feelings of depression will not be limited to night-time. There will be occasions when you want to surrender and simply have it all end, particularly if you are no longer able to perform the daily functions which were once so routine (**146-147**). The important thing to remember when this happens is that even a person who is totally well will have good and bad days. No one remains on a permanent "high." Your challenge is to regain control and proceed on with the fight. One of the tricks which I found successful when I found myself in a deep funk was to compare myself to a prisoner of war. I had been captured by this disease, it had imprisoned me, and was often mistreating me, sometimes even inflicting great pain. With this in mind, I became determined not to surrender, but to continue to fight on, to remain confident that the day would come when I would be rescued.

How you handle these dark moments will be critical. You will have to experiment to find what works best for you. You may benefit from the experience of others who have had your same disease or condition. Once again, membership in a support group can provide access to many who have already traveled this same highway. Do not be shy about asking others how they overcome these difficult periods.

Rather than waiting for these fits of depression to sink upon you, I recommend that you adopt a proactive strategy. Whenever you sense that you may be heading into a prolonged downer, do something that you have not done recently or perhaps ever before. For example, I found that I could immediately lift my spirits by making some silly purchase out of a catalog (always under $25) via an 800 number. One time I actually turned on the television and bought the first thing which appealed to me on the Home Shopper's Network (**221**)!

For me, the most effective antidote against depression was to develop a daily schedule and to follow it closely. This strategy gave me something specific to look forward to each hour. I knew that if it was 10:30 AM I would be reading the newspaper. If it was 3:35 PM, I would be typing on my laptop computer. I did not schedule any moments of "nothing." This does not mean that I did not relax. I simply chose methods of relaxation which involved my mind doing something. The trick is not to allow your mind time to worry. In short, **manage your brain**.

Step 9   Be aggressive.

One of the major concerns during a long-term illness is finances. Unless you are incredibly lucky, you will very quickly learn that you are your only advocate when it comes to paying for the expenses associated with your illness. HMOs, insurance companies, hospitals, medical service providers, and even doctors and nurses cannot continue to provide services unless they have a stream of income. You are the source of their income. Never forget this fact. I assure you that they do not forget it!

Hence you will find that on any given day there will be several organizations attempting to collect money from you, or trying to avoid compensating you for payments which you have already made. These folks are generally not evil; they are simply trying to ensure that they remain in business. Most of these organizations regard you not so much as an ill person, but rather an opportunity for monetary gain. Do not take this personally. You should remain calm and deal with them aggressively. We learned that you can win this battle.

You will find that every hospital and most doctors will ensure that they have received insurance information from you before they admit or treat you (**39-40**). This is the case even in the emergency room. Once we became aware of my disease, we carried our insurance cards with us at all times. If you are fortunate enough to have two or more insurers, make certain that the clerk taking your information has all the information before you leave. Insist that they do all the billing directly to all of your insurance companies and that you receive copies of the bills.

You will need to set up a filing system in your home. Soon you will start receiving copies of bills and "EOBs" (Explanation of Benefits) from insurance companies. For the first three years, we kept track of each service performed by a doctor, lab, or hospital on legal pads (I went through nearly 17 pages!!). The same process can be done on a computer spreadsheet, but we found that we were more comfortable with pencil and paper. Ultimately, however, we found that this procedure was not worth the effort. Now we simply look at each piece of correspondence and file it in an envelope with all the information from that individual provider. If an issue develops, we simply open that envelope and find the documentation. You will probably have to use the trial and error method to find what system works best for you. The important thing is to have a filing system with which you are comfortable. You **will** need it.

You will also find that it pays to call your HMO or insurance company any time that it appears that you will require hospitalization. We learned that it is far easier to receive pre-approval for a procedure than to fight over the issue ex-post-facto. If you do not receive the answer you want to hear, i.e. you are turned down, go to the next person up the chain. You may need to be especially aggressive in this situation; if you need the procedure or treatment, fight for it!

If you encounter a difficult situation, we found that two people are better than one in financial scuffles. Sharry, for example, was our family "bad guy" in dealing with insurance issues. She did not hesitate to use the full range of emotions when dealing with HMOs, insurers, or anyone attempting to do us wrong. At different times she begged, pleaded, screamed, threatened, chastised, flattered, insulted, embarrassed, or "rationally explained" as the situation dictated (**143**). Sometimes she used several of these tactics in the same conversation! The point to remember is the old dictum about the squeaky wheel receiving the grease. Someone in your family needs to be squeaky.

If you do not have insurance coverage, your situation is not hopeless. You should immediately contact as many social services organizations as possible, particularly those at your local hospitals. Although our doctor bills were significant, the bulk of our expenses were associated with hospital stays. I do not want to (nor could I) give everyone a blueprint on how to finance your illness, because everyone's situation is different. What is common is that you must be aggressive. If you sit back hoping that all will go well financially, it probably will not. You can minimize the impact of finances on surviving your illness by taking a very aggressive approach.

Other areas in which an aggressive approach will pay dividends include research and "patient rights." What is current today in terms of information concerning your disease may not be current tomorrow. By definition, any disease for which we do not presently have a cure or effective treatment is one which is probably being heavily researched. AIDS and prostate cancer are two examples which come immediately to mind. The cardiac bypass surgery procedure which I observed the spring after I had received my own transplant operation has now been extensively modified by new techniques. The two defibrillators which were inserted into my abdomen to monitor and respond to tachycardia episodes (**118-119, 138**) have now been replaced by a much smaller, more powerful model. Because of this rapidly changing nature of medicine, you need to be alert for new developments and, more importantly, receptive to suggestions from your medical team to try new procedures/hardware/medicines. Both of my defibrillators were "investigational devices," that is, they did not have final FDA approval. I signed the necessary waivers acknowledging that I was aware of this status, and I am alive today because I did so. This is what I mean by being "aggressive" in terms of research.

Patients rights is another area where you must speak up. Never forget that you are a paying customer. As I said earlier, if you are having difficulties with a particular physician or nurse, find a way to replace them. When a nursing error on a particular floor at my hospital left me unattended in the basement following a midnight x-ray, my doctor had me immediately tr.nsferred to another floor where he felt the nurses were more experienced in handling my condition (**173-174**). On other occasions I refused x-rays until I learned which doctor had written the order and why. In one instance it turned out that an intern who knew nothing about me or my condition had written the order (**108-110**). If you are being bothered by a loud or obnoxious roommate while hospitalized, do not be shy about informing the nursing staff. I assure you that you are paying big bucks for the hospital room, so you should be able to rest (Chapter 11 discusses several of these situations in detail). Finally, always check the medicines which you are given **before** you take them. Although hospitals, physicians, nurses, and care providers take extensive measures to guard against medication errors, Murphy's Law dictates that a mistake may still occur. I was nearly mis-medicated on two occasions, but my review of the medication before I swallowed it prevented the error and possible serious consequences for my survival.

In summary, do not allow yourself or your family to be passive players in your battle to survive. You have the greatest stake in your remaining alive, so **be aggressive.**

Step 10 Have faith.

It is essential that **you** believe that you are going to survive. For some, this level of absolute faith may be a natural reaction to adversity of the worst type, i.e., a doctor telling you that you have a fatal disease. For many others, however, such as myself, the initial reaction may be less optimistic (**5**). I was worried - very worried. In fact, I was terrified.

Fortunately, my wife was stronger. "Don't worry, sweetheart. Somehow or other we will make it through this," were her first words to me after we learned that I had been placed on Life Row (**5**). Throughout the following 3 1/2 years her steady faith that we would somehow find a cure or a solution or a miracle or ....?? kept us going during some of our darkest hours together.

Faith can be expressed in many forms, both secular and religious. Because Sharry and I had been raised in the Christian tradition, we found that prayer was a natural path to focus our faith. At the same time we were both realists. We had both seen many "good Christians" die early in their lives. The theme of our prayers, therefore, became requests for God's will to be done, and to hope that the result would be "the best" for everyone concerned (**23**). Our thoughts were that the Lord had been with us through several other difficult periods and that our decisions as we proceeded along Life Row would be similarly blessed (**74**).

There were times of extreme anxiety, of course, when my prayer became more intense and specific. When I was dying in the E.R., for example, I found myself begging God to "take care of my family" and "Help me, Lord." (**105-106**) I believe that my faith in a divine being has never been stronger than during that terrifying episode. Although I had what some might term an "out-of-body" experience, I never doubted that the Lord wanted me to continue on

Life Row, at least through that night. Another night of intense, directed prayer occurred when my defibrillator was firing frequently at the beginning of my final hospitalization prior to the transplant operation (**171-172**). Throughout what was probably "the worst night of my life," I lay awake praying for God's help. I received no further shocks as I prayed, and the monitor trace the following AM indicated that the arrhythmias had suddenly disappeared.

I do not know that God played a role in either of these situations. But I do know that I had faith that God's will would be done, and that I was sincerely expressing that belief throughout both incidents.

Throughout our struggle I made an effort to set aside time for regular daily prayers of thanksgiving. Each morning I tried to read an appropriate daily devotion to thank the Lord that I had been brought safely through another night (**213**), and each evening I always paused before going to sleep to say a short evening prayer of thanks (**225**). I may have missed a few days, but it was unintentional. My goal was to pause at least twice each day to reflect on some bit of positive news or some pleasant thought which would give me reason to want to live another day.

We also benefited from the prayers of hundreds of friends who were praying for us. Members of our congregation, former students of mine, neighbors, relatives, and family friends were daily expressing their faith through a myriad of denominations and individual beliefs (**234**).

Because I was unconscious and hovering near death throughout most of "The Ordeal," I did little actual praying. Sharry, however, more than picked up the slack during this difficult phase. In fact, my condition was so grave that she felt as if **all** she could do was to pray (**257, 262**). One of my first acts upon regaining consciousness and realizing just how blessed I had been was to pause to thank the Lord (**269**).

Once we arrived home from the hospital, Sharry and I continued to thank our supporters for their prayers. Their faith had been unswerving, and we wanted to take every opportunity to express our gratitude for their generosity and kindness (**291**). Ultimately, of course, our primary benefactor was God. Our first post-transplant Thanksgiving dinner in 1994 was a very special opportunity for us to give thanks for our unique blessing. As we reflected on our good fortune, we also prayed for the soul of my donor and for each member of her family whose gift to us had played such a key role in my survival (**299**).

Our experience with prayer has been thoroughly positive. Nonetheless, I find it difficult to endorse a specific strategy in this very personal area. What I do feel comfortable doing is to extol the benefit of the power of absolute faith and positive thinking. I also encourage each member of any family in a medical crisis, regardless of religious beliefs, to provide as much moral support as possible for the patient (and for each other). Ultimately, however, faith is an individual challenge. My hope is that you will **have faith** and that each of you will be as blessed as we have been.

SUMMARY

Let me again emphasize that each person's health is a very individual, and unique, situation. We believe, however, that using all, or some combination, of the **10 Steps** can help every family to improve the odds of surviving a medical crisis. Use the following list to draft your plan today. As we are so pleased to report, there **can** be a happy ending to your stay on Life Row!

The 10 Steps to Survive

1.	**Know your enemy.**	☐
2.	**Seek professional help.**	☐
3.	**Recruit a support team.**	☐
4.	**Examine all options.**	☐
5.	**Understand yourself.**	☐
6.	**Live for the moment.**	☐
7.	**Use emotional outlets.**	☐
8.	**Manage your brain**	☐
9.	**Be aggressive.**	☐
10.	**Have faith.**	☐

Reader Feedback

We are very interested in hearing the experiences of other families who have been confronted with battling a potentially life-threatening medical situation. We are convinced that we have not been on LIFE ROW alone, and that many others have lived through similarly trying circumstances. It is our hope that the wisdom which many of you have gained can be collected for use by other families when they face their own LIFE ROW challenge.

We are particularly interested in your thoughts on the 10 Steps. Which did you find to be most helpful in your situation? What other techniques/ideas/suggestions would you add? Are there any ideas presented in these 10 Steps with which you disagree?

Please tell us about your experiences. Even if your outcome was not as favorable as ours, others may be able to benefit from your story. It may also be helpful to hear strategies that were not successful, so that others may choose to avoid those approaches. Our goal is to compile a collective wisdom to assist other families when they must face their own LIFE ROW.

The form on the next page is an outline to assist in organizing your thoughts. Please feel free to use your own words. Do not worry about grammar, spelling, or anything other than your own honest feelings. We will attempt to respond to all e-mail correspondence and to as many letters as possible.

Thank you for sharing your thoughts with us.

God Bless!

LIFE ROW **Reader Feedback Form**
(please photocopy)

Patient Name:_____

Other Family Members and relationship:

_____

_____

Address:_____

_____

Telephone(optional):_____

e-mail (optional):_____

Nature of Illness:_____

_____

_____

_____

Time Frame of Illness:_____

Comments concerning LIFE ROW:_____

_____

_____

_____(continue on back)

Suggestions concerning "10 Steps to Survive"_____

_____

_____

_____

_____(continue on back)

What worked best for your family?_____

_____(continue on back)

What did not work for you?_____

_____(continue on back)

May we contact you? (Y/N)_____May we quote you? (Y/N)_____

Please e-mail response to: **exchpub@erols.com** (in subject line, put Life Row Feedback)   or mail to

> **Exchange Publishing**
> **P.O. Box 2394**
> **Springfield, VA 22152**
> **ATTN: Life Row Feedback**

Also please feel free to include a copy of this form or any other comments with any book orders. Thanks and God Bless!

Index

(drug trade names are in bold print, chemical names are in regular type)

Would you like your own copy of Life Row?
Do you know a family who can benefit from reading
10 Steps to Survive an Extended Medical Crisis?

Do you want a *great gift* for a friend or relative?

Order Form (please photocopy)

☎ **Telephone** orders: Call Toll Free: 1(800) 326-2223
(have credit card info ready)

💻 **On-line** orders: **e-mail: exchpub@erols.com**
(send mailing address and quantity, along with credit card info)
or use our internet page
www.iea.com/~adlinkex/liferow.html

⌘ **Fax** orders: (509) 455-7940

✉ **Mail** orders: Exchange Publishing
P.O. Box 2394
Springfield, VA 22152

Name:_____

Address:_____

City:_____State_____Zip:_____

Price: $16.00 U.S. (sales tax included)
********* e-mail orders take $1.00 off !! *********
(Quantity discount available; call Exchange Pub. for info)
Shipping/Handling: $4.00 ($2.00 each additional book)
Payment: Copies ordered_____ Total enclosed $_____
☐ Check (mail orders)
☐ Credit card ☐ VISA ☐ Master Card ☐ Discover
Card Number:_____
Name on card:_____Exp. Date____/____
Call *toll free* or *e-mail* and order now !!

About the Author's Family

Because *Life Row* is a true story involving each member of the Linz family, the reader may find it interesting to know more about the principals involved.

Sharon, Ed's wife, is a graduate of the University of Connecticut. She continues her work as a Public Health Nurse for the Fairfax County (Virginia) Health Department, specializing in maternal and child health and communicable diseases, such as TB and AIDS. She is an avid chair caner, hiker, and reader.

Aaron was a high school senior when his father was placed on Life Row. He has since completed his Masters Degree at University of North Carolina at Chapel Hill (where he was all-ACC in track) and is now an accountant in Greensboro. His free time is spent competing in mountain bicycle racing.

Nelle was 16 when she learned of her father's potentially fatal disease. She will graduate from Indiana University in May 1997 with a dual major in chemistry and East Asian studies. She is a certified EMT and works summers as a nursing assistant on a cardiac floor at Fairfax Hospital. Her current plans are to pursue a career in medicine.

Emily was in 8th grade when Life Row began. She lettered in cross country throughout high school and is now a student at Elon College in North Carolina. Her goals are to combine her love of music with a career in business. Her hobbies include playing the soprano sax and listening to country music.

Sydney, the family dog, remains faithful, lovable, and....bad. Her goals generally do not extend beyond the next meal.

About the Author

Ed Linz is now into his third career. After spending 20 years in nuclear submarines, including a tour as Commanding Officer of the missile submarine, USS KAMEHEMEHA, Ed spent the next nine years teaching mathematics and physics and coaching cross country running at high schools in northern Virginia. "My illness was actually a blessing in disguise," he reports, "because it gave me the free time to pursue my long-held ambition to write and lecture." He now teaches on a part-time basis, coaches cross country each fall season, lectures frequently concerning transplantation and organ donation, and still finds time to write daily. His current projects include *They Never Throw Anything Away*, (an oral history of the Great Depression), and a novel, *Billie Benkie*, involving some of the outrageous characters from his childhood in Kentucky. His hobbies include hiking, winning his annual NFL pool, and bird-watching.

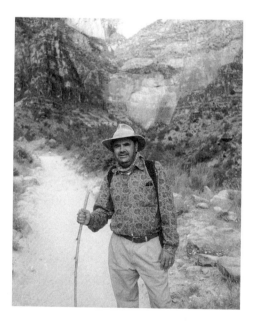

Ed hiking Bright Angel Trail, Grand Canyon, May 1995
(seven months following heart transplant operation)

Would you like your own copy of **Life Row?**
Do you know a family who can benefit from reading
10 Steps to Survive an Extended
Medical Crisis?

Do you want a *great gift* for a friend or relative?

Order Form (please photocopy)

☎   **Telephone** orders: Call Toll Free: 1(800) 326-2223
                          (have credit card info ready)
🖳   **On-line** orders: **e-mail: exchpub@erols.com**
      (send mailing address and quantity, along with credit card info)
                   or use our internet page
              www.iea.com/~adlinkex/liferow.html
⌘   **Fax** orders: (509) 455-7940
✉   **Mail** orders: Exchange Publishing
                          P.O. Box 2394
                          Springfield, VA 22152
Name:_____
Address:_____
City:_____State_____Zip:_____

Price: $16.00 U.S. (sales tax included)
********* **e-mail orders take $1.00 off !! *********
      (Quantity discount available; call Exchange Pub. for info)
Shipping/Handling: $4.00 ($2.00 each additional book)
Payment: Copies ordered_____ Total enclosed $_____
☐ Check (mail orders)
☐ Credit card ☐ VISA ☐ Master Card ☐ Discover
Card Number:_____
Name on card:_____Exp. Date____/____
      Call *toll free* or *e-mail* and order now !!